Praises for The Bragg Heal

These are just a few of the thousands of te receive yearly, praising The Bragg Health Books for the rejuvenation benefits they reap – physically, mentally and spiritually. We look forward to hearing from you also.

Thanks to the Bragg Health Books, they were our introduction to healthy living. We are very grateful to you and your father.
– Marilyn Diamond, Co-Author, "Fit For Life"

Paul Bragg saved my life at age 15 when I attended the Bragg Health Crusade in Oakland. I thank the Bragg Healthy Lifestyle for my long, healthy, active life spreading health and fitness.
– Jack LaLanne, thankful Bragg follower to 96½

Thank you Patricia for our first meeting in London in 1968. You gave me your Fasting Book, it got me exercising, brisk walking and eating more wisely. You were a blessing God-sent.
– Reverend Billy Graham

When I was a young gymnastics coach at Stanford University, Paul Bragg's words and example inspired me to live a healthy lifestyle. I was twenty-three then; now I'm over sixty, and my health and fitness serves as a living testimonial to Paul Bragg's health wisdom, carried on by his health crusading daughter, Dr. Patricia Bragg. Thank you both!
– Dan Millman, Author of "The Way of the Peaceful Warrior"
www.danmillman.com

It was in Hawaii I began to realize that while lifestyle choices can not only be a major negative to health and well-being, but lifestyle can be a winning asset to wellness! My discovery on fitness and health began shortly after I arrived in Hawaii at 19 when I discovered fitness and health pioneer Paul Bragg teaching a free exercise class 6 days a week at Waikiki Beach.
– Kathy Smith, Hollywood, CA • *www.kathysmith.com*

I've read the wonderful Bragg Health Books for over 25 years. They are a blessing to me, my family and to all who read them. These books help make this a healthier, happier world.
– Pastor Mike MacIntosh,
Horizon Christian Fellowship, California

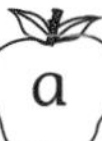

Praises for The Bragg Healthy Lifestyle

Bragg Health Books were my conversion to the healthy way.
– James F. Balch, M.D.,
Co-Author, *Prescription for Nutritional Healing*

As a youth I had a learning disability and was told I would never read, write or communicate normally. At 14 I dropped out of school and at 17 ended up in Hawaii surfing. My road to recovery led me to Paul Bragg who changed my life by giving me one simple affirmation to repeat: "I am a genius and I apply my wisdom." Bragg inspired me to live a healthy lifestyle and go back to school and get my education and from there miracles happened. I've authored 54 training programs and 14 books and love to crusade around the world thanks to Bragg.
– Dr. John Demartini, Author, Dynamic Crusader in *The Secret.*
www.drdemartini.com

For 30 years I've followed the Bragg Healthy Lifestyle. It teaches you how to take control of your health and build a healthy future.
– Mark Victor Hansen,
Co-Producer, *Chicken Soup for The Soul* Series

I've been reading Bragg Books since high school days. I'm thankful for my healthy lifestyle I learned from them and admire their health crusading to make this a healthier world!
– Steve Jobs, Creator & CEO – Apple Computer/iPods

I met Paul Bragg in 1964, at "L" Street Beach in Boston. Both Paul and daughter Patricia are dynamic, energetic and life-changers! They have always been health inspirations to millions around the world, but especially to me! I gave my first lecture with them in April 1964, I was 22, I am over 64 now. Patricia has more energy than any 3 people I know put together and loves traveling the world for Bragg Health Crusades.
– David Carmos and Dr. Shawn Miller, Co-Authors,
You're Never Too Old To Become Young
www.perfecthealthnow.com

Thank you Paul and Patricia Bragg for my simple, easy to follow Bragg Healthy Lifestyle. You make my days healthy!
– Clint Eastwood, Academy Award Winning Film Producer, Director, Actor and Bragg follower for over 55 years

Praises for The Bragg Healthy Lifestyle

Thanks to Paul Bragg and Bragg Books. My teen years of struggling with asthma were cured in only one month with Bragg Healthy Lifestyle Living and Super Power Breathing!
– Paul Wenner, Gardenburger Creator • *gardenburger.com*

Thanks to *Miracle of Fasting* and Bragg Healthy Lifestyle, we are healthy, fit, singing better and staying younger than ever!
– The Beach Boys • *www.beachboysfanclub.com*

I love the Bragg Books and *The Miracle of Fasting.* They are so popular and loved in Russia and the Ukraine. I give thanks for my health and super energy. I just won the famous Honolulu Marathon with the all-time women's race record!
– Lyubov Morgunova, Champion Runner, Moscow, Russia

You've recharged me with hope, encouragement and love which poured from your words. I'm now able to fast and no more cigarettes and coffee for me. The Bragg Healthy Lifestyle has certainly improved my life! – Marie Furia, New Jersey

---

The Bragg Healthy Lifestyle with Fasting has changed my life! I lost weight and my energy levels went through the roof. I look forward to "Fasting" days. I think better and I am a better husband and father. Thank you Patricia, this has been a great blessing in my life. Also, thank you for sharing the Bragg Healthy Lifestyle at our "AOL" Conference.
– Byron H. Elton, VP Entertainment, Time Warner AOL

I give thanks to Health Crusaders Paul Bragg and daughter Patricia for their dedicated years of service spreading health. It has made a difference in my life and millions of others worldwide. – Pat Robertson, Host CBN "700" Club

---

I am a big fan of Paul Bragg. I use the Bragg Liquid Aminos daily on my food. I even take it with me when I travel for my seminars, I wouldn't be without it! The world and I are blessed with the health teachings of Paul and Patricia Bragg!
– Anthony "Tony" Robbins • *www.anthonyrobbins.com*

My uncle, The Dalai Lama, and family are supporters of Bragg health teachings over 40 years. We eat brown rice and healthy meals with delicious Bragg Liquid Aminos. We thank you. – Jigme Norbu, The Dalai Lama's Nephew

Praises for The Bragg Healthy Lifestyle

Your dad, Dr. Paul Bragg, IS the FATHER of the natural health industry and the entire natural health movement. Everything that has been done in natural health and physical culture since has been based on the pioneering vision and principles articulated by Dr. Paul C. Bragg. He gave us all our direction! – Dr. William Wong, Texas

---

I am following the Bragg Healthy Lifestyle which I heard of through a friend. Your books are motivators and have blessed my health and life and are making perfect gifts to inspire my friends to a healthy lifestyle. – Delphine, Singapore

---

In 1975 I was diagnosed with coronary heart disease. I followed the Free Bragg Exercise Classes and Lectures at Fort DeRussy in Waikiki, 6 times a week. Over thirty-three years have passed and I am going strong and healthy. Now I am 84 years young thanks to The Bragg Healthy Lifestyle. In 1932 my father had severe hip arthritis and was hardly able to walk. He followed the Bragg Healthy Lifestyle and the vinegar regime and was cured of his arthritis. – Helen Risk, RN, California

---

I praise Paul Bragg for his strong Health Crusading. The Bragg Healthy Lifestyle Teachings are inspirations to my family. *The Miracle of Fasting* book got me on the health path and cured my asthma and arthritis.
– Cloris Leachman, Actress, an 85 year young vegetarian

We get letters daily at our Santa Barbara headquarters. We would love to receive letters and testimonials from you on any blessings and healings you have experienced after following The Bragg Healthy Lifestyle. It's all within your grasp to be in top health. By following this book, you can reap Super Health and a happy, long, vital life! It's never too late to begin. You can receive miracles with nutritious recipes, exercise and some fasting! Start now!

Daily our prayers & love go out to you, your heart, mind & soul.

Patricia and Paul C. Bragg

3 John 2 **Genesis 6:3**

Miracles can happen daily through guidance and prayer! – Patricia Bragg

BRAGG PHOTO GALLERY

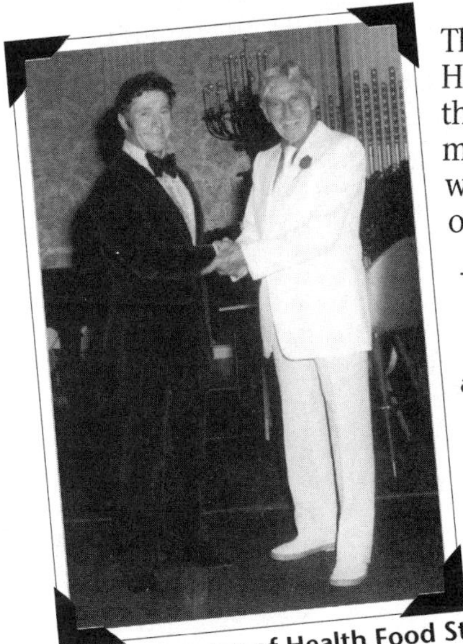

Paul Bragg, Creator of Health Food Stores, with his prize student Jack LaLanne, who thanks Bragg for saving his life at 15.

Thanks for The Bragg Healthy Lifestyle that you shared with me and are sharing with millions of others world-wide.
– John Gray, Ph.D., Author

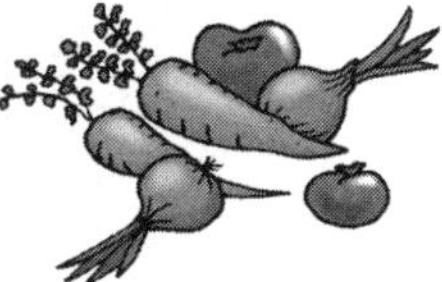

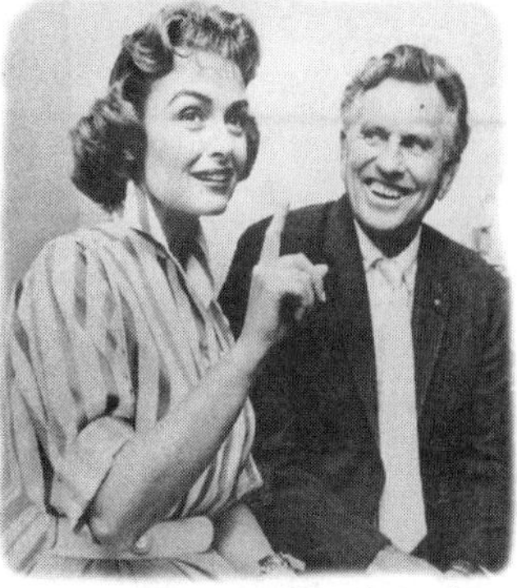

Actress Donna Reed saying "Health First" with Paul Bragg

PAUL C. BRAGG, ND, PhD.

Life Extension Specialist and Originator of Health Food Stores

In Medical School I read Dr. Bragg's Health Books, they changed my way of thinking & the path of my life. I founded Omega Institute. – Stephan Rechtschaffen, M.D.
www.eomega.org • famous since 1977

I love Bragg Products! My family uses Bragg Liquid Aminos, spray on popcorn for treat. You will see it recommended in many of the recipes in my books. – Marilu Henner, Actress and Health Book Author • marilu.com

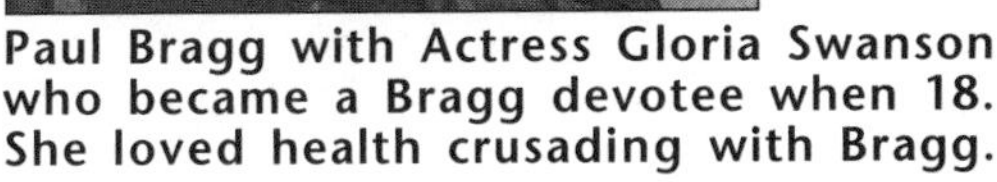

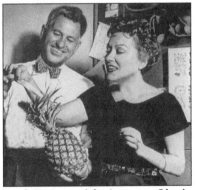

Paul Bragg with Actress Gloria Swanson who became a Bragg devotee when 18. She loved health crusading with Bragg.

I'd like to thank you for teaching me how to take control of my health! I lost 55 pounds and I feel "great"! Bragg books have showed me vitality, happiness and being close to Mother Nature. You both are real "Crusaders for Health for the World".
Thanks. – Leonard Amato

I lost 102 lbs. with Bragg Apple Cider Vinegar and The Bragg Healthy Lifestyle and have kept it off for over 15 years, staying away from white flour, sugar and other processed foods.
– Dee McCaffrey, Chemist & Diet Counselor, Tempe, Arizona

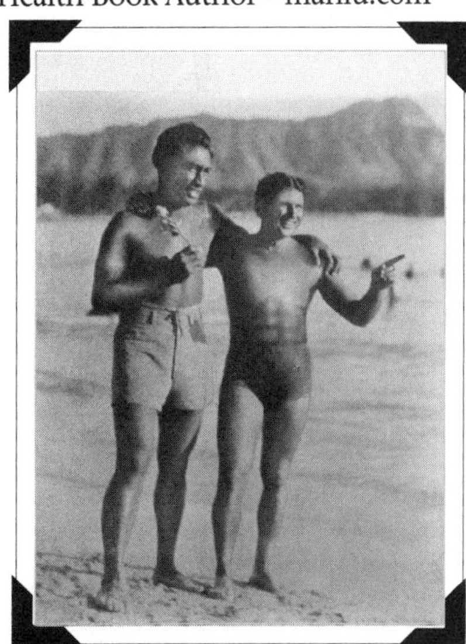

Paul Bragg with Duke Kahanamoku, the Olympic swimmer who taught Paul how to surf. His beautiful wife Nadine was Patricia's godmother.

PHOTO GALLERY

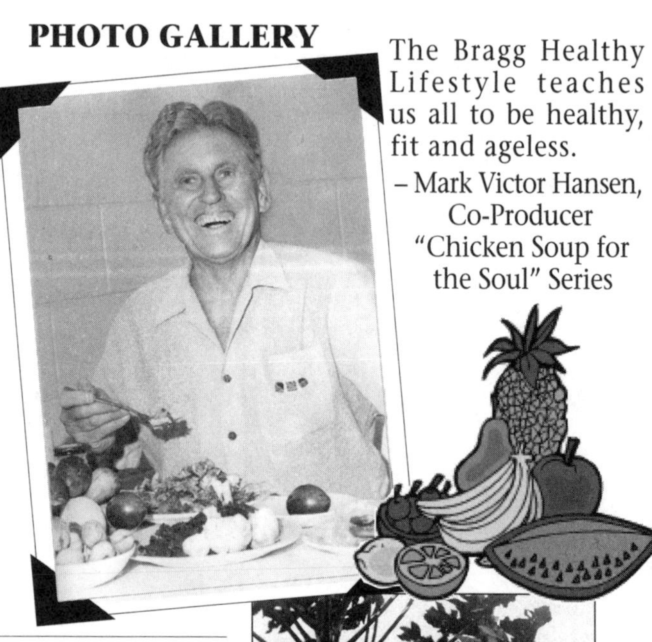

The Bragg Healthy Lifestyle teaches us all to be healthy, fit and ageless.
– Mark Victor Hansen, Co-Producer "Chicken Soup for the Soul" Series

Paul Bragg owes his powerful body and superb health to living exclusively on live, vital, healthy, organic rich foods.

PAUL BRAGG STAYING HEALTHY & FIT!

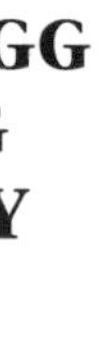

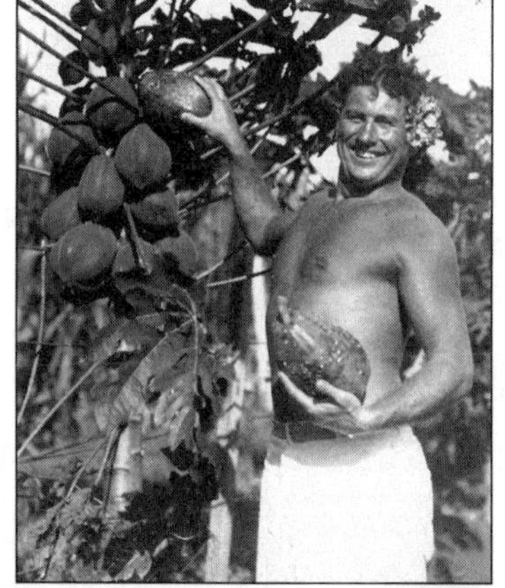

Paul Bragg in Tahiti (1925) gathering tropical papaya fruit.

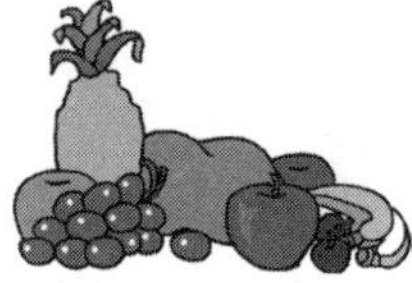

Paul C. Bragg and daughter Patricia were my early guiding inspiration to my health education and health career.
– Jeffery Bland, Ph.D., Famous Food Scientist

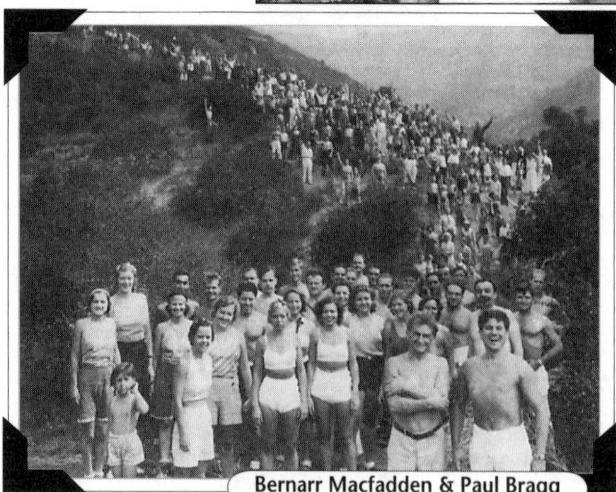

Bernarr Macfadden & Paul Bragg

A thousand happy Bragg Health Students enjoy hiking, exercise and fresh air on the trail to Mount Hollywood (above Griffith Observatory) in beautiful California, summer of 1932.

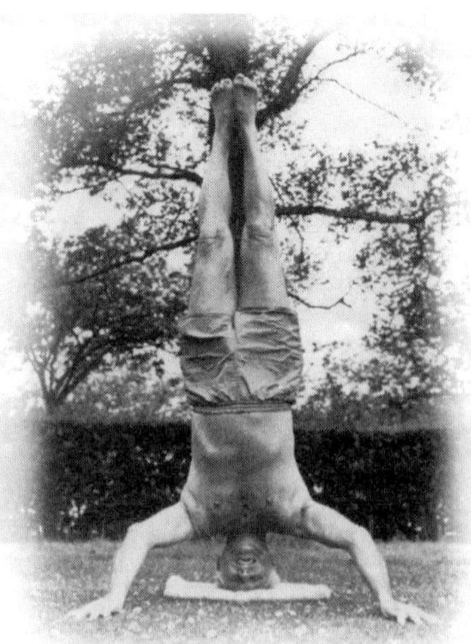

Paul C. Bragg at Regent's Park, London

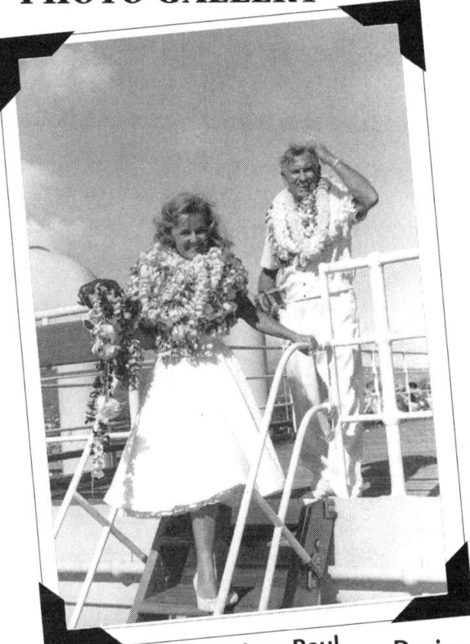

Patricia and father, Paul on world trip in 1950's, during stop in Tahiti.

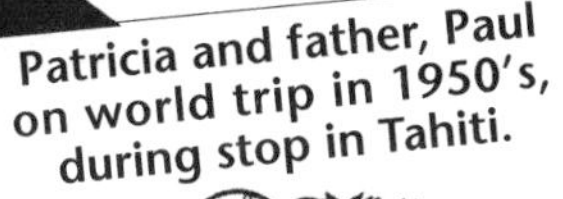

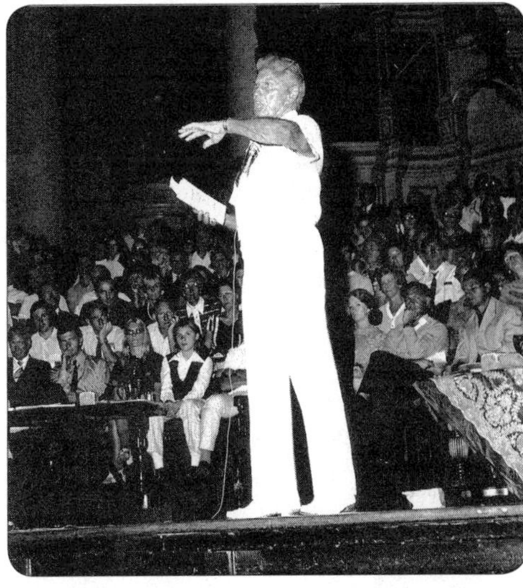

PAUL & PATRICIA BRAGG HEALTH CRUSADING

During the 50-plus years Patricia worked with her father, she was right there beside him, assisting him on the Bragg Health Crusades world-wide. They were a team, when you looked at them, you would see only two people headed in the same healthy direction.

Our lives have completely turned around! Our family is feeling so very healthy, we must tell you about it.– Gene & Joan Zollner, parents of 11, Washington

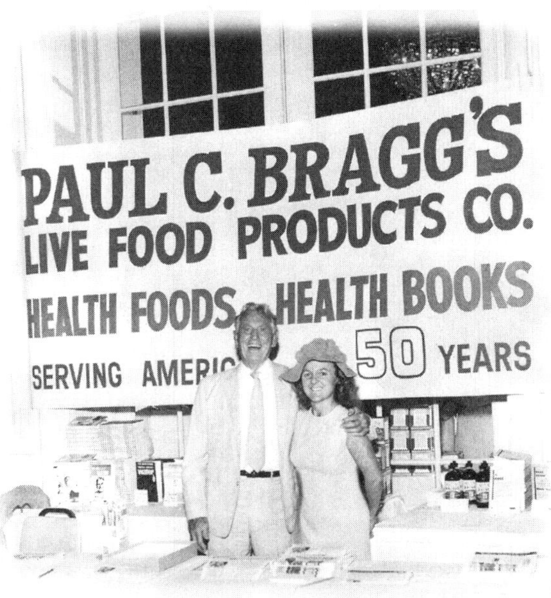

Paul C. Bragg in 1958, with daughter, celebrating here over 50 years of Bragg Health Products, Books & Crusading world-wide, spreading Health around the world.

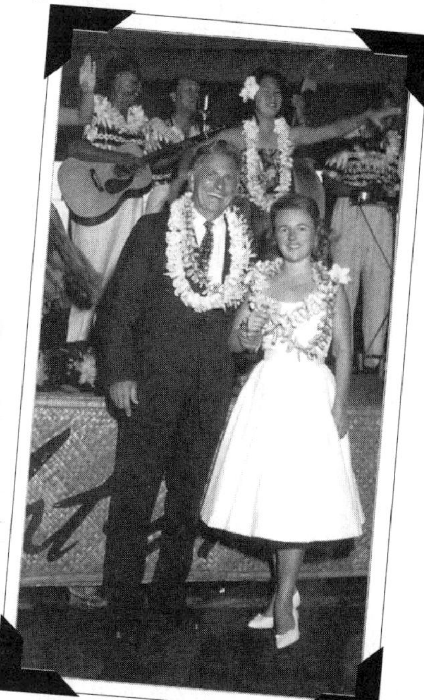

Paul & daughter Patricia, Royal Hawaiian, Honolulu

PHOTO GALLERY

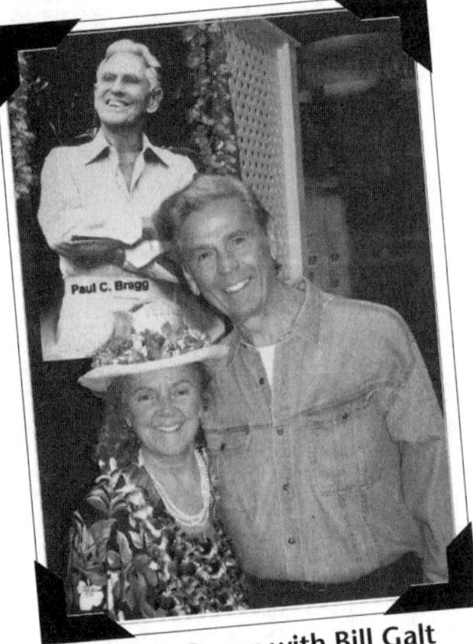

Patricia Bragg with Bill Galt inspired by Bragg Books and founded Good Earth Restaurants

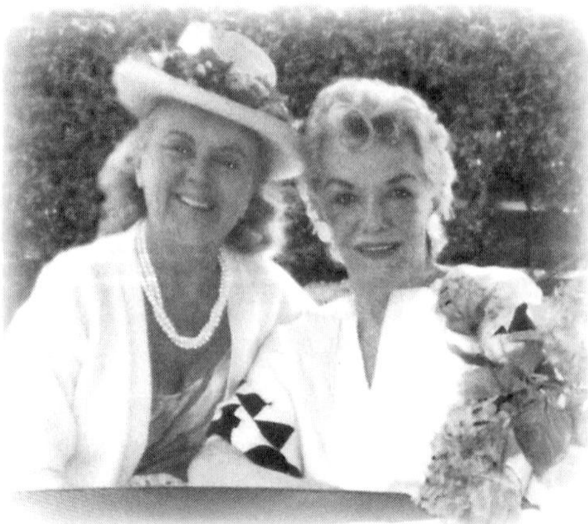

Patricia Bragg with Actress Jane Russell.

PATRICIA BRAGG CONTINUING THE HEALTH CRUSADE!

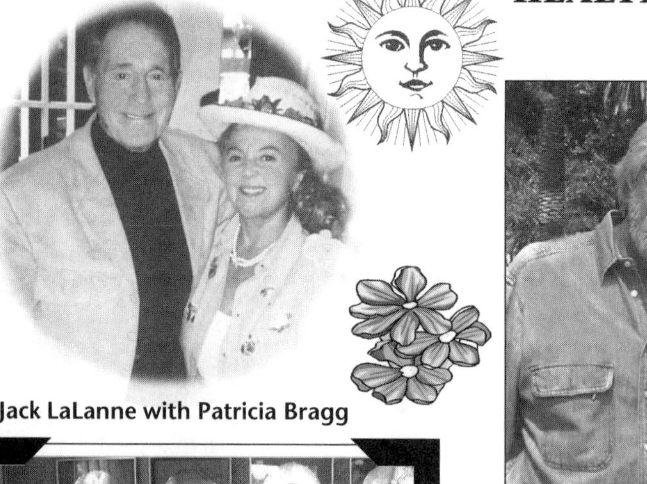

Jack LaLanne with Patricia Bragg

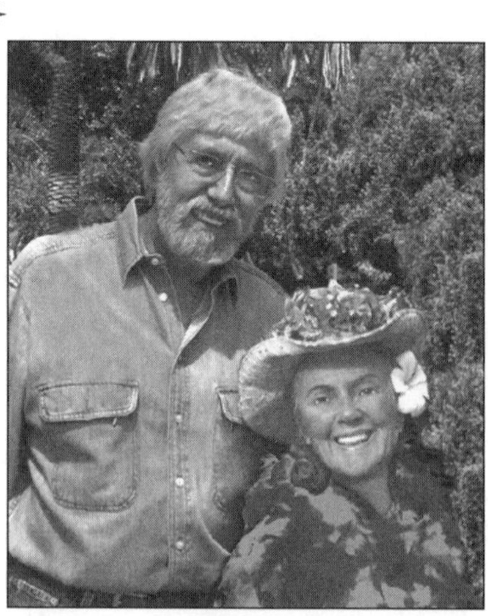

Patricia with Jean-Michel Cousteau Ocean Explorer & Environmentalist

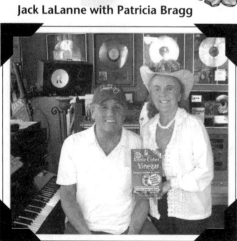

Patricia in studio with famous Beach Boy Bruce Johnson, Bragg follower over 30 years. He played for her his latest records.

Dear Friends – you cannot know how greatly you have already impacted my life and some of my friends! We love your Bragg Health Books, teachings and products and are now living healthier, happier lives. Thanks!
– Winnie Brown, Arizona

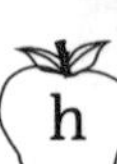

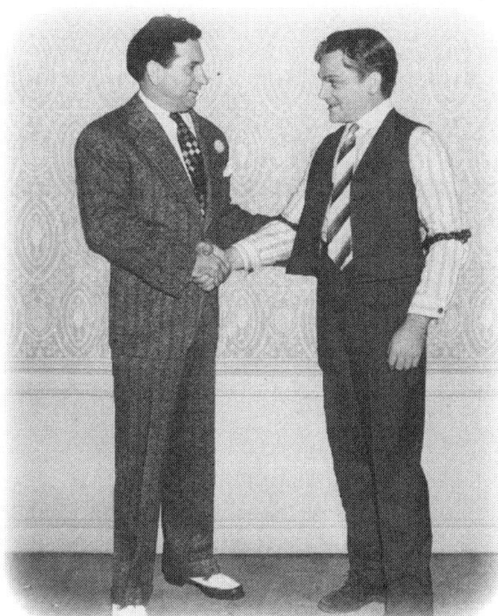

Paul Bragg with James Cagney, American film actor. He won major awards for a wide variety of roles. The American Film institute ranked him 8th among the Greatest Male Stars of All Time.

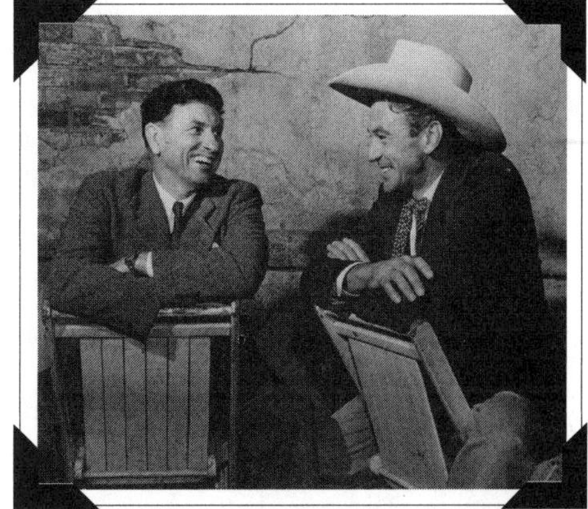

Paul C. Bragg with Gary Cooper, famous American film actor, best known for his many Western films.

Famous Hollywood Actress Cloris Leachman, who sparkles with health, says, "Bragg Fasting is simply wonderful. It is my solution to many problems. It is a miracle cure for sure . . . it cured my asthma." I praise Paul and Patricia Bragg daily for their Health Crusading!

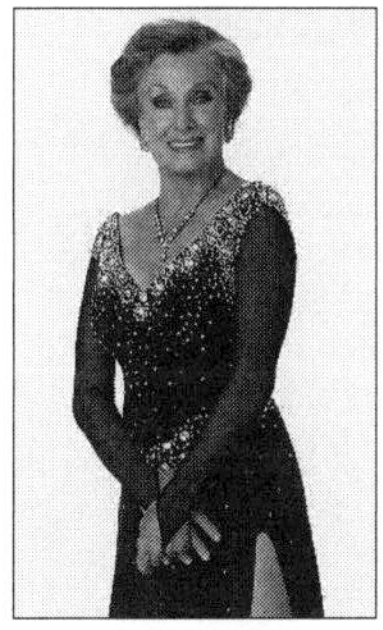

Cloris Leachman on Dancing with the Stars Show

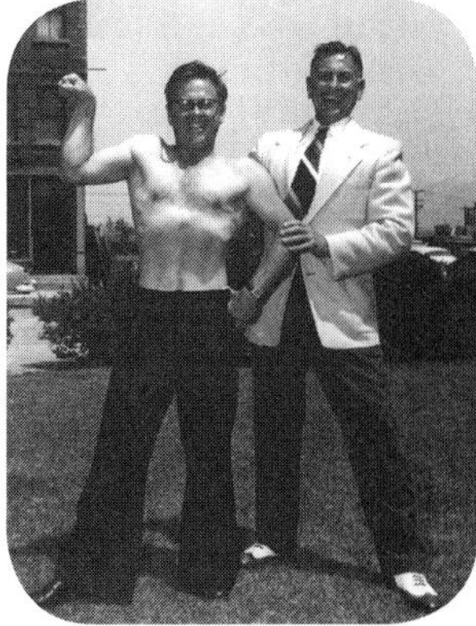

Paul with Mikey Rooney, American film actor and entertainer. He has won multiple awards and has had one of the longest careers of any actor!

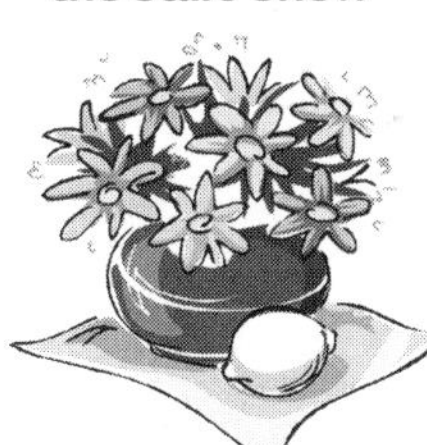

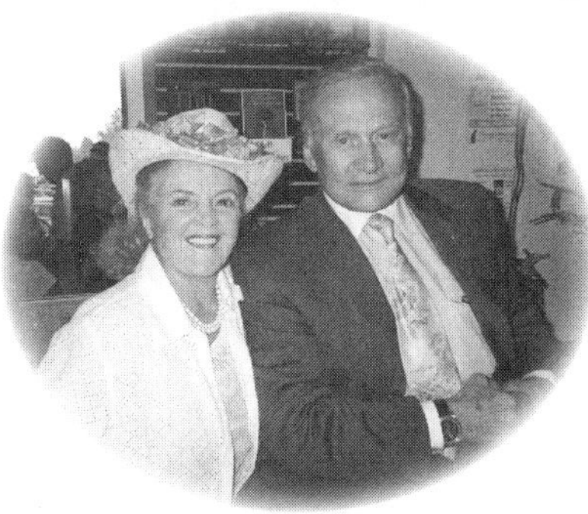

Patricia with Astronaut Buzz Aldrin, celebrating over 40 years since pilot of Apollo 11 first landed on the moon.

Kindness is a frame of mind in which we are alert to every chance: to do, to improve, to give, to share and to cheer. – Patricia Bragg

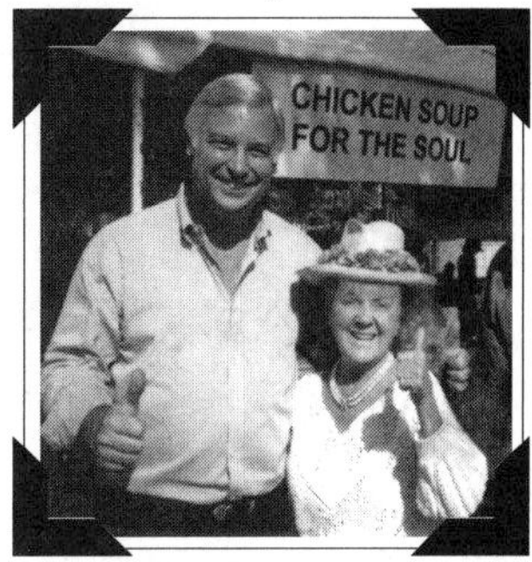

Patricia with Jack Canfield, Bragg follower, Motivational Speaker and Co-Producer of *Chicken Soup for the Soul* Series

I am a big fan of Paul Bragg. I fast and use the Bragg Aminos daily on my food. I even take it with me when I travel for my seminars, I wouldn't be without it! The world and I are blessed with the health teachings of Paul and Patricia Bragg! – Anthony "Tony" Robbins

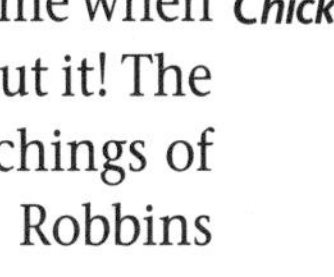

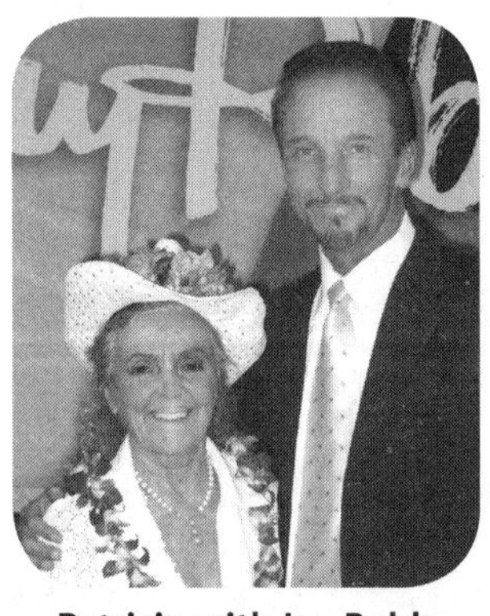

Patricia with Jay Robb

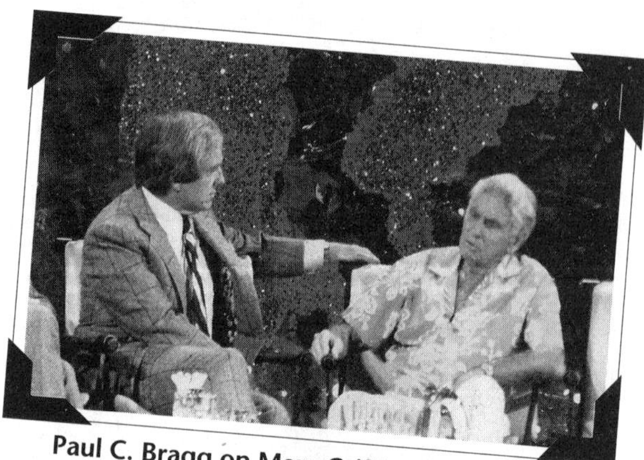

Paul C. Bragg on Merv Griffin Show, 1976

Paul Bragg inspired me many years ago with the *Miracle of Fasting* and with his philosophy on health. His daughter Patricia is a testament to the ageless value of living the Bragg Healthy Lifestyle, – Jay Robb, author of *The Fruit Flush*

PATRICIA & PAUL BRAGG NUTRITIONISTS TO THE HOLLYWOOD STARS

Amazing Duggar Family – "19 Kids and Counting" are big Bragg Fans. Their family relationship is based on respect, love, and Christian family values. We are thrilled the entire Duggar family loves Bragg Liquid Aminos & Apple Cider Vinegar.

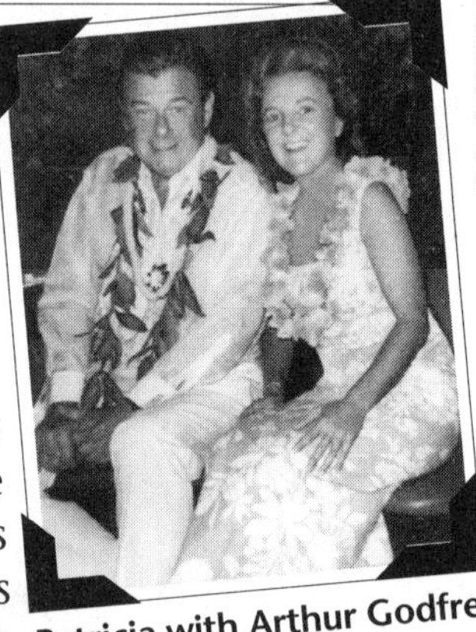

Patricia with Arthur Godfrey

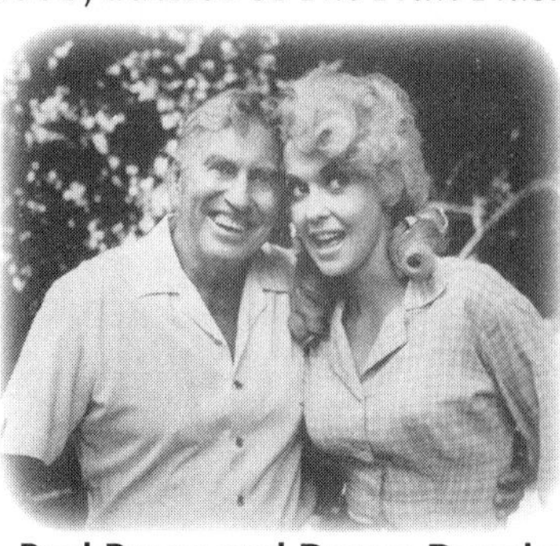

Paul Bragg and Donna Douglas, one Hollywood's most beautiful, talented and best Health Girls. She played the part of "Elly-May" in the Beverly Hillbillies, which became one of the longest-running series in television history and was the #1 show in America in its first 2 years.

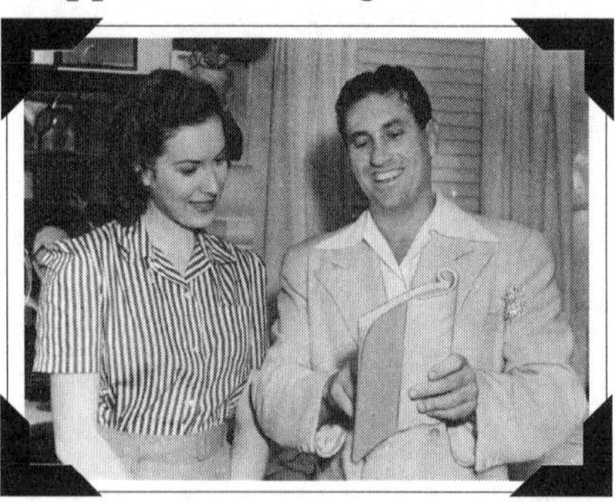

Paul Bragg with Maureen O'Hara, Irish film actress and singer. She was best noted for playing passionate heroines with a highly sensible attitude.

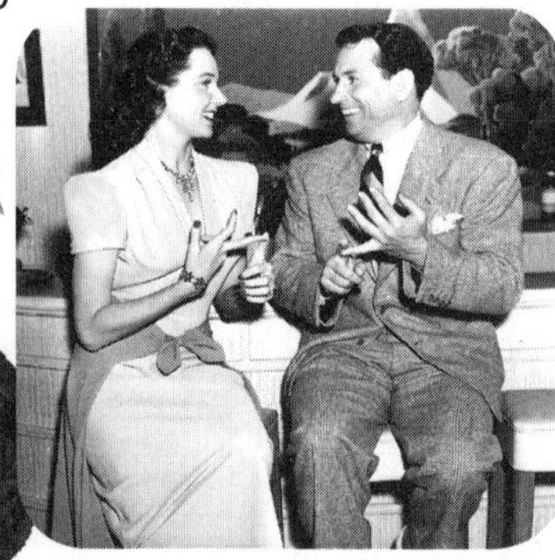

Paul with Actress Jane Wyatt, Emmy award-winning American actress. She is best remembered for her roles in the 1937 film, *Lost Horizon* and the popular TV series *Father Knows Best*.

BRAGG VEGETARIAN HEALTH RECIPES

For Super Energy & Long Life to 120!

Your days shall be 120 years.
Genesis 6:3

PAUL C. BRAGG, N.D., Ph.D.
LIFE EXTENSION SPECIALIST

and

PATRICIA BRAGG, N.D., Ph.D.
HEALTH CRUSADER & LIFESTYLE EDUCATOR

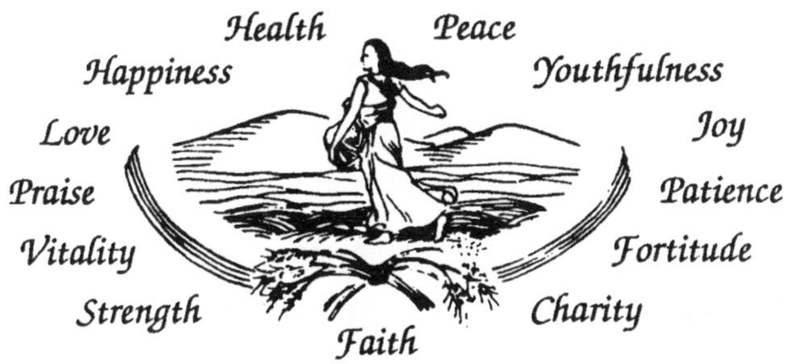

BECOME

A Bragg Health Crusader – for a 100% Healthy World for All!

HEALTH SCIENCE
Box 7, Santa Barbara, California 93102 USA

World Wide Web: www.bragg.com

Notice: Our writings and recipes are to help guide you to live a healthy lifestyle and prevent health problems. If you suspect you have a health problem, please seek qualified health professionals to help you make the healthiest informed choices.

BRAGG

VEGETARIAN HEALTH RECIPES

For Super Energy & Long Life to 120!

Genesis 6:3

PAUL C. BRAGG, N.D., Ph.D.
LIFE EXTENSION SPECIALIST
and
PATRICIA BRAGG, N.D., Ph.D.
HEALTH CRUSADER & LIFESTYLE EDUCATOR

Health Science, Box 7, Santa Barbara, California 93102
Telephone (805) 968-1020, FAX (805) 968-1001
e-mail address: books@bragg.com

Quantity Purchases: Companies, Professional Groups, Churches, Clubs, Fundraisers, etc. Please contact our Special Sales Department.

To See Bragg Books and Product Information on-line, visit our website at: www.bragg.com

This book is printed on recycled, acid-free paper, which saves thousands of trees.

Second Edition MMXI
ISBN: 978-0-87790-027-6

Library of Congress Cataloging-in-Publication Data on file with publisher

Published in the United States
HEALTH SCIENCE, Box 7, Santa Barbara, California 93102 USA

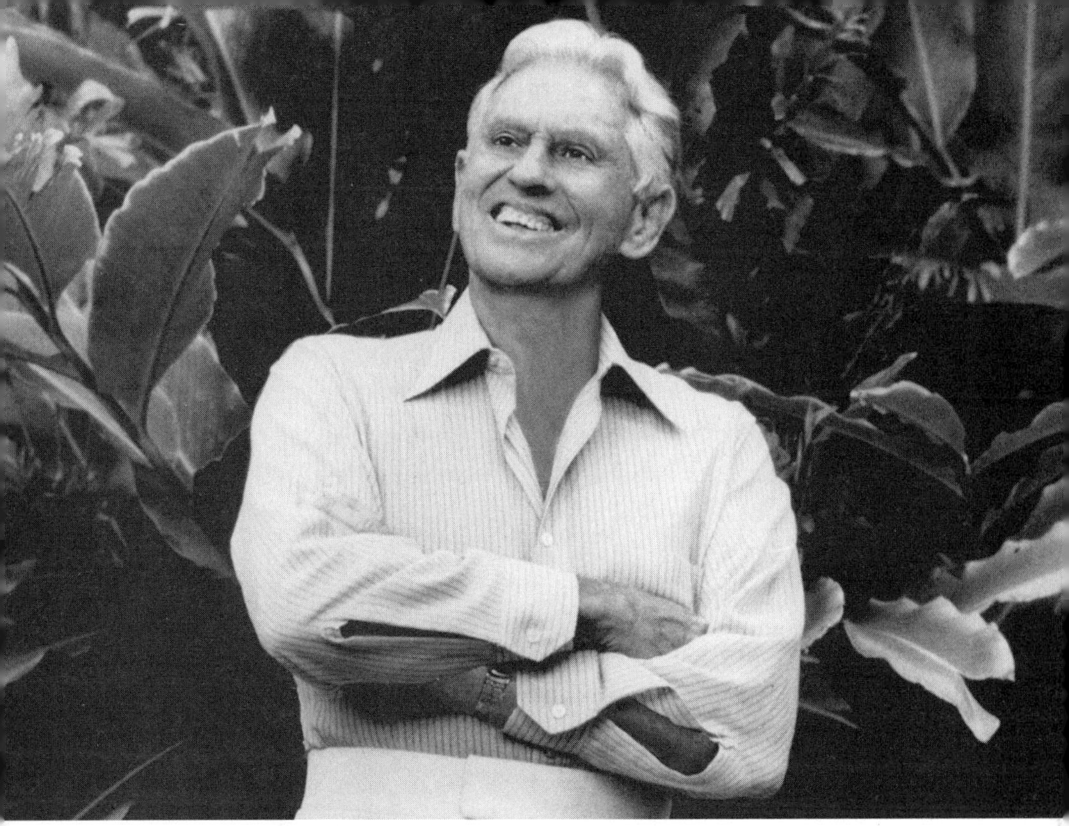

PAUL C. BRAGG, N.D., Ph.D.

World's Leading Healthy Lifestyle Authority

Paul C. Bragg's daughter Patricia and their wonderful, healthy members of the Bragg *Longer Life, Health and Happiness Club* exercise daily on the beautiful Fort DeRussy lawn, at famous Waikiki Beach in Honolulu, Hawaii. View club exercising www.bragg.com. Membership is free and open to everyone to attend any morning – Monday through Saturday, from 9 to 10:30 am – for Bragg Super Power Breathing and Health and Fitness Exercises. On Saturday there are often health lectures on how to live a long, healthy life! The group averages 75 to 125 per day, depending on the season. From December to March it can go up to 150. Its dedicated leaders have been carrying on the class for over 30 years. Thousands have visited the club from around the world and carried the Bragg Health and Fitness Crusade to friends and relatives back home. When you visit Honolulu, Hawaii, Patricia invites you and your friends to join her and the club for wholesome, healthy fellowship. She also recommends visiting the outer Islands (Kauai, Hawaii, Maui, Molokai) for a fulfilling, healthy vacation.

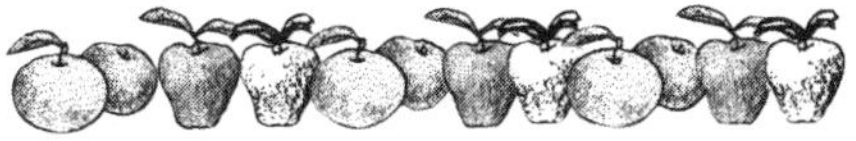

To maintain good health, normal weight and increase the good life of radiant health, joy and happiness, the body must be exercised properly (stretching, walking, jogging, running, biking, swimming, deep breathing, good posture, etc.) and nourished wisely with healthy foods. – Paul C. Bragg

Be a BRAGG Crusader, copy and share with friends, family, co-workers, etc.

Decades of Amazement as Life Rolls By

Where did our years go? They went by so fast.
When we're young they seem to cra-a-wl,
With each decade, they fly past!

At 29 we're the center; At 30 we feel supreme
But 40 strikes terror; Life's not what it seems.
By 50 we've reached maturity; At 60 we accept seniority.
When we're filled with excitement of creative living,
There's no room for depression and despair!

But at 65, wisdom that comes from experience
Then takes over and we learn to accept ourselves as we are.
Each new day is a gift to be treasured,
Enabling us to go far!

At 75, life is for the living
But it is through our sharing, loving and giving
that we reach the Stars of Joy, Peace
and the Possibilities of Eternity!

– by Ruth Lubin, 88 years young & going strong,
who started writing poetry & sculpturing at 80!
PS: Ruth is a fan of the Bragg Healthy Lifestyle for over 58 years!

WITH LOVE PROMISE YOURSELF 

- *Promise yourself to be so strong that nothing can disturb your peace of mind.*
- *To talk health, happiness and prosperity to every person you meet.*
- *To make your friends feel that they are special & appreciated.*
- *To look at the sunny side of everything & make your optimism come true.*
- *To think only of the best, to work only for the best and expect only the best.*
- *To be just as enthusiastic about the success of others as you are about your own.*
- *To forget the mistakes of the past and press on to the greater achievements of the future.*
- *To be too large for worry, too noble for anger, too strong for fear & too happy to permit the presence of trouble.*
- *To give so much time to the improving yourself that you have no time to never criticize others.*
- *To wear a cheerful expression at all times and give a smile to every living creature you meet.*

– Christian D. Larson
Author & Influential Leader

WE NEED YOUR SUPPORT!

With Your Support The Bragg Health Crusades Can Continue to Spread Paul C. Bragg's Teachings

For over 80 years we have been sharing Paul C. Bragg's teachings on healthy living worldwide! Millions are following the Bragg Healthy Lifestyle principles and their lives have been changed forever! Everyday people send us letters, e-mails and call, saying – ***"Paul Bragg saved my life!"***

Former U.S. Surgeon General, Dr. C. Everett Koop said Paul Bragg did more for the Health of America than anyone person he knew of.

OUR MISSION: To spread health worldwide and inspire youth and people of all ages to achieve optimal health – physically, mentally and spiritually and live long, productive, caring, happy lives.

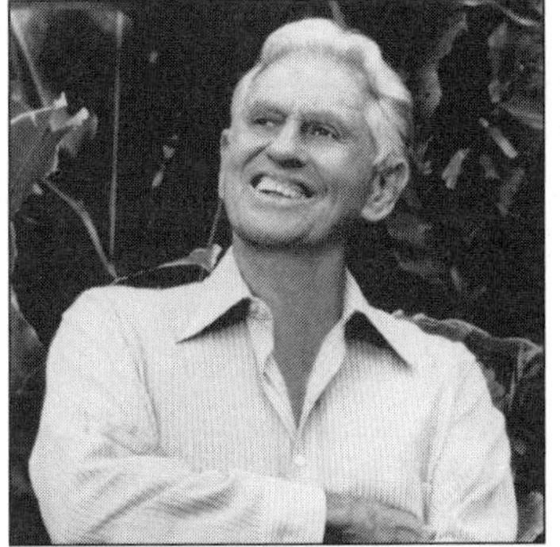

Paul C. Bragg, N.D., Ph.D.
Originator of Health Stores
Life Extension Specialist
Health Crusader to the World

If your life has been touched and helped by Bragg health teachings, please help us carry on the Bragg Legacy into this 21st Century and beyond. Your tax deductible donation to the *Bragg Health Institute* will support our mission to continue the Bragg Message of Health worldwide and inspire future generations.

The non-profit and philanthropic work of the *Bragg Health Institute* funds The *Bragg Health Crusades*, community health, health education lectures, health seminars, and publications on healthy living. The Institute conducts health outreach to youth in schools, also organic gardening teaching programs, and helps sponsor health science research and provides scholarships to worthy students pursuing the natural health science professions.

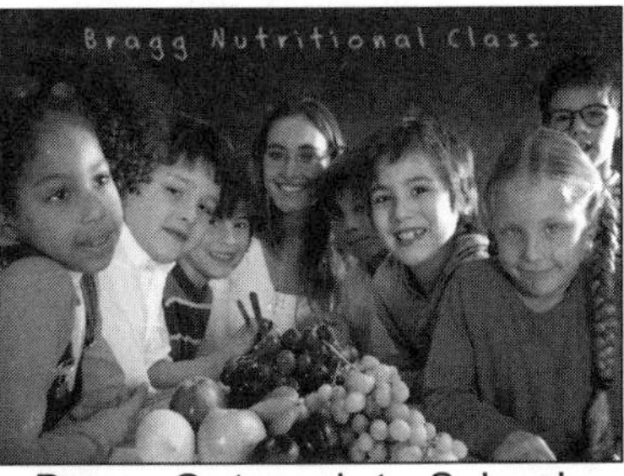

Bragg Outreach to Schools

Please join us in sharing The Bragg Health Legacy!

(Please see next page for more information)

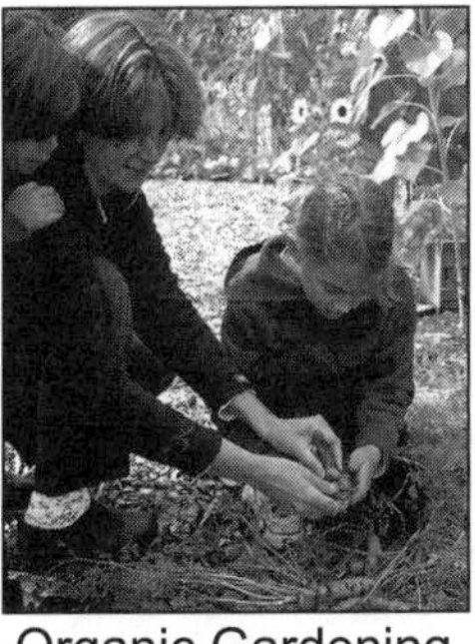

Organic Gardening Teaching Programs

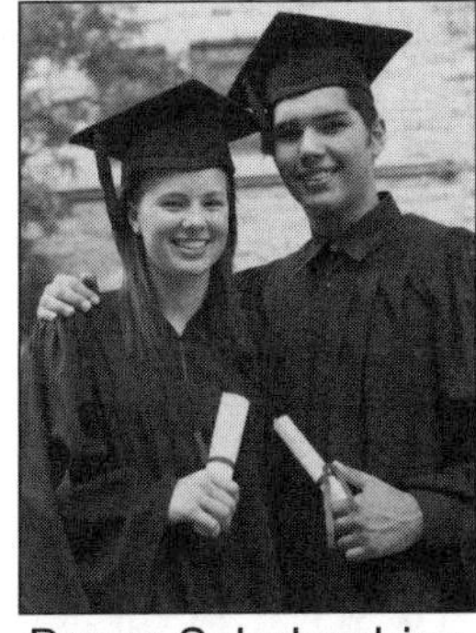

Bragg Scholarships

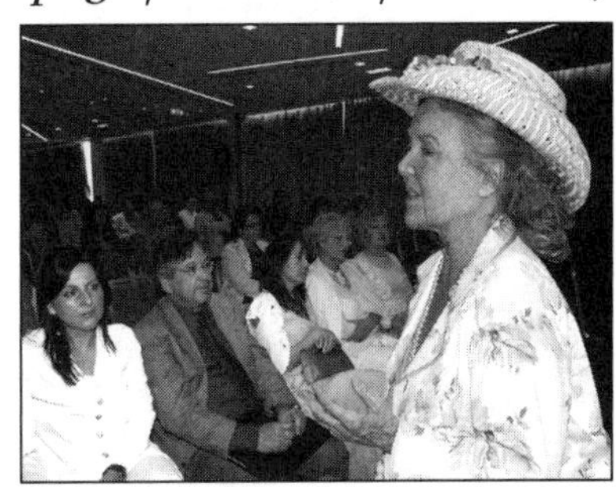

Patricia Bragg lecturing at Bragg Health Seminars

HEALTH DREAM WITH NEW HEALTH VISION

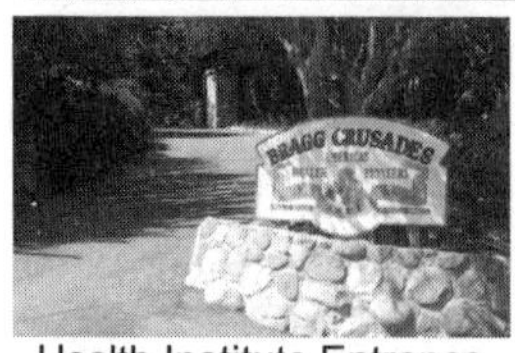

Health Institute Entrance

The Bragg Health Institute is located on a beautiful 120 acre Campus and Organic Farm on the coast of Santa Barbara, California. Patricia Bragg and the Directors of Bragg Health Institute have designated this as the future site of the greatest living tribute to the life of Paul C. Bragg. The new Bragg Health Institute will become a world center for organic and healthy lifestyle education and research. (See our *Mission, Purpose and Vision for the Future* video on *bragghealthinstitute.org*)

You can also be part of Paul Bragg's lasting legacy by having your name permanently inscribed upon one of the educational nature walks or inspirational walls that will enhance the natural beauty of the Bragg Health Institute Campus and Organic Farm. Or you may want to have your name inscribed in the Grand Entrance or one of the rooms in the Bragg Memorial Library or Health Education Center. Your name can be part of your own legacy, as you will be recognized for generations to come as a great Health Crusader because of your financial support of these wonderful health projects. When thousands of visitors see your name each year, they will know that you helped make a difference in the world.

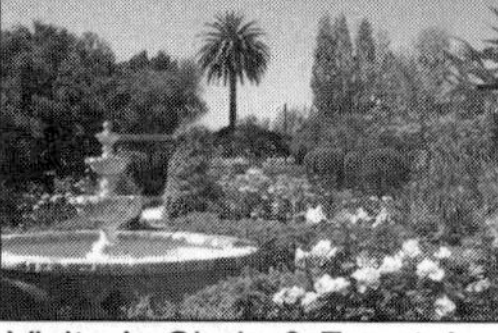
Visitor's Circle & Fountain

Some Special Health Projects You Can Partner with us:

- ❑ Healthy Lifestyle Teaching Videos
- ❑ Paul Bragg Library & Rose Gardens
- ❑ Organic Medicinal Herb Gardens
- ❑ Scholarships for Future Health Doctors
- ❑ Special Health Events & Programs
- ❑ Organic Teaching Gardens
- ❑ Health Teaching Kitchen
- ❑ Health Eco Education Center
- ❑ Bragg Nature & Farm Walks
- ❑ Bragg Health Museum

— — — — — — — — — — — — *COPY AND MAIL* — — — — — — — — — — — —

YES! I would like to help support Bragg Health Crusades by making a contribution to the Bragg Health Institute, a 501(c)(3) non-profit foundation, tax ID# 27-0983248 Your contributions are tax deductible.

❑ Enclosed is my tax-deductible gift of $________ ❍ Check ❍ VISA ❍ MC ❍ Discover

❍ $25 ❍ $50 ❍ $100 ❍ $250 ❍ $500 ❍ $1,000 ❍ $2,500 ❍ $__________

❑ Please send me info on where my name can be permanently inscribed at Bragg Center.

My gift is in honor/memory of ______________________________________

Please send notice of this gift to (name & address):______________________________

____

Credit Card Number:______________________________________ Card Expires: _____/_____ month / year

Signature:______________________________________

● ____

Your Name PLEASE PRINT

● ____ ● ________

Address Apt. No.

● ____________________ ● ____________ ● ____________

City State Zip

● ( ) ____________ ● ______________________________

Phone e-mail

If giving by check, please make check payable to: ***Bragg Health Institute***

Mail To: Box 7, Santa Barbara, CA 93102 USA • (805) 968-1020

For more info check out our web: www.bragghealthinstitute.org

Spreading health worldwide since 1912

VEGETARIAN NUTRITION AND DIET

For Optimal Health, Disease Prevention and Longevity

By John Westerdahl, Ph.D., M.P.H., R.D., C.N.S.

Today scientific research has established that a healthy vegetarian diet can play a major role in preventing disease and achieving optimal health and longevity. There are great health benefits for those who choose to follow a vegetarian lifestyle.

HEART DISEASE – Most health experts agree that vegetarians have the advantage when it comes to heart disease prevention. For the most part, plant-based diets reduce the intake of cholesterol-raising saturated fat and artery-clogging cholesterol. Both saturated fat and cholesterol are two dietary constituents strongly linked to increased coronary heart disease risk. The less we eat of them, the better it is for our heart. Eating a diet with lots of fruits, vegetables, whole grains, and beans can reduce our risk of heart disease in other ways as well. Foods such as beans, oats, and apples are rich sources of soluble fiber. Soluble fiber is effective in helping to lower blood cholesterol.

There is evidence that the B-vitamin, *folic acid,* helps reduce the risk of heart disease by lowering blood levels of a harmful *homocysteine*. Fruits and vegetables are a major source of folic acid, a heart-healthy vitamin, another reason why vegetarian diets help prevent heart disease.

Vegetarian diets have lower levels of iron. Iron, which is concentrated in red meat, promotes cell-destroying free radical activity. Free radicals promote ageing and also oxidize LDL ("bad") cholesterol thereby making it a more harmful substance to the arteries which promotes atherosclerosis. Fruits and vegetables are rich in vital phytochemicals (plant nutrients) that are anti-ageing antioxidants or scavengers of harmful free radicals. Vegetarians have much higher levels of plant antioxidants circulating in their bloodstreams compared to meat eaters. The antioxidants found naturally occurring in plant foods such as vitamins C and E, polyphenols and flavonoids, may help prevent or even reverse free radical damage that leads to heart disease.

Studies have proven that healthy, very low-fat vegetarian diets not only prevent heart disease, but also reverse it! Research confirming this has been conducted by Dean Ornish, M.D., of the Preventive Medicine Research Institute located in Sausalito, California. Dr. Ornish demonstrated that blocked arteries can actually become clearer after a year on a healthy vegetarian diet alone – without the use of cholesterol-lowering drugs! (see web: *www.ornish.com*)

CANCER – There is strong scientific evidence that a diet rich in fruits and vegetables protect us against many forms of cancer. This includes cancers of the lung, colon, stomach, mouth, larynx, esophagus, bladder and prostate. Many scientist believe that natural phytochemicals found in plant foods like carotenoids, vitamin C and E, selenium, indoles, isothiocyanates, flavonoids, phenols, limonene and others are the protective compounds (see page 73).

In addition to phytochemicals, plant foods are rich in healthy fiber. Fiber is beneficial in preventing colon cancer. Studies also show that men who are heavy red-meat eaters have increased risk of getting colon and prostate cancers. This may be related not only to animal fats, but carcinogens created when meat is cooked. The high iron (a pro-oxidant) content of red meat may also be a contributing factor to increasing cancer risk.

STROKE – More and more scientific research is establishing the fact that a diet rich in fruits and vegetables is beneficial in reducing the risk of stroke. Studies show eating more fruits and vegetables are contributing protective factors for the arteries in the brain.

CONSTIPATION AND DIVERTICULOSIS – Vegetarians eat significantly more dietary fiber, which helps prevent these colon problems. Fiber adds bulk to the waste material in the colon, which promotes more rapid elimination that helps prevent constipation and also reduces intestinal pressure preventing diverticulosis.

The vegetarian diet is the optimal diet for the prevention, treatment and even reversal of disease. Physicians and Health Science Researchers have demonstrated this. Well-balanced vegetarian diets also make the optimal anti-ageing diet. Vegetarian and plant-based diet population groups, like the Seventh-Day Adventists, the people of Hunza, and the centenarians of Okinawa, have shown by example that eating a diet based mostly on plant foods, contributes to good health and a long active life. See website: *http://ngm.nationalgeographic.com/ngm/0511/feature1/*

John Westerdahl, Ph.D., M.P.H., R.D., C.N.S., is the Director of the Bragg Health Foundation and the Director of Health Science for Bragg Live Food Products, Inc. Dr. Westerdahl is a nutritionist and registered dietitian and is recognized as one of the nation's leading authorities on vegetarian and vegan nutrition and diets. He is the former nutrition editor for *Veggie Life* magazine. Dr. Westerdahl is an active member of the Vegetarian Nutrition Dietetic Practice Group (*www.vegetariannutrition.net*) of the American Dietetic Association (*www.eatright.org*) and has received national awards for his contributions to the field of vegetarian nutrition.

Dr. John Westerdahl Is A Young Paul C. Bragg Health Crusader

John Westerdahl is a young Paul C. Bragg, for he is a dedicated true Health Crusader. He has spread the message of health throughout Hawaii via his radio talk show "Nutrition and You," and with his lectures and clinics on nutrition, weight control, stop-smoking, stop-drugs and his HEARTBEAT Program, which promoted cardiovascular fitness. John's outreach especially in Hawaii has improved the health of thousands. He continues to reach millions with Bragg world-wide Health Crusades, Radio and TV shows, and magazine articles. (*www.bragg.com*)

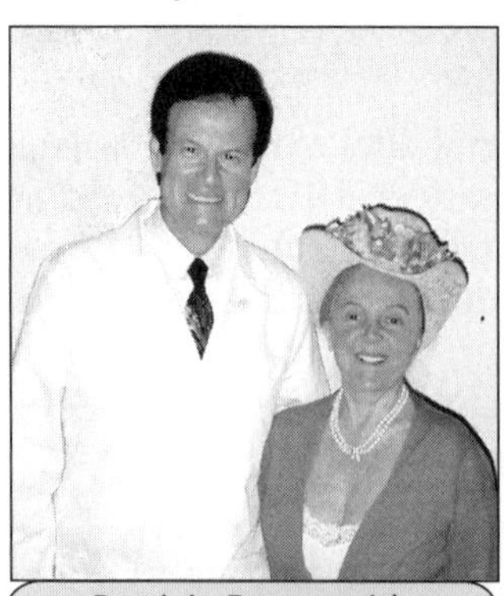

Patricia Bragg with Dr. John Westerdahl Director of Bragg Health Foundation

Dr. John was chosen as one of ten most outstanding young people of Hawaii. He justly deserved this high honor, for he's dedicated and loves being a Health Crusader! We at Health Science are proud of John and welcome him as the new dynamic Director of the Bragg Health Foundation. We encourage more young people into this Wellness Crusade to put America back where we belong, #1 in Health and Fitness instead of way down on the world list. – Patricia Bragg

The 5th International Congress on Vegetarian Nutrition

The Premiere Scientific Conference on the Health Effects of Plant-based Diets held at Loma Linda University

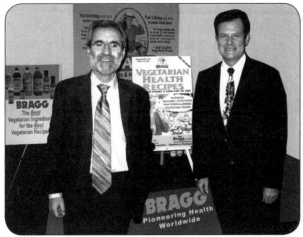

Dr. J. Sabaté and **Dr. John Westerdahl** at the official introduction of Patricia Bragg's new *Bragg Vegetarian Health Recipes* book at the Congress. Dr. J. Sabaté, M.D., Dr.P.H. is the Professor and Chair of the Department of Nutrition at the School of Public Health, Loma Linda University in California and chairman of the 5th International Congress on Vegetarian Nutrition.

How to Live The Bragg Healthy Lifestyle

The Bragg Healthy Lifestyle has many wise components. Here is a list of Do's and Don'ts that Paul C. Bragg developed and Patricia Bragg practices and preaches world-wide:

- ✓ Don't eat refined sugar, salty foods, white rice, white flour, fried foods, saturated fats or hydrogenated oils, coffee or caffeinated teas, sodas and drinks, pork, smoked fish and smoked meats, and all foods preserved with salt, sugar and chemicals.
- ✓ Do allow 4 to 5 hours between meals so the digestive system has time to work, before eating more food.
- ✓ Don't eat a big breakfast because it's too difficult for the body to digest. Fresh fruit and blender energy pep drinks are excellent.
- ✓ Do drink eight glasses of distilled or purified water daily, along with herbal teas and juices.
- ✓ Do fast one day a week to cleanse and detoxify your system to help stay healthy.
- ✓ Don't drink cow's milk and its products.
- ✓ Do enjoy early or late gentle sunshine regularly, it has germ-killing and healing energy.
- ✓ It's best to get your protein from healthy vegetarian sources instead of meat.
- ✓ Do make sure you have regular bowel movements (have ample water, salads, etc.).
- ✓ Don't rely on enemas or high colonics unless sick or extreme constipation.
- ✓ Do exercise regularly, walk, swim, bike, etc.
- ✓ Don't "self-drug"; correct your problems with living a Healthy Lifestyle.
- ✓ Do think positively, cultivating health, cheerfulness, happiness, kindness, charity and the love of family and brotherhood.
- ✓ Don't neglect your sleep, get 8 hours nightly.
- ✓ Do practice deep breathing throughout the day and always maintain good posture.
- ✓ Do make every effort to improve yourself physically, mentally, emotionally and spiritually every day! *– 3 John 2*

You are what you eat, drink, breathe, think, say and do!
– Patricia Bragg, ND, PhD., Pioneer Health Crusader

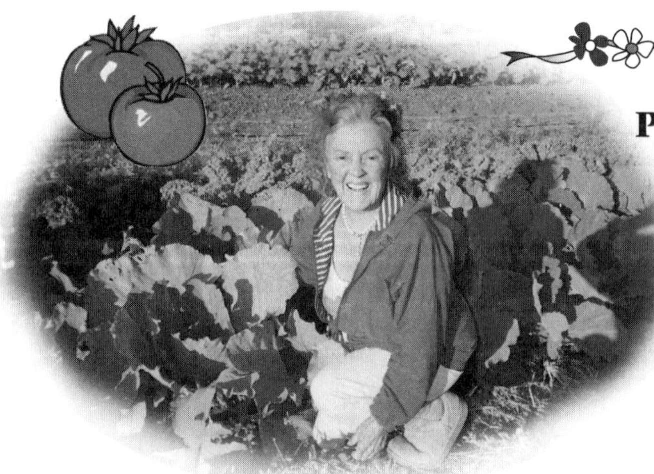

Patricia Bragg in her organic garden,
Santa Barbara, California

PATRICIA BRAGG SPREADING HEALTH, JOY, HAPPINESS, KINDNESS, & LOVE!!

Love is the sun shining in us to sparkle our lives! – Patricia Bragg

Man's body is his vehicle through life, his earthly temple . . . and the Creator wants us filled with joy & health for a long, fruitful life. – Patricia Bragg

Kindness should be a frame of mind in which we are alert to every chance: to do, to give, to share and to cheer. – Patricia Bragg

Create the kind of self you will be happy to live with all your life!!

Anyone who helps you grow is an angel to you.

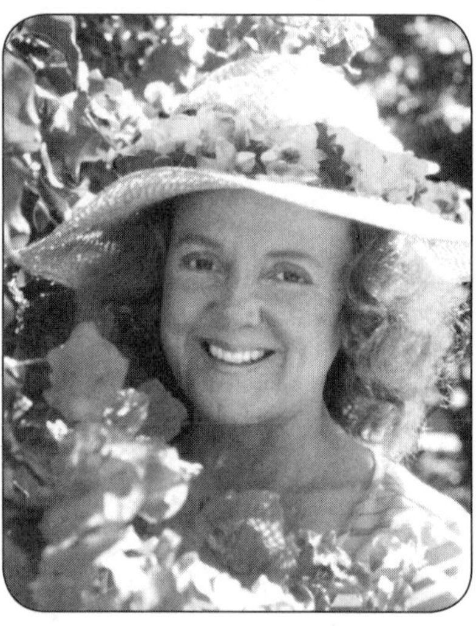

There is a fountain of youth:
it is your mind, your talents,
the creativity you bring to your life
and the lives of people you love.
When you learn to tap this source,
you will have truly defeated age.
– Sophia Loren

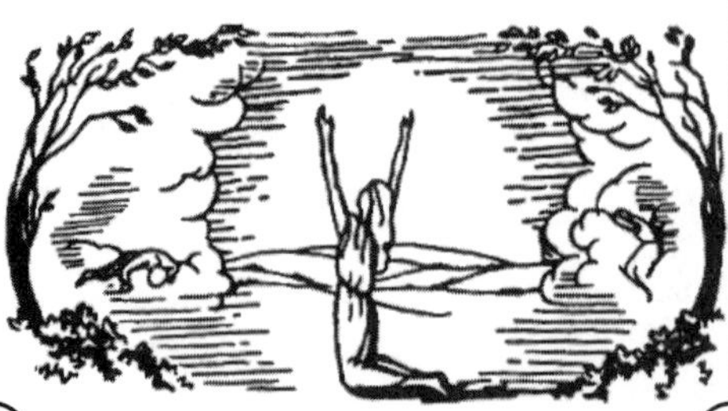

Love makes the world go 'round, and it is everlasting when it is written with caring, loving advice that will improve and enrich your life! This is why my father and I love sharing with you the health wisdoms which can be with you on your life's journey. Our inspiring books on health, fitness and longevity go 'round the world spreading health, peace of mind, joy and love!
– Patricia Bragg, N.D., Ph.D.
World Health Crusader

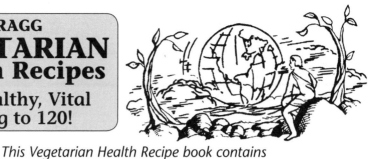

BRAGG
VEGETARIAN Health Recipes
For Healthy, Vital Living to 120!

This Vegetarian Health Recipe book contains both cooked and raw food (RF) vegetarian recipes.
RF *symbol designates recipes are categorized as Raw Food Recipes.*

Table of Contents

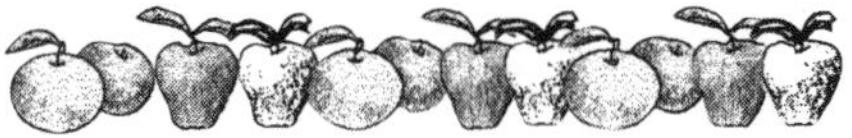

We are blessed and recharged by each one of you reading our teachings. They are filled with health wisdom and love for you – Thank You! – Patricia Bragg

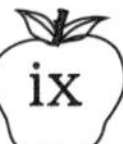

Contents

The grains that are heart-healthy are organic brown rice, organic whole grain breads, cereals, and whole-wheat pastas. Also popcorn, organic corn is a whole grain. My favorite is air-popped and top with Bragg Aminos, Bragg Olive Oil and Bragg Nutritional Yeast (see recipe page 254). There's also bulgur, buckwheat groats, barley, millet, spelt, and quinoa. Quinoa is a complete protein and makes an ideal breakfast cereal.

Contents

In my opinion, a vegetarian (plant-based) diet is preferable to a flesh-meat diet for many reasons. It is more humane. It is conducive to good health and it is more simple and economical. I believe that a vegetarian diet is essential to our civilization, to universal brotherhood, and to the increase of human happiness and health. – Paul C. Bragg, ND, PhD., Life Extension Specialist

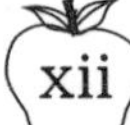

A huge volume of scientific data confirms the protective role of fruits and vegetables on human health. – Life Extension Magazine, www.lef.org

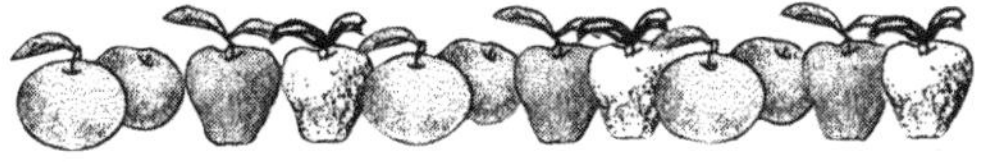

There are dozens of foods that contain almost NO bad fat and avocados and olives, fruits and vegetables have perfect ZERO fat!

Seek out and choose whole foods, organic fruits, vegetables and organic whole grain cereals, breads, etc. rather than the commercial, canned, refined white flour and sugar products and other highly processed goods in the center aisles.

Poor diet & lack of exercise may soon be the leading causes of death in U.S.
See website: www.nutrition.gov for healthy nutritional tips

Contents

Dr. Dean Ornish has been able to reverse heart disease in more than 70% of his patients who follow, among other things, a low-fat vegetarian diet.

Sad Facts: *Many people go throughout life committing partial suicide – destroying their health, heart, youth, beauty, talents, energies and creative qualities. Indeed, to learn how to be good to oneself is often more difficult than to learn how to be good to others.* – Paul C. Bragg, ND, PhD.

For where your treasure is, there will your heart be also. – Matthew 6:21

Reflect upon your blessings, of which every man has plenty,
Not on your past misfortunes, of which all men have some.
– Charles Dickens

Introduction

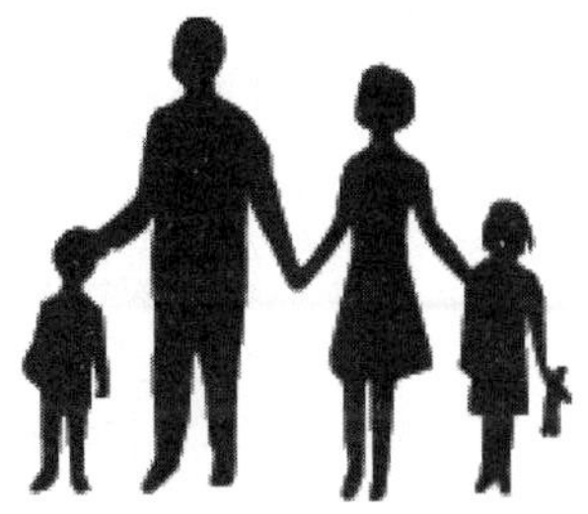

The Art of Eating Healthy For The Whole Family

The person you are today, the person you will be tomorrow, next week, next month, ten years from now depends on what you eat and drink. You are the sum total of the food and liquids you consume. How you look, feel and carry your years all depends on what you eat and drink and the lifestyle you live.

Every part of your body is made from food – the hair on your head, your eyes, teeth, bones, toenails and fingernails, blood and flesh. Even your expression is formed from what you eat, because the healthy person is a well-fed, happy person.

Today, because of economic necessity, our markets are stocked with dead, processed foods. We have milled the life out of our grains and taken the vitamins and minerals out of many foods; processing and preservatives destroy some of our most valuable food factors. If you don't put the healthy foods that contain the basic vitamins and minerals into your body, someday you are going to face a serious deficiency disease. You can't escape this law of biochemistry. Yet for many years "health foods" have been looked upon as unappetizing, tasteless and uninteresting. This is not so! When properly prepared, "health foods" are the most delicious! They are the true essence of healthy food preparation.

Our foods should contribute to physical restoration and sensual enjoyment, tempered with intelligence and the keen satisfaction of enjoying healthy meals. It's not just what we eat that feeds the body; it's what we digest! Digestion is enhanced by giving thanks, chewing food thoroughly and enjoying healthy mealtime foods.

Flavoring must be discreet, must present itself subtly while the appreciative eater is unaware. The intangible sense of pleasant discovery and the enjoyment of an unexpected, harmonious blending of subdued flavors add much to the rhythmic functioning of the physical processes of the body. Food that announces its presence with impressive blasts of flavor may be nutritionally good, but still not good cookery. Both flavoring, herbs and healthy nutrition are important!

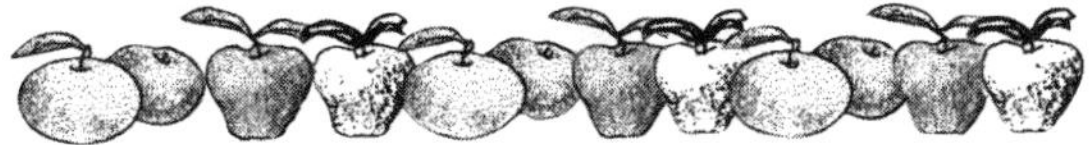

Open your eyes to behold wondrous things out of Thy law. – Psalms 119:18

The greatest wealth is health. – Virgil, famous Roman poet and philosopher

The Foods You Eat Will Minimize or Maximize Your Health

Basically, your food's job is to fill your physical needs; but it can't do it completely unless it gives stimulation to the appetite and delight in the eating, and leaves a feeling of contented satisfaction that makes for better digestion. Remember, the food you eat becomes your body's fuel – and becomes you!

Moderation is closely tied to the art of good eating. Excessive eating dulls the appetite and appreciation. No food remains "good" food when overindulgence governs the appetite, making you sluggish, sleepy and overburdening your digestive system!

Nutritional science alone is not enough. It must be blended with inspiration, art and healthy imagination. For those who have never learned to blend science and art in their everyday eating, this book is written with the hope that it will guide them firmly onto the path of a healthy eating lifestyle, with healthy foods for a long, healthy, happy, fulfilled life! (*Genesis 6:3*)

Why You Need a Health Food Recipe Book

In Health Food Cookery, white flour and white sugar are not used; nor are processed, devitalized, degerminated, demineralized foods. We use the whole-grains, containing all the life element, and natural sweeteners instead of refined white sugars. That's why cooking with whole, natural foods requires special proportions, ingredients and directions.

You will find cooking with natural whole-grain flours and natural sweeteners well worth the trouble; and bringing out the "soul" of foods with natural, healthy herbs and spices is a tremendous thrill and meal adventure you will love!

Most of the good, wholesome, natural foods you need for these recipes can be found in health food stores and whole food supermarkets. Many stores have everything from organically grown fruits and vegetables to 100% organic whole-grains, flours, pastas, pizzas, cereals, vitamin and mineral supplements, natural sweeteners, fresh juices and delicious healthy beverages, un-sulphured sun-dried fruits and thousands of other health products. My father, Paul C. Bragg, named and originated health food stores and now they are found throughout America, and the world, playing a major role in keeping people healthy!

Almost any recipe prepared with dead, demineralized, devitaminized ingredients can be made better with healthful, wholesome foods! As you learn to prepare foods the Bragg Healthy Lifestyle way, you may begin adjusting these recipes to your taste. On the next page are some healthy substitutes.

Healthy Recipe Substitutes

BAKING POWDER, SODA & YEAST: Use non-aluminum baking powders from your health food store. Try: Rumford, Hain or Cellu Baking Powders or you can also use quick rise dry yeast.

CHOCOLATE: Use dark unsweetened chocolate. Carob is a great nutritious chocolate substitute.

CORNSTARCH: For thickening use arrowroot, tapioca, agar agar for baking and desserts. Potato flour for gravies, soups, and stews, etc.

COFFEE, CHINA TEA: Non-caffeine, herbal and grain coffee substitutes, Postum, Cafix, herbal and only non-caffeine green teas.

DAIRY: Organic soy and rice milks (large variety of non-dairy cheeses, yogurts and ice cream are available), and nut milks (almond, cashew, etc.). If you do use dairy: raw certified, chemical and hormone-free cow and goat's milk products are best; use salt-free raw butter, kefir, yogurt, etc. Over-processed milk is dead! See web: *notmilk.com*

EGGS: Egg Replacer is a culinary egg substitute containing no eggs or animal products. This commercial product is made by Ener-G Foods, Inc. (see web: *ener-g.com).* The product is made of potato and tapioca starch and leavening agents. It is designed for use in baking and is used in place of eggs in many recipes in this book.

MEAT: Vegetarian – soybeans, tofu (soybean curd), tempeh, beans, soy cheeses, sprouts, raw nuts and seeds, etc. (See Vegetarian Protein Chart, page 138).

SALT: Herbs, garlic, Bragg Aminos (from organic sodium and non-GMO soy). Also try our delicious Bragg Sprinkle (24 Herbs & Spices) and Bragg Kelp Seasonings. Both perfect replacements for salt.

SHORTENING: Never use hardened lard or unhealthy commercial oils. Use unrefined natural, cold-pressed oils (such as Bragg Organic Extra Virgin Olive Oil, safflower, flaxseed, sunflower, soy or nut oils).

VINEGAR: Most commercial vinegars are dead. Use only Bragg Organic, Raw Apple Cider Vinegar – it can replace any vinegar and has great health benefits. (pg. 202) Read *Bragg Vinegar Book* (see booklist back pages) or visit our interesting, informative web: *bragg.com.*

WHITE FLOURS: Use only 100% organic, whole-grains for bread, rolls, pasta, pizza, etc. and organic pastry flours for baking. Use 20% more liquid with whole-grain flours due to bran and wheat germ.

WHITE SUGAR: Substitute natural sweeteners to your taste. When preparing recipes with raw honey: for each cup of sugar, substitute cup honey. Use herb Stevia powder (see pg. 224) which is safe for diabetics. Also try these for variety: barley malt, brown rice syrups, concentrated fruit juices, 100% maple syrup, molasses, natural raw brown and date sugars. Living the Bragg Healthy Lifestyle you will enjoy more fresh fruits and less sweets.

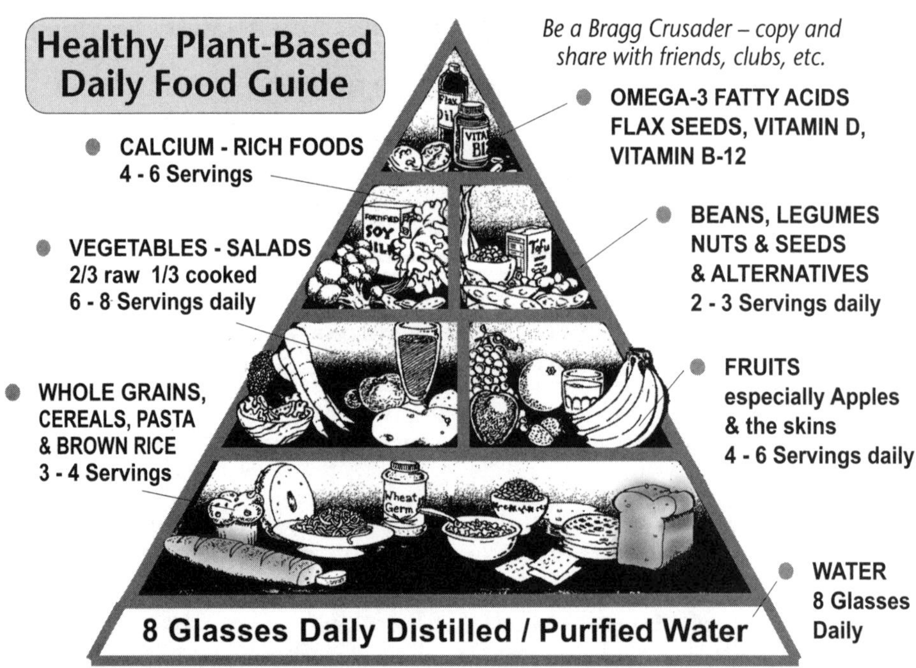

The Healthy Plant-Based Daily Food Guide

The Healthy Plant-Based Daily Food Guide Pyramid is much different than other food guide pyramids you may have seen. This food pyramid is based on a more optimal diet eating plan of healthy vegetarian foods. There are no "junk foods" found in this pyramid. For those wanting to eat a healthful, balanced vegetarian diet, this pyramid provides an excellent guide. It is in harmony with the Bragg Healthy Lifestyle principles of optimal nutrition.

At the foundation of the pyramid is distilled/purified water. We recommend distilled water as the optimal source of water to drink. It is the healthiest and purist type of water. We recommend drinking at least eight glasses of distilled water daily. Recognize that you also "eat your water" by eating healthy plant foods such as raw fruits and vegetables. The eight glasses you drink is in addition to the water you take in from your plant-based foods.

After the water base, the next pyramid level is whole grains. This includes all whole grain foods, including cereals, pasta, and brown rice. We recommend eating three to four servings a day of whole grains. An example of a serving of whole grains is one slice of whole grain bread, one-half cup cooked grains or cereal, or pasta. One ounce of a ready-to-eat whole grain cereal is also a serving in this group.

We next recommend eating at least six to eight servings of vegetables every day. Try to eat two-thirds of these vegetable servings raw and only one-third of your servings lightly cooked for optimal nutrition! Examples of a serving of vegetables are one-half cup of cooked vegetables, one cup of raw vegetables including salad, and three-fourths of a cup of vegetable juice.

We next recommend eating at least four to six servings of fruits daily. Here again we recommend to have most of your fruit servings raw, organic and uncooked. Examples of fruit serving include: one apple, banana, orange or pear; one-half cup of fruit, three-fourths of a cup of fruit juice, and one-fourth cup of dried fruits.

It is important to have at least four to six servings each day of calcium-rich foods. You do not need to get your calcium from dairy products. There are plenty of other non-dairy, vegetarian calcium alternatives. (See chart page 52). These include soymilk, tofu and high calcium greens. Examples of serving sizes for the calcium-rich food group include: one-half cup of soymilk; one-quarter cup of tofu; one cup of raw or cooked calcium-rich greens like kale, collards, broccoli or Chinese greens; and one-quarter cup of almonds.

Beans, legumes, nuts and seeds, and vegetarian meat alternatives are excellent sources of vegetable protein in the vegetarian diet. It is recommended to have two to three servings from this group each day to meet your protein needs. Examples of vegetable protein servings include: one cup of cooked legumes (beans, lentils, dried peas); one-half cup of tofu; one serving of a vegetarian meat substitute such as a soy-based veggie-burger or "veggie" meat slices; three tablespoons of nut butter; or one-quarter cup of raw nuts.

In order for you to get your essential fatty acids we recommend eating healthful fats from foods such as nuts and seeds (flax seeds and walnuts are excellent sources of omega-3 fatty acids), flaxseed oil, and Bragg Organic Extra Virgin Olive Oil. Taking dietary supplements that provide vitamin D and vitamin B12 are also recommended because sometimes these nutrients can be missing or at low levels in certain vegetarian diets if they are not properly balanced.

The Healthy Plant-Based Daily Food Guide Pyramid provides you with nutritional guidelines that can be helpful in preparing healthful, delicious vegetarian meals for you and your family.

Maintaining Nutrient Content in Vegetables

Avoid long storage of perishable vegetables, especially greens. Store vegetables in a cool atmosphere. Stored vegetables, even those not wilted, have lost a large part of their vitamin C and nutrient content. Please remember fresh and organic is best!

Avoid trimming or paring vegetables and fruits *before* cooking if possible. If they must be handled in this manner, cook them as quickly as possible after exposing their surfaces.

Avoid boiling in water that will be discarded later. Most minerals are indestructible; but water-soluble vitamins are lost when cooking water is discarded, so serve with recipe or save for soup stock.

Never add baking soda to nonacid vegetables. It destroys the vitamin B1 and C content. Do not overcook. Most foods are easily digestible and of better color and flavor if cooked moderately tender. Heat is destructive to vitamin B1.

Avoid cooking too large of quantities at a time; reheating leftovers causes vitamin loss! Serve all hot foods promptly. Plunge foods into boiling water quickly whenever possible in the boiling process, rather than starting them in cold water. This avoids oxidation and helps conserve vitamins A and C.

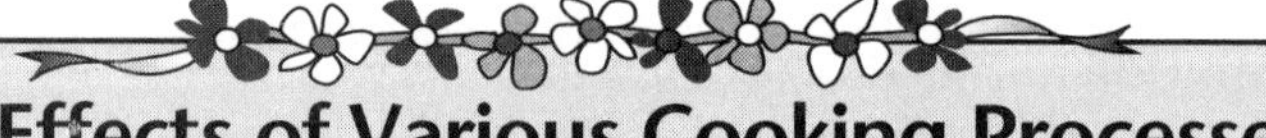

The Effects of Various Cooking Processes

Baking or Roasting. The effect of these methods of cooking varies with the food. For best vitamin retention, baking or roasting should be stopped as soon as food is cooked as desired, never overcooked.

Boiling. If food is added to a small amount of actively boiling water, and all the water is retained, the vitamins can be well conserved. Slow heating from cold water, overcooking, discarding of cooking waters containing soluble nutrients, boiling dry with air exposure, causes high vitamin loss, particularly of vitamin C.

Broiling. The retention of vitamin and mineral content of foods is high during broiling, if it is brief; it is superior to frying and is comparable to light roasting. But if the food is cut thin, permitting a large surface exposure, the vitamin loss may be comparatively high.

Frying. Frying is generally a destructive process for vitamins sensitive to oxidation. Light stir fry or sautéing on low heat is best.

Pressure-Cooking. Carefully-timed pressure cooking with a good atmosphere of steam is satisfactory; but if too much air remains at the start of cooking or if heating is prolonged, there may be heavy losses of both vitamins B1 and C.

Steaming. Theoretically, this is the most desirable process of cooking for vitamin retention (*raw is still the best*).

The Principles of Scientific Nutrition

It is only in recent years that the practice of dietetics has been guided by the modern science of nutrition. Many diet kitchens and diet lists are still dominated by traditions and fads. Many so-called "special diets" are needlessly complex, unscientific and often, if continued over a long period of time, positively dangerous because of a nutritional imbalance that brings about deficiency conditions. Too often, they tend toward the correction of only one particular issue and completely ignore the interrelation of ample quantities of essential foods, organic salads, etc. for healthy, entire body nutrition. Common sense must be used in treating special conditions. Remember you become what you eat and drink.

God has furnished man with abundant means for the gratification of an un-perverted appetite. He has spread before him the products of the earth – a bountiful variety of food that is palatable to the taste and nutritious to the system. Of these our benevolent heavenly Father says we may freely eat.

Grains, fruits, nuts, and vegetables, constitute the diet chosen for us by our Creator. These foods prepared in as simple and natural a manner as possible, are the most healthful and nourishing. They impart strength, endurance and a vigor of intellect that are not produced by a refined and stimulating diet.

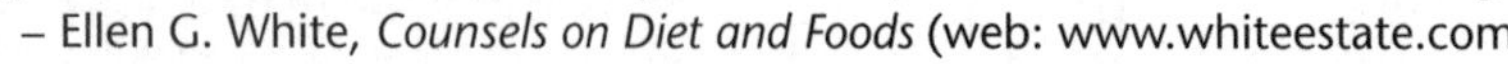
– Ellen G. White, *Counsels on Diet and Foods* (web: www.whiteestate.com)

The Alkaline or Acid Effect of Food

Foods, such as meat and eggs, that are high in proteins tend to exert an acid effect in the body because when they are "burned" in the body, a number of the normal "end products" are acidic, such as uric acid, sulphuric acid and phosphoric acid. However, these acids are rendered harmless when they are balanced with alkaline material from the body, as they then form neutral salts. The neutral salts are eliminated normally by the kidneys.

Fruits and vegetables usually exert an alkaline effect because they contain the alkaline salts, such as calcium, and neutralize the acid products in the body. When we eat fruits and vegetables with free acids such as citric (in lemons), malic (in apples), tartaric (in grapes) and lactic (in sauerkraut), the body burns them up and converts them to carbonic acid, which is easily eliminated in the breath. The body is protected by "buffers" in the blood so it is not subject to sudden changes in its normally slight alkaline reaction.

It is hard for the body to "burn up" oxalic acid when present in rhubarb, chard, kale and cocoa (chocolate). When these foods are eaten, a liberal supply of natural calcium from other sources, such as mustard greens, asparagus, cabbage, tofu, figs and prunes should be provided. A normal, healthy body is equipped to utilize efficiently the healthy foods eaten regardless of alkaline or acid properties, especially when you add raw, organic Bragg Apple Cider Vinegar to salads, green vegetables, etc. This provides a healthy acid–alkaline balance for healthy digestion, see page 202.

Dietary Health Supplements

If we were living strictly according to nature's plan, we would not need supplementary vitamins, minerals or amino acids. If we were able to get meat from animals in the wild that were fed organic, highly mineralized and vitaminized feed, or foraged in rich, fertile pastures or if we were able to obtain organically-grown vegetables and fruits fresh from healthy soil, our problems would be simple. However because of mass distribution, today we get our foods after they have been long in storage and lost much of their high vitamin and mineral content. Some never had a high vitamin and mineral content to lose because they were not grown in rich, organic soil. Thus our foods, vegetables and grains, etc. are not always what they should be, even though we get them in sufficient quantities and prepare them properly. For that reason, health supplements have become a great necessity.

You can obtain vitamin and mineral supplements at your health food store. You can make sure you are getting your nutrients such as vitamins A, B, C, D, E, calcium, iodine, phosphorus, magnesium and all the minerals. These supplements are no substitute for a healthy balanced diet, but they are one way of making certain that your diet is supplemented adequately so that you do not fall prey to vitamin or mineral deficiencies.

With Your Hands You Prepare Either Health or Sickness – It's Up to You

They who provide the food for the world, decide the health of the world! A vast multitude of the human race are slaughtered by incompetent cookery. Though you may have taken lessons in music, painting, etc., you are not well-educated unless you have taken lessons in preparing healthy meals. You can either prepare health or sickness with your two hands. Healthy, nutritional planning and preparation produces healthy, delicious meals and healthy bodies.

Coronary Disease is Preventable & Reversible

Dr. Dean Ornish's book *Reversing Heart Disease* states: ***"Heart problems are not only preventable but are also reversible by changing your lifestyle."*** *(Web: www.ornish.com)* We agree – if people would only eat and exercise properly, coronary disease could be stopped in its tracks! Future heart problems would be prevented and heart disease would begin to reverse! People have the power to take control of their health! Most people never know real physical health. They miss out on the priceless benefits of living the Bragg Healthy Lifestyle.

***Wise Health Advise from Dean Ornish,* M.D.** *www.ornish.com*

We tend to think of advances in medicine as being a new drug, a new surgical technique, a new laser, something high-tech and expensive. We often have a hard time believing that the simple choices that we make each day in our diet and lifestyle can make such a powerful difference in the quality and quantity of our lives, but they most often do. My health program consists of four main components: exercise, nutrition, stress management, love and intimacy and these four promote not only living longer and happier, but living better.

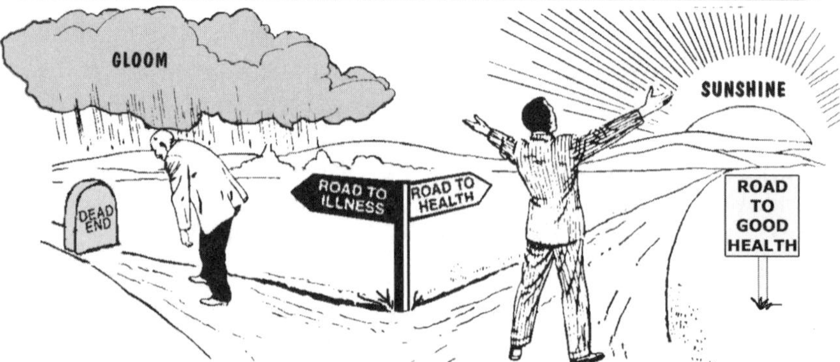

NEGATIVE ← OR → POSITIVE

The choice of which road to take is up to you.

You alone decide whether to reach a dead end or live a healthy lifestyle for a long, healthy, happy, active life. – Paul C. Bragg

Chapter 1

Flavor

the Soul of Food that Excites Your Appetite & Meals

Ordinarily, cookbooks have a stereotyped sequence. First come the tables of measurement, then the soups, salads, etc. To my mind, no recipe book can start without flavor as a basis – and especially no health food recipe book. In cooking for health, the pleasure of well-savored flavor is almost as important as nutritional quality, as it makes mealtime more enjoyable, which also helps with digestion.

Good cooking is the combination of two great fields of human experience: science and art. The science of food tells us what good nutrition is. The art of preparing food requires learning the art of flavor. Using herbs such as Bragg Sprinkle (24 herbs & spices) and Bragg Kelp Seasoning, garlic and 100% whole, fresh, organically grown foods are always the best.

Stock: the Foundation of Flavor

Flavor can only be as good as the stock from which it is based. Good stock, properly used, is the difference between excellent and mediocre cooking. When the stock (or consommé) is excellent, the creation of fine flavor is easy. When food lacks flavor, meals can taste flat and dull.

In foreign lands, mention of stock in a cookbook would be superfluous. However, in our culture it is a little-known and seldom practiced principle of the basic art of cooking. There are several reasons for this: unless a great deal can be prepared at a time, the cooking of stock is time-consuming. You can make three quarts at one time, freeze some in ice cube trays, and transfer to freezer bags to use as-needed for small amounts. Place remaining stock in jars and refrigerate. Put a date on all stored food items!

A stainless steel pressure-cooker is a great time-saver in the preparation of stock. The cooking time can be divided by ten. This means that the Vegetable/Mushroom Stock recipe on the next page, which requires 20 minutes cooking time, can be reduced to 2 minutes. (The pressure takes time to build up before you should start counting cooking minutes.)

VEGETABLE/MUSHROOM STOCK

2 whole leeks, dice
4 shallots, chop
3 medium-sized carrots, dice
3 cloves garlic, chop
8-10 basil leaves
2 bay leaves
2 sprigs cilantro (optional)
1 Tbsp Bragg Liquid Aminos
1 sprig thyme
3 sprigs parsley
2 sprigs chervil
2 celery ribs, dice
1 large tomato, dice
10 fresh or dried mushrooms of your choice, dice
½ tsp Bragg Sprinkle

Combine all ingredients with 10 cups distilled water. Bring to a boil. Reduce and simmer for 30 minutes, remove from heat, cover and let stand for an hour. Add Bragg Aminos. Strain through strainer lined with cheesecloth. Remove solids and store cooled consommé, covered in refrigerator for 3 days. Freeze unused portion in ice cube tray and next day store stacked cubes in dated freezer bags for future seasoning use. Makes 2 quarts.

GINGER BROTH

1 large red onion, quarter
2 plum tomatoes, quarter
3-4 cilantro sprigs (optional)
1½ cups Bragg Apple Cider Vinegar
1-3 tsps Bragg Liquid Aminos
6-7 slices fresh ginger
3 large carrots, chop
⅓ tsp cayenne pepper
2 qts distilled water
½ tsp Bragg Sprinkle

Bring all ingredients except the Bragg Aminos to boil in stockpot. Reduce the heat and simmer, covered for 20 minutes. Remove from heat and let stand 20 minutes, then add Bragg Aminos to taste. Blend ingredients and strain. The broth can be used immediately or refrigerated up to 2 days or frozen up to 3 months. Makes about 10 cups of broth.

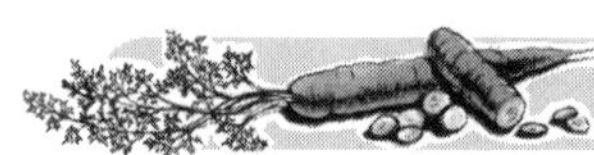

VEGETABLE STOCK

2 carrots, slice
4 leeks, chop
2 Tbsps Bragg Organic Olive Oil
2 tsps Bragg Sprinkle
2 red onions, slice
2 celery ribs, chop
10 cups distilled water
Bragg Liquid Aminos to taste

Sauté vegetables in olive oil until soft, but not brown, about 4 minutes. Add distilled water and bring to boil. Add Sprinkle seasoning and simmer covered for 2 hours. Remove from heat and let stand 10 minutes. Now add Bragg Aminos to taste. Blend and strain. Discard solids. Store, covered, in refrigerator. Use within 24 hours. This stock does not freeze well.

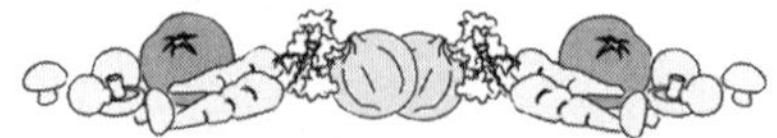

Wake up and say, "Today I am going to be happier, healthier and wiser in my daily living as I am the captain of my life and am going to steer it for 100% healthy lifestyle living!" Fact: Happy people look younger, live longer, are happier and have fewer health and life problems!
– Patricia Bragg, N.D., Ph.D., Healthy Lifestyle Educator

Herbs and Spices

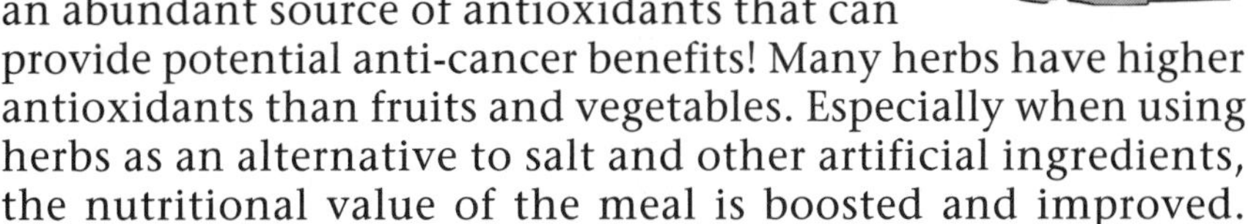

Along with adding flavor to your dishes, herbs have health benefits as well. Herbs are an abundant source of antioxidants that can provide potential anti-cancer benefits! Many herbs have higher antioxidants than fruits and vegetables. Especially when using herbs as an alternative to salt and other artificial ingredients, the nutritional value of the meal is boosted and improved.

Use of Herbs and Spices for Taste Delights

For real adventure in food, one need not go to China, Borneo, Malaysia or Egypt. With a good stock of choice herbs on the kitchen shelf, the wise cook can transform ordinary foods into exquisite delicacies. Dishes can be prepared that have come to us from far away countries and times, and have been translated into the true style of modern health cookery. Herbs were the first medicine of humanity, and although they are a seldom practiced art today, they still give hints of luscious feasts and dishes with aromatic fragrances, which is their real function. They are true vegetable substances with pungent quality, and belong in all good nutritional health cookery.

Few modern kitchens rely upon the old-fashion herb garden. Fresh herbs are a great treat, and you can even have a kitchen window sill with herb plants – plus stock your pantry with Bragg Sprinkle (24 herbs & spices) for delicious herb flavors and stock a variety of dried herbs. Many stores now have fresh herbs in the vegetable section.

Bragg Sprinkle - 24 Herbs & Spices

Bragg Sprinkle Seasoning is an original blend of 24 all natural herbs & spices and is salt free. Created in 1931 by Health Pioneer Paul C. Bragg. It adds health and delicious flavors to most all recipes.

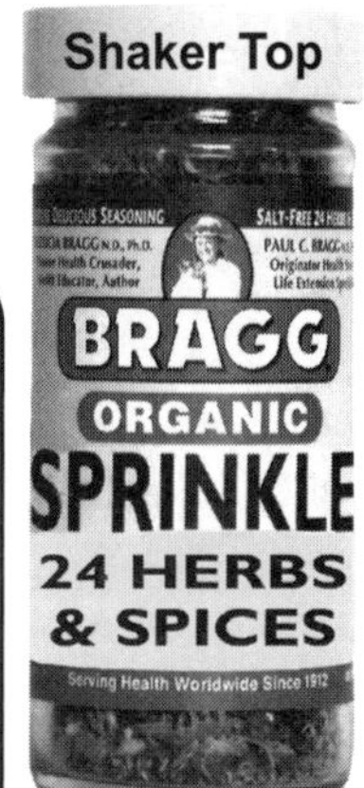

Bragg Sprinkle Contains 24 Organic Herbs & Spices:

Rosemary	Thyme	Parsley	Pepper
Sweet Basil	Celery Seed	Sage	Oregano
Orange Peel	Coriander	Ginger	Onion
Bay Leaves	Garlic	Savory	Carrot
Citric Acid	Sunflower Oil	Tarragon	Tomato
Lemon Oil	Red Bell Pepper	Kelp	Dill Seed
Granulated Bragg Liquid Aminos			

Bragg Sprinkle, a delicious, versatile 24 organic herbs & spice seasoning used in many health recipes throughout this book.

Herbs should be used lightly and cautiously at first! The hint of delicate flavor they impart is better than combinations of strong, predominant flavors. The finest herb cookery is characterized by the subtle use and blending of flavors, so that the specific herbs remain a mystery. If the flavor is so strong and distinct that it can be detected instantly, the dish is not a complete success. There are exceptions to this rule, such as dishes where more tarragon or dill, etc. are used. A good general rule for the experimenter is to use extreme caution to avoid over-flavoring!

To Remember When Using Herbs

Average Quantities. The warning to use herbs cautiously must again be emphasized. It is not always wise to exactly follow recipes calling for herbs. So much depends on the strength of herbs. When you buy a new container of dried herbs, they are "full strength." The longer you keep them on the shelf after you have broken the seal of the package, the weaker they become. Herbs of greater strength must obviously be used with more caution than the older, more exposed, weaker herbs. A good guide, although one to be used with discretion, is to use about ½ to one teaspoon of dried herbs in a dish designed to serve 8 people, decreasing or increasing according to the number of desired servings. If you are fortunate enough to be able to use fresh herbs and your recipe is written in terms of the dried variety, increase the amount of fresh herbs to four times the suggested dry amount. Herbs and spices should enhance, but not over power the flavor of your food.

To Prevent Herb Specks in Food. Flecks of herbs can be very attractive in some dishes, but undesirable in others. If you want to have the finished dish clear, use a stainless steel herb ball packet or tie the required herbs in a bit of cheese cloth. Remove packet before serving.

To Use in Uncooked Food. Herbs should be placed in the liquid long in advance. It is sometimes best to let them stand overnight to obtain the full release of flavor.

To Use in Cooked Food. Herbs should be added during the last hour of cooking unless recipe states differently.

Moistening Herbs. If herbs are to "kiss" the dish – that is, to be used only for a short time in preparation – they should be pre-moistened. Do this by allowing them to stand for 45 minutes slightly moistened by distilled water, a little Bragg Olive Oil, or a drop of soy milk. Herbs need not float in liquid, but simply be dampened. If time is short, a similar effect of quicker flavor-releasing may be obtained by putting the herbs in a herb ball holder and dipping for a few seconds into boiling water and then into ice-cold distilled water. Drain before using.

And thou shall eat the herbs of the field. – Genesis 3:18

Herb Infused Oils

Flavored oils have become part of the vocabulary of contemporary cooking, providing a means of packing deep, vibrant flavors into dishes from which excessive amounts of butter, cream, eggs or hydrogenated oils have been deleted in the interest of good health. Just a few drops of an herb or spice infused oil may be all that's necessary to season a whole dish. Herbed oils can be substituted for butter or cream; added to soup stocks, stir-fried vegetables or sautés; or to make exceptional dressings and sauces. Oils infused with mint, basil or cilantro are the subtlest and most versatile, while thyme, rosemary and oregano should be used sparingly. There are many infused oils on the market today at health food stores and gourmet shops. Make your own by adding herbs like garlic or lemon peel to our delicious Bragg Organic Extra Virgin Olive Oil.

How to Store Herbs

When storing spices, keep them in a cool, dark place. Humidity, light and heat will cause herbs and spices to lose their flavor more quickly. Dried herbs and ground spices will retain their best flavors for a year. Whole spices may last longer, 3-5 years. Proper storage should result in longer freshness. To keep larger quantities of spices fresh, store them in the freezer in tightly sealed containers.

The Herb Packet

Certain herbs blend more desirably than others. There are many combinations for different flavor purposes. These combinations can be placed in little packets so that they are easily available to the busy chef. These little packets are small cheesecloth bags, about the size of a nutmeg, tied with a string. One end of the string should be left about 3 or 4 inches long, and looped to make the packet easy to remove with a fork or cooking utensil at the precise moment the desired flavor of the dish is achieved. They can be tossed into a soup or other dishes while cooking, and removed before serving.

Herbs for Seasoning

When using herbs to flavor foods, add sparingly to avoid an overwhelming flavor. Be creative and enjoy using herbs and spices. In time you will find herb mixtures you prefer for these recipes. When using in long-cooking dishes, add herbs and spices an hour or less before serving. Cooking spices too long may result in overly strong flavors.

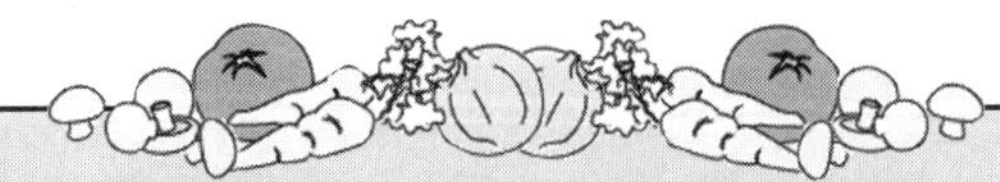

Delicious Herbs – Food Combinations:

Beans (dried): Sweet basil, oregano, dill, savory, mint, cumin, garlic, parsley, bay leaf

Beets: Tarragon, dill, sweet basil, thyme, bay leaf, cardamom seed

Broccoli: Tarragon, marjoram, garlic, oregano

Brussels Sprouts: Sweet basil, dill, savory, caraway, thyme

Cabbage: Caraway, celery seed, savory, tarragon, dill

Carrots: Sweet basil, dill, marjoram, thyme, parsley

Cauliflower: Rosemary, savory, dill, garlic, tarragon

Cucumbers: Dill, tarragon, sweet basil, savory

Eggplant: Sweet basil, thyme, garlic, oregano, rosemary

Green Beans: Sweet basil, dill, marjoram, rosemary, thyme, oregano, garlic, savory

Lima Beans: Sweet basil, chives, garlic, marjoram, savory

Onions: Oregano, thyme, sweet basil

Peas: Sweet basil, mint, savory, oregano, dill

Potatoes: Dill, chives, sweet basil, marjoram, mint, garlic, savory, garlic, parsley

Spinach: Tarragon, thyme, oregano, rosemary

Squash: Sweet basil, dill, oregano, savory

Green Salads: Basil, parsley, chives, garlic, tarragon, lemon, thyme

Tomatoes: Basil, oregano, dill, garlic, savory, bay leaf, parsley

Dressings: Dill, marjoram, oregano, rosemary, garlic, savory, mint

Coleslaw: Dill, marjoram, caraway seed, garlic, savory, mint

Fruit Salads: Mint, rosemary, lemon balm

Spaghetti Sauces: Sweet basil, garlic, oregano, tarragon

Chili Sauces: Cayenne, garlic, cumin, oregano

Few BRAGG Shakes Gives Flavor Delights

Add fresh herbs towards end of cooking so flavors will last. Add dried herbs (Bragg Sprinkle and Kelp) usually at start of cooking so flavors can enhance recipe. Add fresh herbs about 15 minutes before serving to make fresh fragrance last longer. When using dried (stronger) herbs, use 3-4 times less than called for in fresh herbs. When using fresh herbs, clean and cut herbs, then gently crush them by hand to release their flavor.

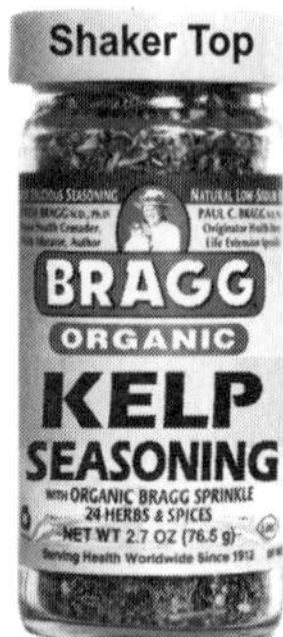

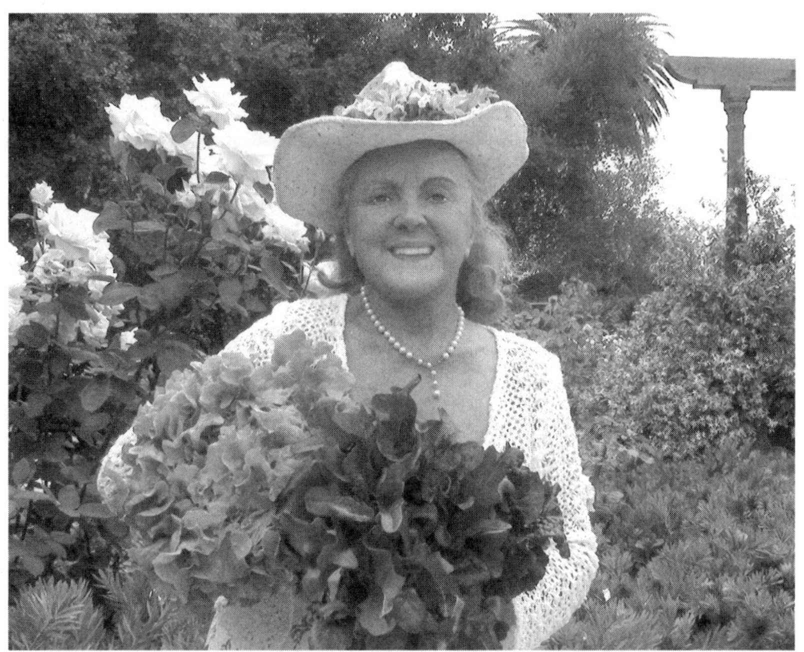

Patricia Bragg, N.D., Ph.D., Health Crusader & Lifestyle Educator

PATRICIA BRAGG, Life Extension Nutritionist and Author, lives on an Organic Farm that includes roses, flowers, vegetables and fruit trees, with many varieties of apples, avocados, bananas, persimmons, pomegranates, apricots, mangos and many other tropical fruit trees in Santa Barbara, Hawaii, and Australia.

The Bragg motto is "Live Foods Make Live People!"

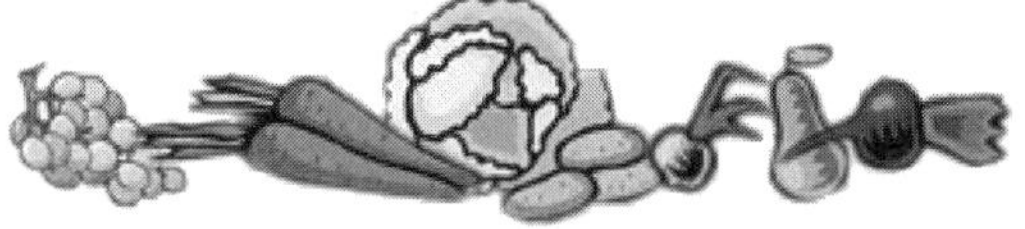

Bragg Healthy Lifestyle Promotes Super-Health & Longevity

Bragg Healthy Lifestyle consists of eating 70-80% of your diet from live organic foods, raw vegetables, salads, sprouts, fresh fruits and juices, raw seeds and nuts, the all-natural 100% whole-grain breads, pastas and cereals and the nutritious beans, seeds and legumes. These foods are the no-cholesterol, no-fat, no-salt, just "live foods" body fuel for more health that makes live people! This is the reason people become revitalized and reborn into a fresh new life filled with Joy, Health, Vitality, Youthfulness and Longevity! There are millions of healthy Bragg followers around the world proving this works miracles!

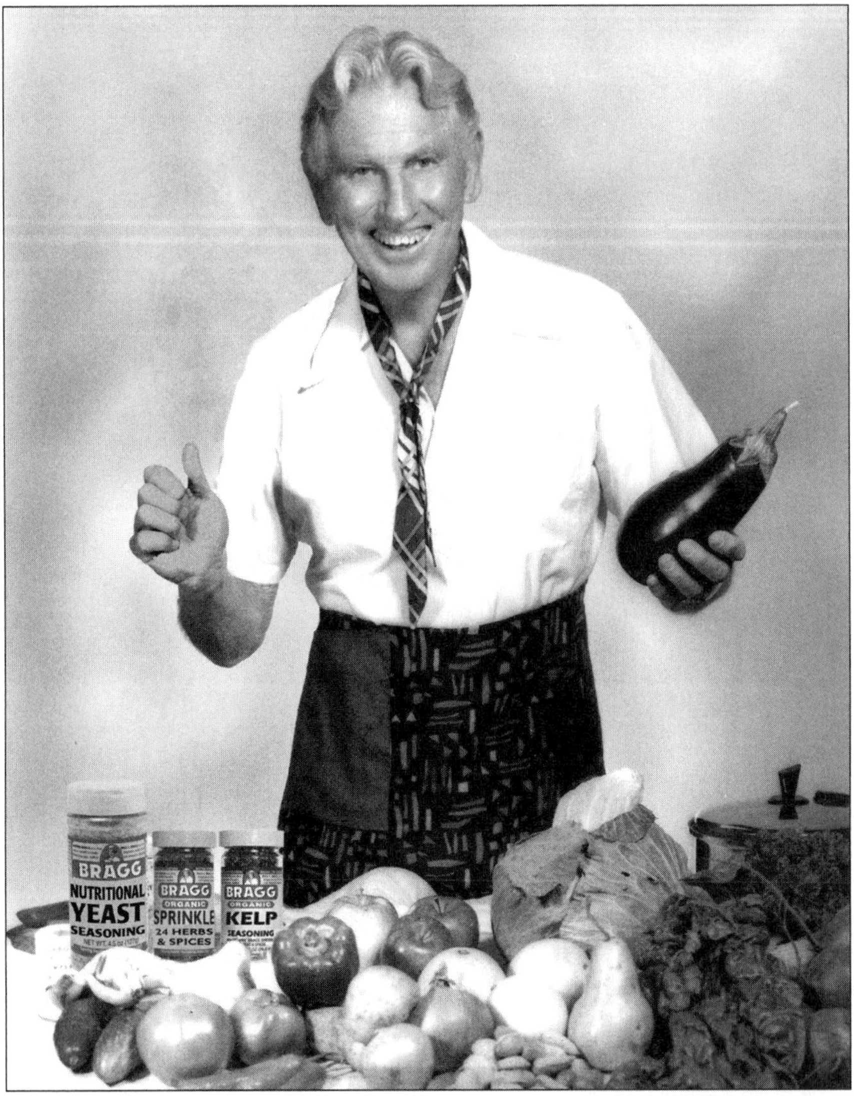

Paul C. Bragg, N.D., Ph.D., Life Extension Specialist

Having fun in the kitchen preparing nutritious, delicious, healthy raw foods and cooked vegetarian recipes.

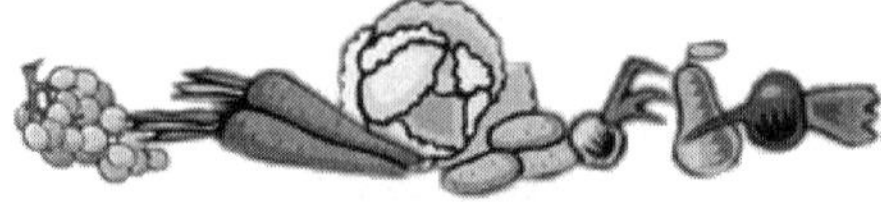

Vegetables as well as fruit, both raw in salads and properly cooked, are among the "protective" foods, and should represent the majority of the diet. They add variety, color, flavor, texture and health to meals. – Paul C. Bragg, N.D., Ph.D.

Many people go through life committing partial suicide – destroying their health, youth, beauty, talents, energies and creative qualities. Indeed, to learn how to be good to oneself is often more difficult than to learn how to be good to others.
– Paul C. Bragg, N.D., Ph.D., Originator of Health Food Stores

Chapter 2

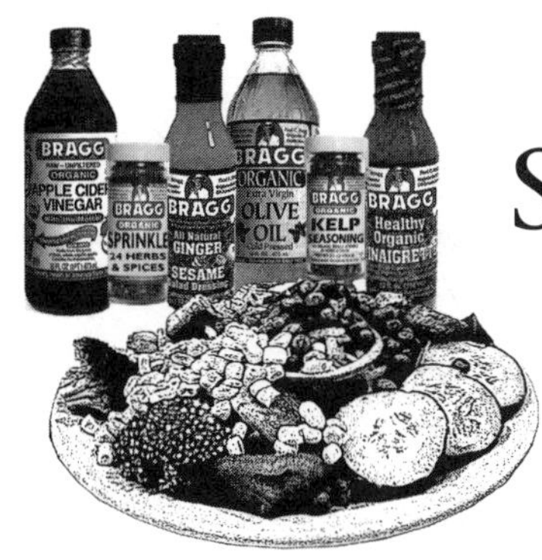

Salad Dressings & Salads

Healthy & Delicious

Today, many people make the mistake of concluding that salad is only lettuce. More adventuresome cooks will go so far as romaine, and perhaps cabbage once in a while; but, after that, often they have exhausted their full repertoire of salad-making.

Nature has almost as many variations of the salad leaf as she has variety in plant life. As a nation, we have trained our grocers and vegetable stores into carrying only the more commonly accepted types of salad leaves; but it is possible at some markets to purchase more variety of delicious leaves, and perhaps you can also grow a small garden of delicious herbs and salad plants for your own kitchen garden. Examples of some of these leaves are the unique sorrel, fennel, and cresses – they are delectable salads in themselves. Also, the escarole, dandelion greens, nasturtium leaves, tender young leaves of the buckwheat, purslane, chicory, and the many varieties of lettuces and romaine, can make up a nutritious variety of healthy, delicious salads.

We have many fascinating health salads for you: vegetable salads, fruit salads – but the king of all salads is the green leaf salad with its cousins, the wild and cultivated seasoning herbs.

Do not cut your vegetables too fine, as the cut portions, when exposed to air, lose vitamin content. Serve as fresh and crisp as possible, not only to preserve the fresh taste and appearance, but for nutritional preservation as well.

Vegetarians are Healthier and Live Longer

Most uninformed nutritionists call meat the #1 source of protein. Those proteins coming from the vegetable kingdom are referred to as the #2 proteins. This is a sad and terrible mistake! It should be the other way around! In this day and age, almost all meat is laden with herbicides, fungicides, pesticides and other chemicals that are sprayed on or poured into the feed which these animals consume. They are also pumped full of hormones, antibiotics, growth stimulators and toxic drugs to fatten them up and keep them from dying from the unhealthy conditions they live in! Beware of animal products!

THE GREEN LEAFY SALAD

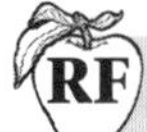

SPRING SALAD BOWL

1 clove garlic
1 large head of leaf lettuce
½ cup radishes, slice
½ cup carrots, grate
3 green onions, finely cut
2 large ripe tomatoes, slice
1 cucumber, slice
2 celery stalks, chop
Bragg Ginger & Sesame or Organic Vinaigrette Dressing (to taste)

Rub salad bowl with garlic clove cut in half. Wash and dry head of lettuce thoroughly, separating and tearing leaves into bowl. Add radishes, carrots, celery and green onions. Slice tomatoes and cucumbers, retaining the skins: skins are not only nutritious, but colorful when serving. Use Bragg Ginger & Sesame Dressing or Organic Hawaiian Dressing. Serves 4.

ROMAINE WITH GARLIC CROUTONS

2 heads romaine lettuce
3 cloves garlic
1 Tbsp lemon juice
4 thick slices whole-grain bread
2 Tbsps Bragg Organic Olive Oil
2 ripe tomatoes, slice

Break romaine into salad bowl. Add tomato slices. Prepare garlic bread as follows: crush garlic cloves into mixture of lemon and olive oil. Allow to stand for several minutes to infuse flavors. Meanwhile, toast whole-grain bread in oven until dry. Then brush with olive oil mixture and cut into small cubes and toss into salad. Add Bragg Organic Vinaigrette or our delicious Braggberry Dressing. Serves 4.

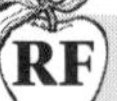

COLESLAW GARDEN SALAD

1 head green cabbage, slice
1 cup red cabbage, slice
1 apple, core and slice
2 green onions, slice
1 large carrot, grate
20 raisins (optional)
Bragg Organic Braggberry or Ginger Sesame Dressing (to taste)

Mix all together (try raisins). Toss with dressing. Serves 4.

SUMMER HERB SALAD

Combine mustard greens, watercress, spinach and lettuce leaves with summer savory, tarragon, rosemary, and celery seed. Add shake of Bragg Sprinkle and Vinaigrette Dressing and toss.

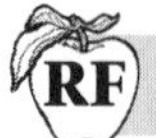

BUCKWHEAT TENDERLEAF SALAD

Use only tender young leaves by themselves. Add Bragg Organic Vinaigrette Dressing and toss. The young, tender, delicious buckwheat leaf has a delightfully distinctive flavor when served alone.

Eat plenty of vegetables and fruits. Aim for at least five servings of raw greens and vegetables daily. Mix and match selections to get healthy amounts of nutrients. – The Health Nutrition Bible

DANDELION SALAD

½ head of leaf lettuce, tear
½ head romaine lettuce, tear
½ cup dandelion leaves, tear
¼ cup dandelion stems, chop
a few fresh mint leaves
1 cup apple, grated (optional)
Bragg Healthy Organic Hawaiian or Ginger & Sesame Dressing

Toss all torn leaves, dandelion stems, mint and grated apple together with Bragg Hawaiian or Ginger Dressing. Serves 4.

LAMB'S LETTUCE SALAD

2 cups lamb's lettuce, tear
Braggberry Dressing
¼ cup soy cheese, grate
1 cup celery, chop

Toss ingredients apply dressing and serve. Serves 4.

NASTURTIUM SALAD

½ head of leaf lettuce, tear
1 full head romaine lettuce
Bragg Hawaiian Dressing
6 or 7 nasturtium flowers
1 cup nasturtium leaves, tear
1 cup apple, grated (optional)

Tear (do not cut) lettuce and nasturtium leaves into small pieces. Cutting with knife or kitchen shears often gives bitter flavor to salad leaf. Toss salad with grated apples and nasturtium flowers, saving several flowers to garnish top of salad. Add Hawaiian Dressing and toss together. Serves 3-4.

PURSLANE SALAD

Use the purslane leaves alone for best flavor. If desired, however, it can be combined with romaine lettuce. Top with Bragg Salad Dressing of choice or juice of orange and serve.

SPRING HERBS – MIXED GREENS SALAD

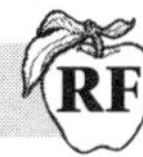

Use any combination of the tender young top leaves of mustard greens, beets, kale, bok choy, Swiss chard, endive, escarole and all lettuces or young greens peeking up through the ground in your garden. Don't be afraid to use wildflower leaves if you know how to identify edible plants. Look for shepherd's purse, wild rocket, sour dock, even the fresh young sprouts of spring milkweed, dandelion, oxalis, wood sorrel and, of course, all the fresh new arrivals from the vegetable garden: turnip and beet greens, radishes and mustard greens. Use as many combinations as you can find, and toss with Bragg Organic Vinaigrette or Braggberry Dressing.

CABBAGE SALAD BOWL

½ head cabbage, either red or green, or mixed makes a colorful salad, slice
other veggies or raisins if desired
shake of Bragg Sprinkle
1 apple, core and chop
1 red onion, mince
Bragg Ginger & Sesame Dressing

Combine cabbage, onion, apple and raisins or other veggies desired. Add Sprinkle and Bragg Ginger Dressing. Serves 2-4.

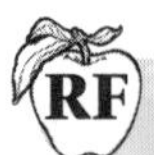

GOURMET MIXED GREEN SALAD

The mixed green salads offered in restaurants are often less nutritious and less flavorful than desired. Here is a healthy mixed green salad that will delight any salad gourmet.

All leaves should be thoroughly washed, dried and crisped in a cool place, then torn into small pieces. It's best not to cut the leaves with a knife or kitchen shears.

1 cup green leaf lettuce, tear
1 cup mixed baby lettuce leaves
¼ cup dandelion greens
½ cup young, spinach leaves
½ cup fresh mint leaves
1 cup watercress
½ cup escarole
1 cup purslane
1 cup sorrel leaves
¼ cup chives, chop
1 cup romaine lettuce
olives, sliced (optional)

Toss all greens with Bragg Organic Vinaigrette Dressing; add some sliced black olives, if desired, before tossing with dressing. It is difficult to assemble all these greens at one time, but the trick of this salad is to use as many leafy greens as you can possibly obtain. Add cherry tomatoes, artichoke hearts, and any other healthy additions desired. Serves 6.

HEALTHY VEGETABLE SALADS

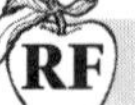

BRAGG FAMOUS RAW GARDEN SALAD

2 stalks celery, slice
½ bell pepper & seeds, chop
½ cucumber, slice
2 carrots, grate
1 raw beet, grate
1 cup green cabbage, chop
½ cup alfalfa or sunflower sprouts
2 spring onions & green tops, chop
½ cup red cabbage, chop
3 medium tomatoes
1 turnip, grate
1 ripe avocado
Try Braggberry, Vinaigrette or Ginger & Sesame Dressing

Dice avocado and tomato and serve in separate bowl for topping. Chop, slice or grate all veggies fine to medium for a variety in size. Mix veggies and serve on bed of romaine, butter or leaf lettuce. For variety add raw zucchini, greenbeans, peas, radishes, mushrooms, broccoli, cauliflower, kale, etc. Serves 4-6.

LENTIL SALAD

2 cups cooked lentils
2 cups cooked brown rice
1 cup red onion, chop
1 tomato, dice
2 cucumbers, dice
1 cup parsley, finely chop
1 Tbsp Bragg Organic Olive Oil
1 Tbsp Bragg Apple Cider Vinegar
½ tsp Bragg Sprinkle
½ tsp paprika
2 cloves garlic, crush
Juice of 1 lemon, about 3 Tbsps

Combine the lentils, rice, onion, cucumber and parsley in a salad bowl. Mix the lemon juice, olive oil, vinegar, paprika, garlic and a shake of Bragg Sprinkle (24 herbs & spices) in a small bowl, then pour over salad and toss gently to mix. Serves 3-5.

CABBAGE AND CHINESE NOODLE SALAD

⅓ cup cashew pieces
2 Tbsps un-hulled sesame seeds
3 cups green cabbage, shred/chop
2 cups red cabbage, shred/chop
3 green onions, chop
sesame seed oil
1 pkg whole grain, ramen noodles, crush
Bragg Ginger & Sesame Dressing
Bragg Liquid Aminos
cilantro sprigs (optional)

Toast cashews and sesame seeds with light spray of Bragg Aminos in 375°F oven until slightly browned, about 10 minutes. Set aside to cool. Place the shredded cabbage in a salad bowl and add chopped onions and cooled nuts. Coarsely crush ramen noodles and add them to salad. Pour ramen seasoning packet into small bowl and stir in Ginger and Sesame or Braggberry Dressing. For crunchy noodles, eat salad immediately. For soft noodles, let salad stand 30 minutes or more before serving. Garnish if desired, with fresh cilantro or Bragg Nutritional Yeast just before serving. Serves 4.

COUSCOUS VEGGIE SALAD

1 cup whole-grain couscous
1 cup boiling distilled water
1 small red onion, mince
1 red bell pepper, dice
1 carrot, grate
½ cup red cabbage, finely shred
½ cup green peas, fresh or frozen
½ cup raisins or currants
⅓ tsp mustard powder
⅓ tsp curry powder
1 tsp sesame oil
1 tsp Bragg Liquid Aminos
shake of Bragg Sprinkle
2 Tbsps Bragg Apple Cider Vinegar

Place couscous in bowl and pour boiling water over it. Stir until mixed, then cover, let stand until cooled. Fluff lightly with fork. Add onion, bell pepper, carrot, cabbage, peas and raisins or currants to couscous. Combine vinegar, sesame oil, Bragg Aminos, Sprinkle, mustard and curry powder. Mix well. Pour over salad and mix. Garnish with Bragg Nutritional Yeast. Serves 4.

GREEN BEANS AND SPROUT SALAD

3 Tbsps Bragg Organic Olive Oil
3 cups cooked whole green beans
2 cups sprouts
2 scallions, chop
2 Tbsps Bragg Apple Cider Vinegar
1 tsp whole-grain flour
¼ cup warm distilled water
1 tsp Bragg Liquid Aminos
shake of Bragg Kelp Seasoning
shake of Bragg Sprinkle

Heat drained beans for two minutes in one tablespoon of olive oil. Place beans in casserole or other serving dish. Heat sprouts and scallions for two minutes in one tablespoon of olive oil. Stir into casserole. Clean skillet with paper towel. Add one tablespoon olive oil. Heat. Stir in flour, vinegar and distilled water. Add Bragg Aminos, stir until boiling. Pour sauce over sprouts and beans. Season with Bragg Kelp and Sprinkle to taste. Keep warm until ready to serve. Serves 4.

Green beans are full of vitamin K, C, A, dietary fiber, potassium, folate & iron

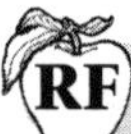

CARROT, APPLE & RAISIN SALAD

½ cup fresh or dried coconut, grate
½ cup raw almonds, slice (optional)
¼ cup fresh lemon or orange juice
3-4 organic apples, core, chop
½ cup raisins or currants
4 cups carrots, grate
1¼ tsp raw honey
Braggberry Dressing

Mix carrots and apples with fresh lemon or orange juice and honey. Add grated coconut, almonds, raisins or currants. Mix thoroughly. Add Braggberry. Always eat salad first. Serves 4-6.

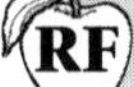

SKIN BEAUTIFUL SALAD

1 carrot, grate
1 turnip, grate
3 radishes, slice
2 apples, core, chop
Fresh lemon juice (to taste)
Bragg Sprinkle (to taste)
2 Tbsps green peas, shelled
1 tomato
1 cup mixed baby lettuce, torn
Bragg Ginger & Sesame Dressing

Put carrot, turnip, apple and sliced radishes in salad bowl. Add lettuce leaves and green peas. Cut un-peeled tomato into small pieces. Mix in with vegetables and lettuce. Add Sprinkle and lemon juice. Toss with Ginger Dressing (to taste). Serves 2-4.

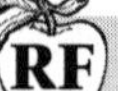

AVOCADO AND TOMATO SALAD BOWL

2 Tbsps Bragg Organic Olive Oil
3 Tbsps fresh lemon juice
4 tomatoes, cut into eighths
2 ripe avocados, chop
2 cups mixed lettuce greens
1 clove garlic, mash
shake of Bragg Sprinkle
½ bunch watercress
Bragg Ginger & Sesame Dressing (to taste)

Pour olive oil, Sprinkle, garlic and lemon juice over tomatoes, and chill. Cut avocados lengthwise in half, remove pit, and chop. Toss salad greens with tomatoes and avocados. Add Ginger & Sesame Dressing or Braggberry (to taste). Serves 2-4.

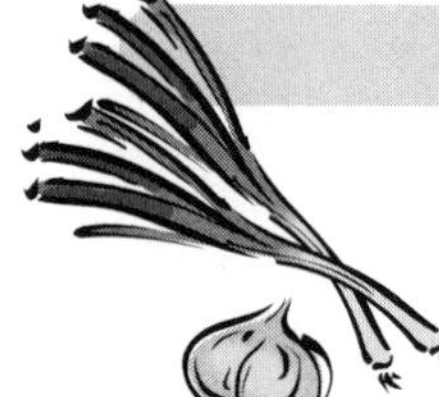

GREEN BEAN – ONION SALAD

1 pound fresh cooked green beans, french slice
1 cup green onions, and stems, finely chop
2 Tbsps Bragg Organic Apple Cider Vinegar
¼ tsp Bragg Sprinkle (24 herbs & spices)
2 Tbsps Bragg Organic Olive Oil

Mix all ingredients. Chill one hour and serve. Serves 4-6.

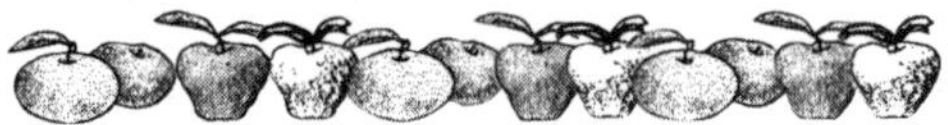

Avoid chopping, peeling, tearing, etc. fresh fruits, vegetables and salads until the last possible minute before eating, as cut and exposed surfaces lose nutrients, vitamin C and begin to oxidize. – The Health Nutrition Bible

---

Before there was medicine, there was food.
– Howard Murad, M.D., famous skincare specialist

Try calling upon God's Calming Angels of Peace . . .
and spending time outdoors with God's masterful creations . . .
and enjoy the oasis of divine stillness within your heart, mind and life.

SPROUTED SOYBEAN SALAD

½ head of leaf lettuce, tear
¼ head of cabbage, chop
2 tomatoes, slice
Bragg Liquid Aminos
1 cup soybean or sunflower sprouts
¼ cup red onion, mince
¼ cup red or green bell pepper, chop
Bragg Ginger & Sesame Dressing
Bragg Sprinkle (24 herbs & spices) & Bragg Sea Kelp Seasoning

Tear lettuce, add chopped cabbage, bell pepper, onions and tomatoes. Add raw sprouts of choice. Toss with dash of Bragg Aminos, and a dash of Bragg Sprinkle and Kelp Seasoning. Add Bragg Organic Hawaiian or Ginger Dressing. Serves 2-4.

MEXICAN GUACAMOLE SALAD OR DIP

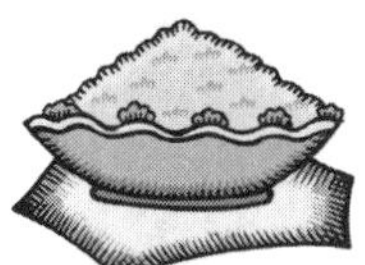

3 avocados, mash
2 cloves garlic, mash
6 green onions, chop
juice of 1 lemon
shake of Bragg Sea Kelp
shake of Bragg Sprinkle
1 tsp tofunaise (page 139)
leaf lettuce or cabbage, slice
6 tomatoes, quarter
dash of Bragg Liquid Aminos

Mix avocados and garlic. Mix in chopped green onions, lemon juice, Bragg Aminos and Sprinkle. Place mixture on bed of leaf lettuce or sliced cabbage, side garnish with tomatoes, any fresh sliced vegetables desired (carrots, celery, etc.) Serves 4-6.

FRESH MUSHROOM SALAD

8-10 fresh mushrooms, of your choice, slice
2-3 tomatoes, slice
1 head romaine lettuce, tear
½ red onion, chop
½ tsp Bragg Liquid Aminos
shake of Bragg Sprinkle and Bragg Sea Kelp Seasoning

Toss ingredients in bowl. Add desired dressing. Serves 4.

SPINACH, APPLE AND RED ONION SALAD

1-2 bunches of spinach, tear
2 apples, core, chop
1 red onion, chop thin
raw honey (optional)
3 cloves garlic, mince
½ tsp Bragg Liquid Aminos
shake of Bragg Sprinkle
3 Tbsps Bragg Organic Olive Oil
3 Tbsps freshly squeezed lemon juice or orange juice

For dressing: combine garlic, lemon juice, olive oil, Bragg Aminos, honey (optional) and Sprinkle. In salad bowl, toss spinach, onion and apples and add this dressing. Serves 4.

SPINACH TOFU SALAD

1-2 bunches fresh spinach
½ red onion, thinly slice
2 cups raw mushrooms, slice
½ cup firm tofu, crumble
Bragg Vinaigrette, Ginger or Braggberry Dressing

Combine and toss salad with dressing to taste. Serves 4.

Raw Spinach is a healthy source of dietary fiber, protein, Vitamin A, C, E, K, niacin, zinc, thiamin, riboflavin, vitamin B6, folate, calcium, magnesium, phosphorus & iron. See website: nutritiondata.self.com/facts

COUSCOUS AND ORANGE SALAD

2 cups couscous
1 bunch scallions, chop
1 small bell pepper, dice
½ cucumber, chop
7 oz can garbanzo beans, drain
⅔ cup raisins
Bragg Liquid Aminos to taste
lettuce leaves & sprigs of mint to garnish
2 oranges to garnish, slice

DRESSING:
grated rind from organic orange
⅔ cup silken tofu, mash
1 Tbsp fresh mint, mince

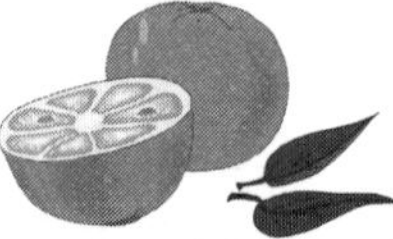

Put the couscous into a bowl and cover with boiling distilled water. Let soak for 5-10 minutes, stir with fork to separate grains. Add scallions, bell pepper, cucumber, garbanzo beans and raisins to the couscous, stir. Season with the Bragg Aminos. Mix dressing ingredients and toss. Arrange on lettuce or sliced cabbage with orange sections and mint sprigs. Serves 4-6.

BEET AND PASTA SALAD

8 oz whole-grain pasta shells, cook
⅔ cup pine, hazel or walnuts, chop
3 Tbsps Bragg Organic Apple Cider Vinegar
Bragg Liquid Aminos (to taste)
2 beets, steam, then chop
3 scallions, slice
2 celery stalks, chop
⅓ cup raisins or currants
1 apple, core and slice

DRESSING:
2 tsps soy milk
2 tsps horseradish
4 Tbsps tofunaise (page 139)

GARNISH:
curly leaf lettuce
watercress
2 ripe avocados, slice

Halve beets, cook in steamer basket 15 minutes. Drain, cool, and chop. Cook pasta; drain and toss with vinegar and Bragg Aminos. Cool mixture. Mix pasta with beets, celery, onions, nuts and apples. Add raisins (optional). Stir all ingredients and dressing together and mix into salad bowl. Chill. To serve, place salad mixture in center of the lettuce and top with avocado slices and watercress. Serves 4-6.

SPINACH - MUSHROOM SALAD WITH WARM DRESSING

2 tsps Bragg Liquid Aminos
¼ cup Bragg Apple Cider Vinegar
1 Tbsp Bragg Organic Olive Oil
1 tsp raw honey or pinch of Stevia
2 bunches fresh spinach, tear
8 fresh mushrooms, thinly slice
1½ Tbsps sesame seeds, toasted
shake of Bragg Sprinkle

Combine Bragg Aminos, vinegar, olive oil, Bragg Sprinkle and honey (or Stevia powder) in saucepan. Simmer 5 minutes. Tear spinach into bite-sized pieces; put in salad bowl with sliced mushrooms. Toss with the warm dressing. Sprinkle with sesame seeds and Bragg Nutritional Yeast. Serve at once. Serves 4.

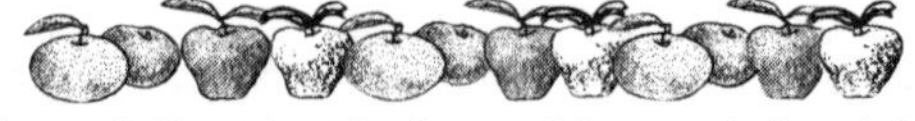

Who wisely satisfies thy desires with good (healthy) things is wise; so that thy youth is renewed like the soaring eagle. – Psalms 103:5

HEALTHY ORGANIC GRAND SLAM SALAD

The purpose of this salad is to see how many varieties of organic vegetables you can put into one salad. Not only does serving almost all vegetables give a delightful flavor but, more importantly, it provides for your family a variety of vegetables they heartily need. Each vegetable in nature's galaxy has its own purpose. They are rich in healthy nutrients. Some pique the appetite. Others add light, porous bulk to the diet. Each has a specialty in the nutritional field. A rich, well-rounded combination of vegetables in a salad can make any meal healthy and nutritious. If it is impossible to include all the vegetables named below, don't worry; however, the more varieties you can work in, the higher the nutritional health value.

3 cups salad greens (make this a wide variety: lettuce, romaine, or: chicory, watercress, endive, escarole, chives, spinach, purslane, kale, nasturtium, buckwheat, lamb's lettuce, cabbage, dandelion greens, sorrel leaves, vegetable tops, and any wild salad leaves you can gather)
¼ cup edible green pea pods, chop
½ cup of any or all of the following: broccoli, cauliflower, fresh corn, chop green beans, tender asparagus
⅓ cup turnips, grate
1 un-peeled cucumber, slice
3 radishes, slice
2 ripe tomatoes, chop
1 cup cabbage, slice
3 stalks celery, chop
2 or 3 artichoke hearts, chop
½ green bell pepper, chop
½ cup tender beets, grate
½ cup carrots, chop or shred
½ cup raw, tender new peas
1 avocado, slice
shake of Bragg Sprinkle and Bragg Kelp Seasoning
Bragg Vinaigrette, Ginger or Braggberry Dressing

You may use the above vegetables raw. You will find this salad adventure can be a delicious, healthy experience. Serves 6-10.

BLACK BEAN SALAD

1 cup black beans
2 cloves garlic, mince
½ red bell pepper, chop
1 small chili pepper, mince
½ cup green onions, chop
1 cup fresh or frozen corn
2 Tbsps fresh lemon juice
2 Tbsps Bragg Organic Olive Oil
shake of Bragg Sprinkle
shake of Bragg Kelp
1 tsp Bragg Liquid Aminos
Bragg Apple Cider Vinegar (to taste)
Optional: chopped cilantro, apples and avocado slices (if desired)

Soak beans overnight. Drain well, rinse and cover with distilled water. Cook for 45 minutes or until tender. Drain well and save liquid for soup. Cool and mix beans with all ingredients. Make dressing with lemon juice, olive oil and Bragg Aminos. Mix thoroughly and add vinegar to taste. Top with chopped cilantro, apples and avocado slices as desired. Serves 4.

We can change and improve if we set our will to improve. – Robert Benson

---

The future depends on what we do in the present. – Mahatma Gandhi

LENTIL SALAD, PITA OR TOSTADA

2 cups leaf lettuce, tear
1/3 cup celery, chop
1/3 cup green onions, chop
1/3 cup cucumbers, slice
1/4 cup fresh parsley, chop
1 cup salsa
diced tomatoes
1 Tbsp lemon juice
1/8 tsp garlic powder
1/4 tsp Bragg Sea Kelp Seasoning
shake of Bragg Sprinkle (24 herbs/spices)
6 whole-grain toast slices, pita bread or corn tortillas
3 cups cooked lentils

Mix lettuce, celery, green onions, cucumbers and parsley together in bowl. Add lemon juice, garlic powder, Bragg Sprinkle and Kelp and mix well. Set aside. Toast whole-grain bread, pita bread or heat corn tortillas, then spread with salsa and spoon hot lentils on top, now cover with chopped veggies and salad greens. Top with tomato, sliced avocados, salsa and sprinkle of Bragg Nutritional Yeast. Serves 6.

RAW BEETS DELIGHT

2 cloves garlic, crush
1/2 cup Bragg Organic Olive Oil
1/2 cup Bragg Organic Apple Cider Vinegar
2 Tbsps raw honey to taste
1/2 cup fresh orange juice
1 1/2 tsps organic orange peel, grate
6 beets, slice thin or grate
2 red onions, chop
1/2 cup parsley, chop
shake of Bragg Kelp
shake of Bragg Sprinkle

Blend garlic in olive oil, vinegar, honey, orange juice, orange peel. Place beets in sauce. Add red onion, parsley, Sprinkle and Kelp Seasoning to taste. Marinate one hour. Serves 4-6.

TUSCAN BEAN SALAD

1 1/2 cups cannellini beans
1/4 cup red pepper, chop
1/4 cup green onions, slice
1/4 cup parsley, chop
3 Tbsps Bragg Organic Olive Oil
1/2 cup black pitted olives, slice
1 Tbsp Dijon mustard
1 Tbsp Bragg Apple Cider Vinegar
1/2 tsp Bragg Sprinkle
1 tsp Bragg Liquid Aminos

Soak cannellini beans overnight. Drain well, rinse and cover with distilled water. Cook 30-40 minutes until tender. Drain well and cool (save liquid for soup). Mix with vegetables and olives. Mix together remaining ingredients for dressing. Toss all together and chill. Serve over bed of sliced cabbage or lettuce. Serves 4-6.

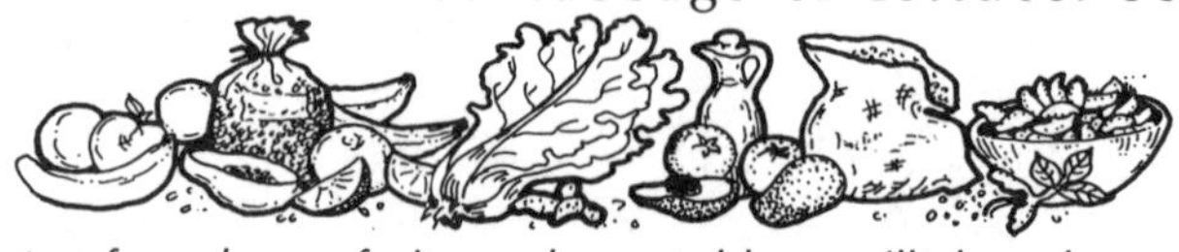

Eating plenty of produce - fruits and vegetables - will slow down ageing. The ageing process that goes on under the skin, and chronic age-associated diseases, including heart disease, cancer and degenerative brain diseases, can be slowed down, and even reversed in some cases, with a change in diet. Adding lots of fruits and vegetables and garlic, taking vitamin and mineral supplements, and avoiding saturated fat will add years to your life and increase your energy. Exercise is also very important in delaying ageing. – Nanci Hellmich, *USA Today*

ASIAN SALAD

8-oz pkg rice noodles
½ lb snap peas, slice diagonally
1 red bell pepper, thinly slice
1 cup red cabbage, thinly slice
2 green onions, slice diagonally
1 clove garlic, mince
1 Tbsp ginger, mince
2 Tbsps Bragg Liquid Aminos
2 Tbsps Bragg Apple Cider Vinegar
1 Tbsp rice vinegar
½ tsp raw honey
⅛ tsp crushed red pepper
3 Tbsps Bragg Organic Olive Oil
1 Tbsp sesame seeds, toast

Pour boiling distilled water over noodles, cover, let stand while preparing vegetables. Mix garlic and ginger with remaining ingredients, except veggies and sesame seeds and set aside. Drain noodles thoroughly and mix with vegetables. Add dressing and mix well. Top with sesame seeds. Serves 4-6.

ASIAN COLESLAW

1 cup Chinese cabbage, thin slice
½ cucumber, peel, slice
½ cup water chestnuts, slice
½ cup carrots, grate
½ red bell pepper
½ cup apple, grate
2 green onions, slice thin diagonally

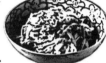

TRY BRAGGBERRY DRESSING OR DRESSING BELOW:

1 Tbsp tofunaise (page 139)
1 Tbsp distilled water
1 tsp prepared mustard
1 tsp Bragg Liquid Aminos
⅛ tsp black or red pepper
1 tsp Bragg Apple Cider Vinegar

Cut cucumber, water chestnuts, and red pepper into julienne strips and mix with carrots, cabbage and onions. Mix dressing of choice and toss with salad. Serve chilled. Serves 4-6.

HIJIKI SEAWEED SALAD

RF

4-oz hijiki seaweed
½ cucumber, thinly slice
8 radishes, thinly slice
1 cup sunflower sprouts
2 cups mixed salad greens
1 small zucchini, cut in matchsticks

MARINADE:

3 Tbsps fresh lime juice
1 Tbsp fresh mint, mince
2 Tbsps fresh cilantro, mince
1 inch fresh ginger, mince
1 Tbsp Bragg Liquid Aminos
1 Tbsp raw honey
4 Tbsps Bragg Organic Olive Oil
½ tsp Bragg Sprinkle

Soak seaweed for 2 hours, drain and finely shred or tear. Mix with vegetables, marinade and let sit at room temperature for one hour. Tasty served over salad greens of choice. Serves 4-6.

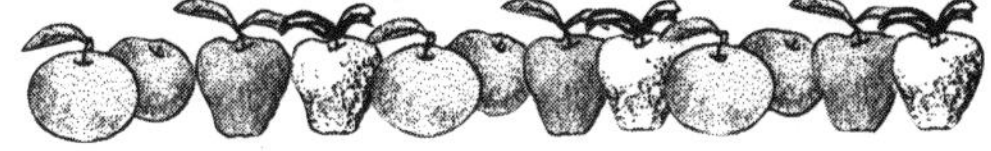

Carrots, a primary source of beta-carotene, are packed with nutrients – vitamins B1, B2, B3, B6, folic acid, potassium, vitamin C, iron, magnesium, and calcium. Carrots promote eye health, helps lower cholesterol and soothes indigestion. Raw organic carrots offer the best nutrition.

Of all the knowledge, the one most worth having is knowledge about health! The first requisite of a good life is to be a healthy person. – Herbert Spencer

VIETNAMESE SALAD ROLLS

½ lb firm tofu, drain and crumble
1 carrot, finely grate
1 cup bean sprouts
roasted peanuts (to taste), chop
½ cup bok choy, finely chop
½ yellow bell pepper, dice
½ cup sweet onion, grate
6 - 8 lettuce leaves

TRY BRAGGBERRY DRESSING OR DRESSING BELOW:

1 Tbsp peanut oil
2 tsps lime juice
1 tsp Bragg Apple Cider Vinegar
1 Tbsp chives, mince
¼ tsp Bragg Liquid Aminos
1 inch fresh ginger, mince

Combine tofu and vegetables and mix with the dressing. On a large leaf of lettuce, place one-sixth of the mixture and roll, tucking in the sides as you go. Place rolls on a platter and top with chopped peanuts or nuts of choice. Serves 4.

GREEN BEAN SALAD OR GARNISH

2 cups green beans, slice, cook
½ cup onion, finely chop
1 Tbsp raw honey
3 Tbsps Bragg Organic Olive Oil
2 Tbsps Bragg Apple Cider Vinegar
shake of Bragg Sprinkle
1 Tbsp Bragg Liquid Aminos
½ tsp mustard powder
1 cup thin strips of soy cheese

Cook green beans for 5 minutes and sprinkle onion and honey over them. Mix well. Cover tightly and chill. In a small jar shake together olive oil, vinegar, Sprinkle, Bragg Aminos and mustard powder. Set aside. When serving, turn the beans into a salad bowl and add oil mixture and toss well. Sprinkle soy cheese strips over top, also makes a tasty garnish for other salads. Serves 4.

DELICIOUS FRUIT SALADS

The following fresh fruits can be combined into delicious, all-fruit salads: apple, banana, cherry, fig, currant, grape, grapefruit, orange, mango, papaya, mulberry, peach, pear, apricot, tangerine, plum, nectarine, pineapple, prune, kiwi, strawberry, blueberries, boysenberry and blackberry. Cantaloupe, and melons of all kinds may be used alone or mixed within the melon family, independent of other fruits. Almost any fruit can be used in a fruit salad or combined with either crumbled soft tofu, shredded coconut, raw honey or soy yogurt.

BERRY HEALTHY SALAD

1 pint blackberries
1 pint raspberries
1 pint boysenberries
1 pint blueberries
1½ cups soft tofu, crumble
2 Tbsps raw nuts of choice, chop
1 head of leaf lettuce
soy yogurt and honey, to taste

Wash berries and dry thoroughly. Mix with tofu and nuts in a bowl. Serve on lettuce leaf and garnish with soy yogurt and honey to taste, if desired. Serves 6.

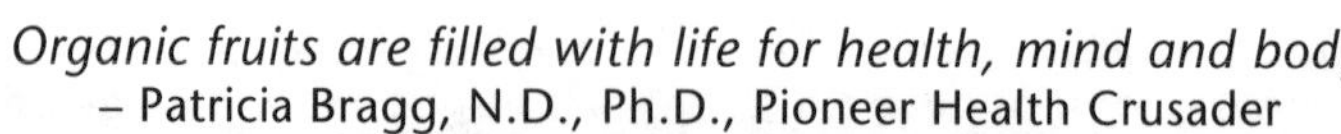

Organic fruits are filled with life for health, mind and body.
– Patricia Bragg, N.D., Ph.D., Pioneer Health Crusader

AMBROSIA

RF

7 bananas, slice
3 oranges, slice
raw honey (to taste)
1 sliced fresh pineapple
1 cup coconut, grate
soy yogurt (optional)
1 cup raw pecans, walnuts or nuts of choice, chop

Mix fruits, pecans and coconut. Add raw honey to taste. Serve in chilled bowl. Top with Braggberry or soy yogurt, if desired. Serves 6.

TROPICAL HAWAIIAN DELIGHT

RF

Any mix of tropical fresh fruit: papaya, mango, kiwi, guava, etc
1 large fresh pineapple
1 Tbsp raw macadamia nuts, chop
1 pint fresh strawberries
soy yogurt (optional)

Quarter pineapple lengthwise. Do not peel. Cut away hard core. Scoop out inside. Chop finely. Mix sliced kiwi, guava, mango or any tropical fruit in season and refill shells. Hull strawberries and slice. Lay on top of pineapple to cover top. Garnish with raw chopped nuts and soy yogurt or try delicious Braggberry. Serves 4.

PAPAYA HAWAIIAN SALAD

RF

2 cups papaya, dice
1½ cups fresh pineapple, dice
2 Tbsps soy yogurt
4-6 lettuce leaves
¾ cup celery, dice
6 dates, pit, chop
1½ Tbsps finely chopped mixed raw nuts or seeds of choice (almonds, sunflower, peanuts, pine nuts, walnuts, etc.)

Combine fruit, celery, yogurt and Braggberry. Add raw nuts, seeds, chopped dates. Serve on crisp lettuce leaves. Serves 4-6.

RAW CRANBERRY DELIGHT

RF

3 cups raw, organic cranberries
¼ cup freshly squeezed lemon juice
1 tsp arrowroot powder (dissolve in ¼ cup hot distilled water)
½ cup raw honey (or Stevia to taste)
⅓ cup almonds, slice
¼ cup apple juice
¼ tsp cinnamon
½ cup soy cheese, dice
soy yogurt and Braggberry

Cover raw organic cranberries in distilled water, soak for 2 hours. Then blend until smooth. Add lemon juice, dissolved arrowroot powder, honey, apple juice, cinnamon and almonds. Chill. Then add soy cheese. Pour into wet molds and freeze (15 minutes to harden). When hardened and ready to serve, cut small squares, place on bed of shredded lettuce or sliced cabbage and top with soy yogurt and Braggberry. Serves 4-6.

Fruit bears the closest relation to light. The sun pours a continuous flood of light into the fruits, and they furnish the best portion of food a human being requires for the sustenance of mind and body. – Louisa May Alcott

---

The pigments that give berries their beautiful blue and red hues are also good for your health. Berries contain phytochemicals and flavonoids that may help to prevent some forms of cancer. Blueberries and raspberries also contain lutein, which is important for healthy vision. See web: nutrition.about.com

PEAR AND GRAPE SALAD

6 lettuce leaves
6 pear halves, fresh or canned
1½ lbs organic seedless grapes, of your choice
2 oz soy yogurt
2 oz soy cheese or soft tofu

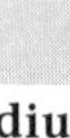

Cover salad plates with lettuce leaves. Place a pear half on each leaf, flat side up. Blend soy cheese or soft tofu with soy yogurt and dash of Braggberry Dressing; generously spread on pears. Cut grapes into halves and arrange flat side-down on the covered pear (please close together to resemble a bunch of grapes). Serves 6.

FRESH FRUIT BOUQUET

1 medium pineapple, dice
3 oranges
2 grapefruits
1 cup grapes, whole
2 fresh pears, cube
soy yogurt (optional)

Chill all fruits. Dice fresh pineapple. Peel and section the oranges and grapefruits. Remove grapes from stems. Cut un-peeled fresh pears into cubes. Combine all fruits and serve in chilled sherbet dishes. Garnish with soy yogurt, if desired. Serves 4.

RHYTHM SALAD

¾ cup stewed prunes
¾ cup stewed apricots
3 apples, core, chop
½ cup raw carrots, shred
¼ cup raisins or currants
1 cup cabbage, slice
lemon tofunaise (pg. 36), to taste
¼ cup peanuts or pine nuts, chop

Remove pits from stewed prunes and apricots, then slice; mix with apples, carrots, raisins or currants and sliced cabbage. Toss with lemon tofunaise, or Braggberry. Sprinkle chopped peanuts or raw pine nuts over the top. Serves 4-6.

SUMMER FRUIT SALAD

1 pear, chop
1 peach, chop
1 nectarine, chop
1 cup fresh blueberries
2 apples, core, chop
1 cup seedless grapes
2 bananas, slice
2 oranges, section, cut in half
nuts, coconut or organic granola
1 cup soy yogurt, dash of Braggberry

Mix fruit. Top with soy yogurt and Braggberry, chopped raw nuts, grated coconut and your favorite organic granola. Serves 4.

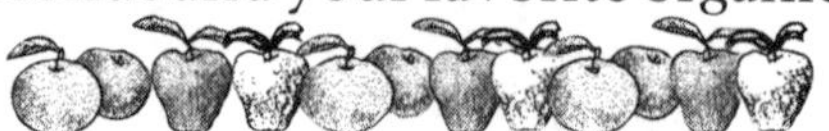

Health is a state of complete physical, mental, and social well-being and not merely the absence of disease or infirmity. – The World Health Organization

Your choice of diet can influence your long term health prospects more than any other action you might take!
– Dr. C. Everett Koop, Former U.S. Surgeon General
Dr. Koop said, "Paul Bragg did more for the health of America than any one person I've known!"

TOFU SALADS

TOFU AND VEGGIE SALAD

2 cups celery, dice
2 green onions, chop
¼ cup parsley, chop
½ cup bell peppers, dice
1 cup firm tofu, crumble
2 Tbsps Bragg Apple Cider Vinegar
Lettuce, cabbage or watercress
1 cup carrots, grate
1 garlic clove, mince
½ tsp Bragg Liquid Aminos
pinch of mustard powder
shake of Bragg Sprinkle
3 Tbsps Bragg Olive Oil
shake of Bragg Sea Kelp

Mix ingredients, chill. Serve on bed of lettuce, sliced cabbage or watercress. Sprinkle on Nutritional Yeast. Serves 2-4.

CURRIED TOFU SALAD

1 cup firm tofu, cut into ½" pieces
shake of Bragg Sprinkle
½ cup apple, core, dice
½ cup carrots, grate
¼ cup currants or raisins
½ tsp curry powder
pinch cayenne (to taste)
¼ tsp tumeric
½ tsp raw honey
⅓ cup tofunaise (page 139)
¼ cup roasted peanuts, or nuts of choice, chop

Mix all ingredients, chill. Spread on lettuce. Serves 2-3.

TOFU AND BEET SALAD

1 cup firm tofu, crumble
shake of Bragg Sprinkle
⅓ cup tofunaise (page 139)
¼ cup chives, mince
1 cup cooked beets, dice
Lettuce or cabbage leaves

Mix tofu, beets, Sprinkle and chives with tofunaise dressing and arrange on lettuce or cabbage leaves. Serves 2-4.

TOFU MOCK EGG SALAD

8 oz soft tofu, crumble
¼ cup mushrooms, mince
¼ cup bell pepper, mince
½ cup celery, mince
⅓ cup red onion, mince
2 Tbsps tofunaise (page 139)
dash of each: garlic powder, ground cumin, and paprika
shake of Bragg Sprinkle
Bragg Liquid Aminos to taste

Crumble tofu, and then add finely minced raw vegetables, seasonings, Bragg Aminos and tofunaise. Mix all together. Serve mixture in bell pepper halves, celery stalks, lettuce leaves, or use as sandwich filling or salad topping. Serves 2-4.

Nothing will benefit human health or increase the chances for survival of life on earth as the changes to a vegetarian diet. It is my view that the vegetarian manner of living, by its purely physical effect on the human temperament, would most beneficially influence all mankind and the world.
– Albert Einstein, German physicist, discovered theory of general relativity

---

Happiness is not being pained in body or troubled in mind.
– Thomas Jefferson, U.S. 3rd President (1801-1809)
Principal author of the Declaration of Independence

SALAD DRESSINGS

HONEY FRENCH DRESSING

- ⅔ cup Bragg Organic Olive Oil
- 2 Tbsps fresh lemon juice
- ½ tsp Bragg Liquid Aminos
- 1 Tbsp raw honey
- 3 Tbsps Bragg Apple Cider Vinegar
- pinch of mustard powder
- a dash of cayenne
- shake of Bragg Sprinkle

Mix all ingredients except raw honey. Add honey to mixture slowly and beat vigorously. Makes 1 cup.

FRENCH DRESSING WITH TOMATO JUICE

- ⅓ cup fresh lemon juice
- ⅓ cup Bragg Organic Olive Oil
- ½ tsp Bragg Liquid Aminos
- 2 tsps Bragg Apple Cider Vinegar
- 1 cup tomato juice, salt-free
- 1½ Tbsps raw honey
- 1 clove garlic, crush
- shake of Bragg Sprinkle

Blend ingredients well. Allow to stand 30 minutes. Makes 2 cups.

GRAPEFRUIT FRENCH DRESSING

- 4 Tbsps Bragg Organic Olive Oil
- 1 cup freshly squeezed grapefruit juice
- 2 tsps freshly squeezed lemon juice
- 1 Tbsp soy cheese, finely crumbled
- shake Bragg Sprinkle

Blend ingredients, (optional 1 Tbsp honey), beat vigorously. Allow dressing to stand hour before serving. Makes 1¼ cups.

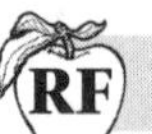

FRENCH DRESSING WITH ONION SAUCE

- ½ cup Bragg Organic Olive Oil
- ½ tsp Bragg Liquid Aminos
- ¼ cup fresh lemon juice
- 1 tsp onion, mince
- shake of Bragg Sprinkle (24 herbs & spices)

Blend all ingredients except oil; then beat oil vigorously into mixture and let stand one hour before serving. Makes ¾ cup.

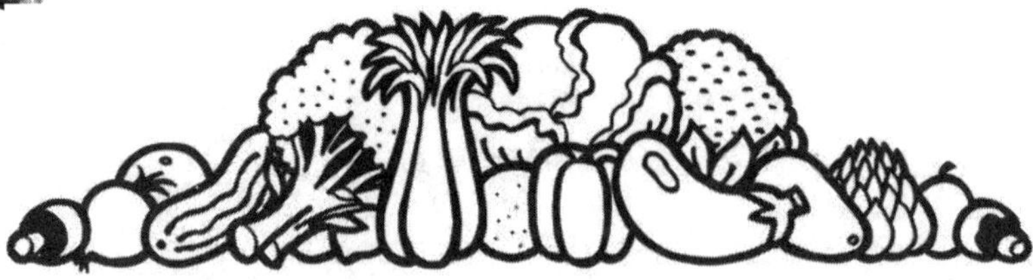

If you would be loved, love and be lovable. – Benjamin Franklin

---

Cow's milk has become a point of controversy among doctors and nutritionists worldwide. There was a time when it was considered very desirable, but research has forced us to rethink this recommendation. Dairy products contribute to a surprising number of health problems. – Benjamin Spock, M.D., *Dr. Spock's Baby and Child Care* • www.notmilk.com

---

He who has health has hope;
and he who has hope has everything. – Arabic Proverb

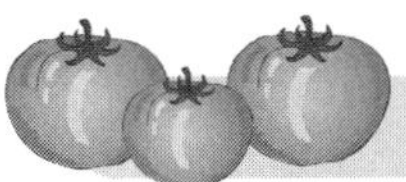

TOMATO JUICE DRESSING

1 cup tomato juice, fresh or can
1 tsp chives, mince
shake of Bragg Kelp
3 Tbsps fresh lemon or orange juice
⅓ cup Bragg Olive Oil
½ tsp Bragg Liquid Aminos
1 tsp red onion, mince
1 clove garlic, crush
shake of Bragg Sprinkle (24 herbs & spices)

Mix all the ingredients and blend well in a blender, Vitamix or Jack LaLanne's HealthMaster 100 (see page 51 for blender list). Then refrigerate 4 hours before using. Makes 1½ cups.

QUICK TOFU TOPPING & DRESSING

For raw vegetable salads, cooked vegetables and sandwiches: Add juice from fresh lemon or lime to cup soft tofu, add teaspoon raw honey or Stevia to taste. Add shake Braggberry. Blend well. Delicious as topping on salads and cooked vegetables.

TOFU DELIGHT DRESSING, TOPPING & SPREAD

For salads, vegetables and sandwiches. Blend or mash two pounds well-drained soft tofu, two tablespoons Bragg Organic Olive Oil, two tablespoons Bragg Apple Cider Vinegar, a tablespoon of honey, a shake Bragg Sprinkle (24 herbs & spices) and one teaspoon Bragg Aminos. Mix all ingredients until smooth and creamy. For variety, add one tablespoon unsweetened pineapple or fruit juice and flaked coconut.

MUSTARD DRESSING

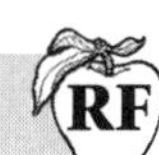

⅓ cup freshly squeezed lemon juice or Bragg Apple Cider Vinegar
shake of Bragg Sprinkle
½ cup Bragg Olive Oil
1 Tbsp raw honey
1½ tsp mustard powder

Blend ingredients well and allow dressing to stand for one hour before serving. Makes 1 cup.

GARLIC SALAD DRESSING

½ cup Bragg Apple Cider Vinegar
2 Tbsps garlic, crush
spray of Bragg Liquid Aminos
1 tsp raw honey
shake of Bragg Sprinkle
1 cup Bragg Organic Olive Oil

Put all ingredients in blender and blend. Refrigerate. Perfect over most salads and veggie dishes. Makes 1½ cups.

FRENCH TOFU DRESSING

1 cup soft tofu
¼ cup French Dressing with Tomato Juice (see page 32)

This is a great dressing for salads and sandwiches. Blend soft tofu with French Dressing. For variety, add minced chives, ripe olives, watercress and freshly blended peeled cucumber.

Tofu is low in fat, high in protein, iron & calcium. – www.vegetarian.about.com

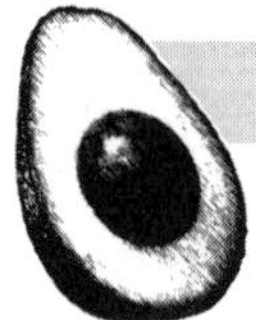

AVOCADO – TOFU DRESSING AND DIP

2 avocados, mash
juice from 1 lemon
1 cup soft tofu, crumble
a dash of Bragg Liquid Aminos
Braggberry and Sprinkle (24 herbs & spices), to taste

Mix mashed avocados and tofu thoroughly. Add Bragg Aminos, lemon juice, Sprinkle and Braggberry to taste. Mix to creamy consistency. A delicious dressing, dip or garnish for salads, vegetables and rice dishes. Makes 2 cups.

LIME DRESSING

4 Tbsps Bragg Olive Oil
2 tsps raw honey
2 Tbsps freshly squeezed lime juice
pinch of celery seed
shake of Bragg Sprinkle (24 herbs & spices)

Blend ingredients. Let dressing stand one hour before serving. *Optional:* Substitute Bragg Apple Cider Vinegar for the fresh lime juice. Makes 1 cup.

PINEAPPLE DELIGHT DRESSING

½ cup pineapple juice, unsweetened
1 cup soy yogurt
raw honey, maple syrup, Stevia, or sweetener of your choice

Gradually add enough pineapple juice to soy yogurt to give the consistency of whipped cream. Sweeten to taste. This is a delicious fruit topping and salad dressing. Makes 1½ cup.

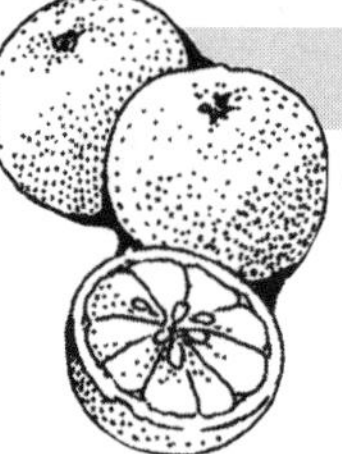

ORANGE TOFU DRESSING

3 oz well-drained soft tofu
1 tsp raw honey (optional)
or Stevia powder to taste
juice from 1 orange
juice from 1 lemon

Blend tofu, lemon and orange juice and honey or Stevia powder until creamy. Makes 1 cup.

TAPENADE VINAIGRETTE DRESSING

This dressing can be green or purple: the green made with green olives, purple (classic version) made with black olives.

2 cloves garlic
3 Tbsps Bragg Apple Cider Vinegar
3 Tbsps tapenade (recipe follows)
⅔ cup Bragg Organic Olive Oil
2 Tbsps capers, drained
Bragg Liquid Aminos (to taste)

Rub garlic thoroughly around inside of a wooden salad bowl; then discard garlic. In the bottom of the bowl, combine the oil, vinegar, capers and tapenade; whisk together until emulsified. Season to taste with Bragg Aminos. Delicious for salad greens, sprouts and veggie salads. Makes 1½ cups.

If families could be induced to substitute the healthy organic apple, sound, ripe and luscious, in place of white sugar, white flour pies, cakes, candies and other sweets with which children are too often stuffed, doctor bills would diminish enough in a single year to lay up a stock of this delicious fruit for a season's use.

OLIVE TAPENADE

RF

½ cup black pitted olives
1 clove garlic, mince
1 Tbsp fresh lemon juice
Bragg Liquid Aminos to taste
½ cup green pitted olives
2 Tbsps capers
¼ cup Bragg Olive Oil
shake of Bragg Sprinkle

In a blender or food processor, combine the olives, garlic, capers and lemon juice. Blend until smooth. With motor running, add the olive oil, little by little to make a thick sauce. Add Bragg Aminos and Sprinkle to taste. Store in airtight container in the refrigerator up to one week. Makes 1 cup.

HONEY CELERY SEED DRESSING

RF

pinch of mustard powder
¼ tsp paprika
⅓ cup raw honey
Bragg Sprinkle (to taste)
1 medium onion, grate
⅓ cup Bragg Apple Cider Vinegar
1 cup soy or Bragg Olive Oil
1 Tbsp celery seed
1 tsp Bragg Liquid Aminos (or to taste)

Measure the mustard powder and paprika into a small bowl. Add honey, Bragg Sprinkle and Bragg Aminos (to taste), and blend thoroughly. Add grated onion and a small amount of vinegar. Beat mixture. Add oil of choice and the remaining vinegar alternately. Celery seed should be added last. Store in a cool place in a covered jar. Makes about 2 cups.

HONEY OLIVE OIL DRESSING

¼ medium onion, grate
1 cup Bragg Olive Oil
pinch of mustard powder
shake of Bragg Sprinkle
½ cup raw honey
6 Tbsps fresh lemon juice
½ tsp celery seed
pinch of paprika

Measure the mustard powder and paprika into small mixing bowl. Add honey (or pinch of Stevia powder) and blend thoroughly. Add grated onion and half the lemon juice. Beat mixture; add olive oil and remaining lemon juice alternately and then celery seed. Store in a covered jar in a cool place. Makes 1½ cups.

SESAME SOY DRESSING

1-2 Tbsps tan sesame seeds, rinse and drain well
½ cup distilled water
Bragg Liquid Aminos, to taste
2 Tbsps brown rice vinegar
2 tsps brown rice syrup
1 tsp sesame oil
2 cloves garlic, mince
½ tsp powdered ginger
shake of Bragg Sprinkle

Dry-roast seeds in a small skillet, 2-3 minutes over medium heat until slightly puffy and fragrant. Simmer remaining ingredients in a small saucepan over low heat 4-5 minutes to help flavors develop. Remove from heat and stir in seeds. Serve dressing warm or at room temperature. Makes about ¾ cup.

LEMON TOFUNAISE

2 cups Bragg Organic Olive Oil
½ cup freshly squeezed lemon juice
shake of Bragg Sprinkle
½ cup soft tofu
1 tsp mustard powder
shake of Bragg Kelp

Combine mustard powder, Bragg Sprinkle and Bragg Kelp with tofu in mixing bowl. Beat together until stiff. Add part of the olive oil, beating it into the mixture drop by drop at first, then proceeding more rapidly, keeping the mixture firm. When it begins to thicken, add a little lemon juice alternately with the remaining olive oil. Makes 2½ cups.

RUSSIAN DRESSING

½ cup lemon tofunaise (above)
¼ cup chili sauce
½ tsp celery seed
1 Tbsp green pepper, mince
1 Tbsp pimientos, chop
⅓ tsp anise seeds
1 garlic clove, crush
1 tsp raw honey

Blend ingredients; beat vigorously and allow to stand for one hour before serving. Makes 1 cup.

INDIAN SALAD DRESSING

1 Tbsp green bell pepper, mince
1 Tbsp red bell pepper, mince
1 Tbsp fresh grapefruit juice
½ cup Bragg Organic Olive Oil
shake of Bragg Sprinkle
2 tsps raw honey
⅓ cup firm tofu
2 tsps parsley, mince
2 Tbsps lemon juice
½ tsp paprika

Press tofu through a strainer and drain off any liquid; combine all ingredients. Now blend dressing well. Good with avocado salads and vegetable salads. Makes about 1½ cups.

AN OLD ENGLISH PRAYER

Give us Lord, a bit of sun,
a bit of work and a bit of fun.

Give us, in all struggle and sputter,
our daily whole grain bread and water.

Give us health, our keep to make
and a bit to spare for others' sake.

Give us too, a bit of song
and a tale and a book, to help us along.

Give us Lord, a chance to be
our goodly best for ourselves and others,
until we learn to live as sisters and brothers
in peace and harmony.

Create the kind of self you will be happy to live with all your life. – Foster C. McClellan

SPICY AVOCADO AND TOFU DRESSING

2 avocados, mash
1 cup soft tofu
shake of Bragg Sprinkle
juice of one lemon
chili powder (to taste)
½ tsp Bragg Liquid Aminos

Thoroughly mix mashed avocados and soft tofu. Add lemon juice, Bragg Sprinkle and Bragg Aminos. Beat to a creamy consistency. Add chili powder as desired. Makes 2 cups.

SOY CHEESE DRESSING

1 cup soy cheese
⅓ cup firm tofu
½ tsp raw honey or to taste
1 tsp fresh squeezed lemon juice

Press tofu through strainer to remove liquid, blend in soy cheese. Add lemon juice and honey to taste. Makes 1⅓ cups.

GRAPEFRUIT VINAIGRETTE

RF

½ cup fresh grapefruit juice
½ cup Bragg Apple Cider Vinegar
shake of Bragg Sprinkle
2 tsps fresh parsley, finely chop
shake of Bragg Sea Kelp
¼ cup cold distilled water
1 garlic clove, mince
1 Tbsp raw honey (to taste)

BRAGG APPLE CIDER VINEGAR
SPRINKLE
KELP

Whisk together grapefruit juice, vinegar and water in bowl. Add garlic, Sprinkle, Kelp, honey (or pinch of Stevia powder to taste), and parsley. Mix and chill until ready to use. Will keep in refrigerator for 4 to 5 days. Makes 1½ cups.

RASPBERRY VINAIGRETTE

RF

2 Tbsps raspberry vinegar
1 tsp fresh rosemary, crush
2 Tbsps Bragg Apple Cider Vinegar
1 tsp fresh tarragon, crush
raw honey to taste
shake of Bragg Sprinkle

Whisk ingredients together with 2 Tbsps of distilled water. Store in refrigerator in tightly sealed container.

ROSEMARY

ITALIAN HERB SEASONING

1 tsp thyme
1 tsp paprika
2 Tbsps sweet basil
1 Tbsp rosemary
1 tsp tarragon
2 Tbsps oregano
1 tsp garlic powder (optional)
shake of Bragg Sprinkle & Sea Kelp

Place all ingredients in an airtight container. Cover and shake thoroughly to blend. Makes approximately 2 cup.

The American Heart Association estimates one out of every four adults has high blood pressure (65 million Americans). Many don't realize this. Studies show during early and middle-adult years, men are more likely to suffer from hypertension. Evidence proves that an unhealthy lifestyle and excess weight can negatively influence blood pressure. www.americanheart.org

---

Salad dressings were made from scratch in home kitchens until the 19th century when restaurant owners began packaging and selling their own dressings.

EAT A RAINBOW OF COLORS EVERY DAY
to Keep Healthy, More Fit & Youthful

By John Westerdahl, Ph.D., M.P.H., R.D., C.N.S
Director, Bragg Health Foundation
Director, Bragg Live Foods, Inc.

In order to achieve optimal nutrition for health, wellness, longevity and a beautiful and more youthful, ageless appearance, it is critical to eat a wide variety of colorful fruits and vegetables everyday. The more colorful the fruits and vegetables, the better they are for you! They contain an abundance of life-giving nutrients and other healthful phytochemical compounds that nourish your body, fight against disease and even give you a more slim and youthful appearance! Try to eat as many of your fruits and vegetables organic, raw and uncooked as possible for optimal health!

Enjoy more health with these colorful, delicious fruits and vegetables recommended by David Heber, M.D., Ph.D., Director, of the UCLA Center for Human Nutrition:

RED: Tomatoes, tomato sauce, tomato-based juices and tomato-based soups, health ketchup, watermelon, pink grapefruit

RED-PURPLE: Grapes, grape juice, red peppers, fresh and dried plums, cherries, cranberries, eggplant, red beets, raisins, red apples, blueberries, blackberries, strawberries

ORANGE: Apricots, carrots, cantaloupes, pumpkins, winter squash, sweet potatoes, mangoes

ORANGE-YELLOW: Oranges, orange juice, tangerines, yellow and pink grapefruit, peaches, lemons, limes, and papayas, pineapples and nectarines

YELLOW-GREEN: Green peas, green beans, spinach, green, red and yellow peppers, cucumbers, mustard greens, kiwi, turnip greens, avocados

GREEN: Broccoli, brussel sprouts, cauliflower, cabbage, Chinese cabbage, kale, bok choy, chard

WHITE-GREEN: Garlic, onions, celery, leeks, asparagus, pears, artichokes, endive, mushrooms, chives

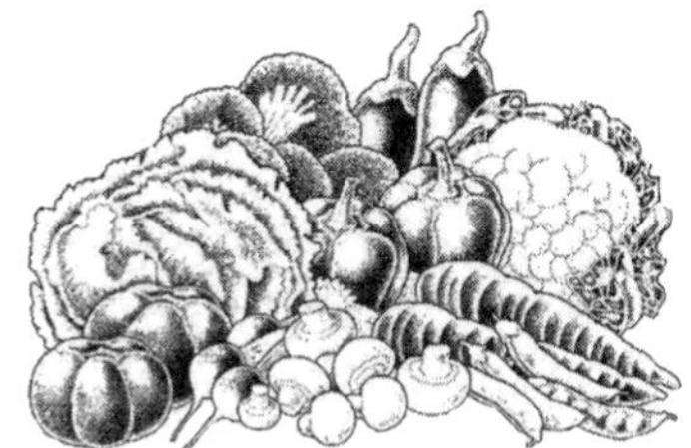

Chapter 3

Nutritious Raw Foods

This chapter is dedicated to the Raw Food Recipes. You can also find Raw Food Recipes throughout the pages of this book.

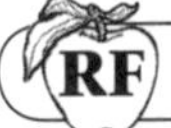

RF *symbolizes the Raw Food Recipes in this book.*

APPETIZERS

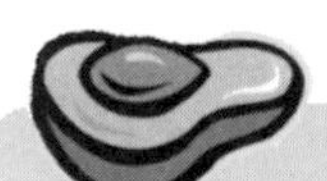

AVOCADO DIP

RF

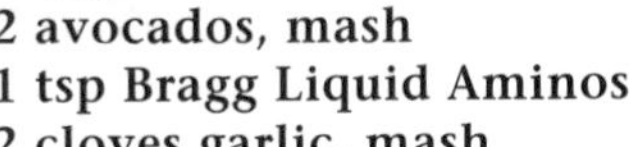

2 avocados, mash
1 tsp Bragg Liquid Aminos
2 cloves garlic, mash
celery stalks
1 Tbsp Bragg Olive Oil
tomato, carrots and zucchini

Combine avocado, Bragg Aminos, Sprinkle, olive oil and garlic. Put mixture on celery stalks. Serve with carrots, zucchini and tomato wedges for dip and on bed of lettuce if desired.

RAW TABOULEH

RF

1 cup wheat berries, soak in water 2 hours, then wash
1 Tbsp lemon juice
2 celery stalks, finely chop
1 medium cucumber, mince
½ cup red onion, finely chop
1 Tbsp Bragg Liquid Aminos
½ cup parsley, finely chop
1½ cups tomatoes, finely chop
Bragg Sprinkle (to taste)

Soften wheat berries, soak 2 hours in water. Drain well and press out excess moisture. Mix wheat berries, onions and seasonings (Bragg Aminos and Sprinkle) and crush all together with fork. Add lemon juice, parsley, tomatoes and cucumbers. Mix thoroughly. Serve on lettuce leaves or as salad topping.

MOCK SUSHI

RF

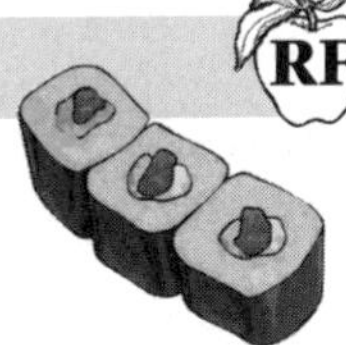

1 head Romaine lettuce
1 cup lentil sprouts
1-2 avocados, mash
1 tsp Bragg Liquid Aminos
2 cups alfalfa sprouts
½ cup wheat sprouts
1 garlic clove, mince
juice of 1 lemon

Thoroughly blend all ingredients except Romaine lettuce. Strip the center core from each lettuce leaf. Overlap the two halves and spread a layer of filling on top. Roll up and secure with a toothpick. Refrigerate 1-2 hours. Serve rolls whole or sliced.

NUT BUTTER DELIGHTS

RF

apple, banana, carrot slices
celery stalks
any fresh fruit and veggie slices
raw almond or creamy peanut butter

Dip banana, celery, carrot and apple slices and fruit and veggie slices in nut butter. Variation: sprinkle with sesame seeds.

RAW VEGETABLE SPREAD

Grind ¼ cup raisins and ½ cup each of shredded cabbage, carrots, and apples. Add 1 tablespoon lemon juice and season to taste. Moisten with Bragg Organic Olive Oil. Makes 1½ cups.

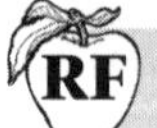

RAW VEGETABLE PATÉ

1 cup ground almonds	**1 cup ground walnuts**
1 cup ground pumpkin seeds	**1 cup raw sesame seeds**
½ cup bell pepper, chop	**1 cup fresh cut corn**
½ cup raw cashew butter	**6 tomatoes, chop**
4 scallions, chop	**2 Tbsps Bragg Liquid Aminos**
juice of 1 lemon	**2 Tbsp Bragg Olive Oil**
¼ cup distilled water	**shake of Bragg Sprinkle**

Mix all ingredients together and press firmly into a jello mold. Chill until firm, serve on bed of lettuce. Makes 6-8 servings.

SOUPS

AVOCADO SOUP

4 ripened avocados	**4 cups distilled water**
1 small red onion	**1 clove garlic**
2 stalks celery, grate	**2 ripe tomatoes**
shake of Bragg Sprinkle	**shake of Bragg Kelp**

Liquefy smooth. Garnish with alfalfa sprouts. Serves 4.

AVOCADO – TOMATO SOUP

2 whole avocados, dice	**½ cup carrots, grate**
4 medium tomatoes	**½ cup cabbage, chop**
½ cup celery, chop	**3 green onions, chop**
1 Tbsp Bragg Liquid Aminos	**1 small bell pepper, chop**
For variation: lemon juice	**shake of Bragg Sprinkle**

Blend tomatoes and avocados first. Then add other ingredients and blend to thick consistency. For variation add lemon juice. See blender information on page 51. Serves 2-3.

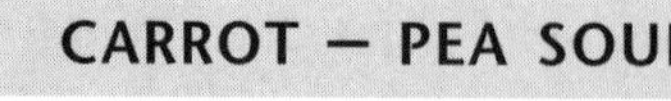

CARROT – PEA SOUP

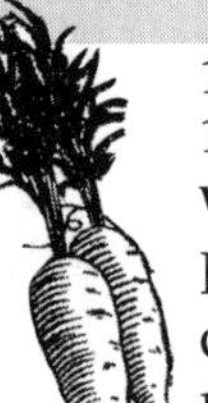

1 cup carrot juice	**1 cup fresh peas**
1 cup celery, chop	**½ cup raw almond butter**
watercress (for garnish)	

Blend all ingredients except watercress to desired consistency. Garnish with watercress. See blender recommendations on page 51. Serves 2-3.

Thanks be to God, since the time I gave up use of meat & wine, I have been delivered from all physical ills. – John Wesley, Letter to Bishop of London, 1747

The word soup originates from "sop" a dish originally consisting of a thick stew which was soaked up with pieces of bread. – See web: www.ifood.tv

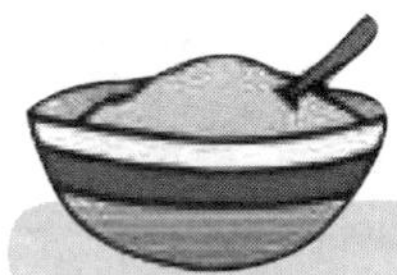

CEREALS

BREAKFAST SEED CEREAL

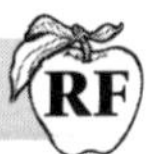

1 cup sesame seeds
1 cup sunflower seeds
1 cup pumpkins seeds
1 cup chia seeds

Mix above seeds in jar with wide opening. Grind fresh each morning ⅓ to ½ cup per serving. Do not grind all the seeds at one time, only grind what you need each time! You can top cereal with Almond Milk or Cashew Milk (see recipes below) and sliced fresh fruit if desired. Store seeds in refrigerator.

NUT MILKS

ALMOND MILK

1 cup raw almonds, (soak overnight)
1 quart distilled or purified water
3 dates, pit, chop (optional)
raw honey or stevia powder to taste

Put rinsed raw almonds, honey, dates and 1½ to 2 cups of distilled or purified water in blender and blend until smooth. Pour into container and add remaining water. Always shake well before pouring, as contents will settle. Makes 4 cups.

CASHEW MILK

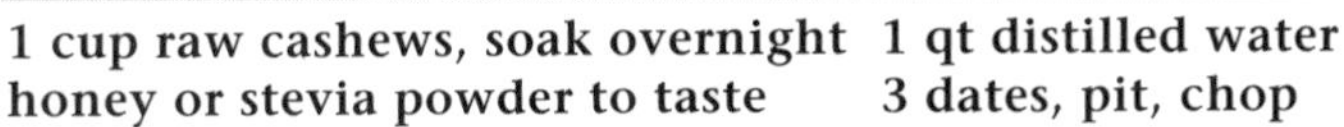

1 cup raw cashews, soak overnight
honey or stevia powder to taste
1 qt distilled water
3 dates, pit, chop

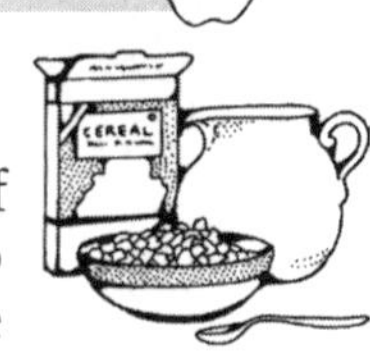

Put rinsed nuts, honey, dates, and 1½ - 2 cups of water in blender and blend until smooth. Pour into container and add remaining water. Always shake well before pouring, as contents will settle. Makes 4 cups.

ENTREÉS

RAW LENTIL BURGERS

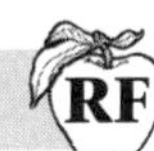

1 cup raw lentils, soak
1 green onion, chop
1 cup celery, chop
1 Tbsp garlic powder
1 cup fresh corn
½ cup raw peanut butter
1 Tbsp Bragg Liquid Aminos
shake of Bragg Sprinkle

Soak lentils in warm water for 4 hours or overnight. Put lentils, corn, onion and celery through food grinder. Add other ingredients and mix together. Form into patties. Serves 4.

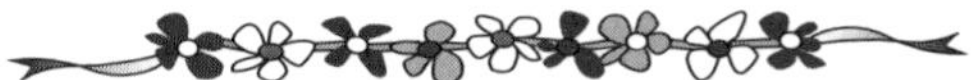

Raw food nutrition is the best way to increase your eating pleasure, improve your health, skin and save energy. – Pascale Corbin, *Your Health Magazine*

Raw foods cuisine is not only easy, but it tastes best and results in feeling better than you ever have before! – Juliano, famous raw food chef

BROCCOLI - MUSHROOM PATTIES

2 cups broccoli, chop
½ cup celery, finely chop
½ cup raw peanut butter
lettuce/parsley (as garnish)
1 cup mushrooms, dice
3 green onions, finely chop
1 tsp Bragg Liquid Aminos
shake of Bragg Sprinkle

Put broccoli through food grinder then add mushrooms, onions and celery. Add remaining ingredients except lettuce and parsley. Form into patties. Serve on bed of lettuce and garnish with parsley or watercress. Serves 4.

SPROUT - NUT - LENTIL PATTIES

3 cups lentil sprouts
2 cups fresh cut corn
3 green onions, mince
2 carrots, slice (as garnish)
2 cups celery, mince
1 cup yellow pea sprouts
1 tsp Bragg Liquid Aminos
shake of Bragg Sprinkle
1 cup raw almond or creamy peanut butter

Put sprouts, corn, celery and onions in food grinder. Add almond or peanut butter, Bragg Aminos and Sprinkle. Mix well. Form into patties, garnish with carrot slices. Serves 4-6.

NUT PATTIES

1 cup almonds, ground
1 cup raw cashew butter
1 cup walnuts, ground
parsley, mince (as garnish)
1 cup pecans, ground
1 Tbsp Bragg Liquid Aminos
1 cup peanuts, ground
walnut halves (as garnish)

Combine ground almonds, walnuts, pecans, peanuts, cashew butter and Bragg Aminos to make patties. Cover each patty with parsley and place a walnut half on top center of each patty. Serve on bed of lettuce. Can be served with slices of avocado, zucchini, onion, tomato and cucumber. Serves 6.

OATMEAL PATTIES

2 cups ground raw pecans
2 cloves garlic, mince
1 tsp Bragg Liquid Aminos
1 cup oatmeal flour
1 small red onion, mince
2 zucchini, cut into wedges

Combine all ingredients except zucchini. Form into patties. Place on platter with zucchini wedges as garnish. Serves 4.

RAW "SALMON-LIKE" PATTIES

2 cups carrots, ground
3 Tbsps raw peanut butter
garlic and onion powder (to taste)
¼ cup sunflower seed meal
2 stalks celery, ground
Bragg Liquid Aminos
Bragg Sprinkle, to taste
turnips or beets (optional)

Combine carrots, celery, peanut butter, and sunflower seed meal. Then add onion powder, garlic powder, Bragg Sprinkle and Bragg Aminos to taste. Form into patties. Garnish with sliced beets, turnips, jicama, or apples, etc. Serves 4.

MUSHROOM BALLS

3 cups mushrooms, mince
1 Tbsp garlic, mince
raw sesame seeds
1 cup raw almond butter
1 Tbsp Bragg Liquid Aminos
shake of Bragg Sprinkle

Combine all ingredients except sesame seeds and form into balls. Roll each ball on sesame seeds. Serve on a bed of lettuce with either sliced tomato halves or sliced red radishes.

SPROUTED "CHICKEN-LIKE" PATTIES

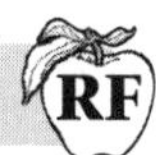

3 cups lentil sprouts
1 cup raw peanut butter
2 cups fresh cut corn
3 green onions, mince
2 carrots, slice
1 cup raw almond butter
2 cups celery, mince
1 cup yellow pea sprouts
1 Tbsp Bragg Liquid Aminos
shake of Bragg Sprinkle

Put sprouts, corn, celery and onions in food processor. Add almond and peanut butter, Aminos and Sprinkle. Mix and form into patties. Garnish with carrot or celery slices. Serves 6.

STUFFED ZUCCHINI

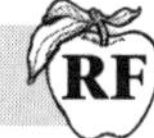

2 to 3 large zucchini

STUFFING:
2 cups sprouted wheat
1 small red onion
½ cup celery, dice
½ cup carrots, shred
1 cup raw almond butter
2 ripe tomatoes

SAUCE:
2 ripe tomatoes
1 cucumber
raw sesame seeds
1 tsp garlic powder
shake of Bragg Sprinkle
1 Tbsp Bragg Liquid Aminos

Cut zucchini length-wise and hollow out. Blend stuffing ingredients and pat into each zucchini "boat." Blend sauce items and pour over each zucchini. Serves 4-6.

DESSERTS

FRUIT ICE CREAM, BLUEBERRY, ETC.

2-4 frozen bananas
1 cup cashew milk (page 41)
1 pint frozen blueberries or frozen organic fruit as desired

Place blueberries or other organic fruit as desired, in bottom of food processor. Add frozen bananas and cashew milk. Blend. Serve and enjoy! Serves 2.

CAROB - NUT FROZEN BANANAS

carob powder
bananas, firm, ripe
raw peanut or raw cashew butter
chopped raw nuts (of choice)

Peel firm bananas. Place on cookie sheet and freeze. Mix carob powder with peanut or cashew butter to taste. Remove frozen bananas and cover with nut butter mixture. Roll covered bananas in chopped nuts of choice and refreeze until ready to serve.

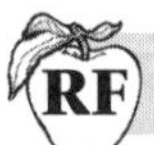

CARROT CAKE

#1 INGREDIENTS:

- 1 cup rolled oats
- ½ cup rice bran
- ½ cup sunflower seed meal
- 1 tsp cinnamon
- ⅓ tsp allspice
- ⅓ tsp nutmeg
- ½ cup unsweetened shredded coconut

#2 INGREDIENTS:

- ¼ cup raw honey
- 3 Tbsp distilled water
- ½ cup raw almond butter
- 3 Tbsp raw apple sauce (see recipe below)
- 3 cups carrots, shredded
- ½ cup dates,
- ½ cup raisins or currants

Mix #1 ingredients in a bowl and keep separate. Put #2 ingredients through the food processor. Add #1 ingredients to #2 ingredients and run through food processor a second time. Form into a loaf. Refrigerate two hours and garnish with coconut and ground nuts.

APPLE SAUCE

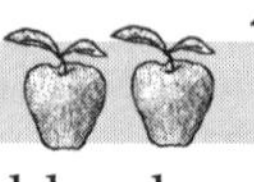
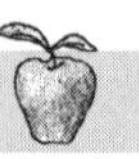
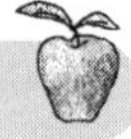

Cut apples into small pieces. Liquefy in blender using raw unfiltered apple juice to make into apple sauce consistency. Can add honey, cinnamon or nutmeg to add more flavor if desired.

BLUEBERRY PIE

- 3 cups fresh or frozen blueberries
- ¼ cup dates, pit
- ½ cup prune juice
- 1 raw pie crust (pg. 203)
- ½ cup raw pecan meal
- ¼ cup raw almond butter
- pinch of nutmeg

Soften dates by placing dates in jar which is set in bowl of warm water. Mash with fork. Gradually add prune juice until mixture is of right consistency to make a medium thick filling. Add pecan meal and mix until smooth. Fold in blueberries. Fill raw pie crust and put in freezer for two hours. Serve chilled.

BANANA CREAM PIE

- 2 bananas, peel
- ½ cup fresh raw apple juice
- 1 Tbsp raw honey
- 1 raw pie crust (recipe page 203)
- ½ cup shredded coconut
- 4 bananas, peel, slice
- 2 dates, pitted

Blend the two peeled bananas and other ingredients (except coconut) in blender, then put into a raw pie crust (pg. 203). Now gently place the thinly sliced bananas and shredded coconut over pie top. Chill to set before serving. Serves 4-6.

APPLE PIE

- 4 cups apples, grate
- pinch of cinnamon
- ½ cup raw cashew butter
- ¼ cup raw honey
- pinch of nutmeg
- 1 raw pie crust (page 203)

Mix all ingredients. Put in raw pie crust. Top with thinly sliced apples and grated coconut if desired. Serves 4-6.

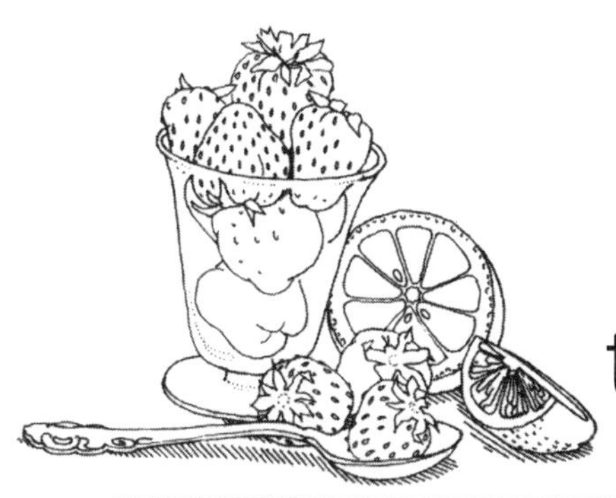

Chapter 4

Drink Health the Juice Way

Enjoy Raw Live Juices for Health Power

All over the United States, we have "cocktail hours," where fancy alcoholic creations are used to produce new thrills, stimulate jaded appetites and bolster failing spirits.

We have a new kind of "cocktail," thanks to my father, Paul C. Bragg. It is not made of whisky, gin, rum or other alcoholic substances. There are no toxic maraschino cherries to be found in any of them. These live, recharging juices are made from fresh, organically-grown vegetables and ripe fruits – the very life-blood of the plant – to boost your energy and immune levels! Dad imported the first hand-juicers from Europe and at the Bragg Crusades introduced juice therapy across America. There is no liquid on Earth so satisfying as the fresh live juice drink. Not only is it delicious, but there is something far greater: the satisfaction and nourishment for the billions of cells that make up your body. When people take to the health cocktail habit, they are putting the plants' liquid life into their bodies, to supercharge their health!

Consider that fruits and vegetables have been grown naturally by solar energy (sunshine). They contain all of the elements that the sun and earth have buried deep into their fibrous cells; they are live-cell foods. Juicing is a convenient, inexpensive way to obtain the most concentrated form of nutrition available from live whole plant and fruit foods.

Select & Prepare Organic Foods for Juicing

Demand and buy organically-grown fruits and vegetables whenever possible, because commercial produce can contain deadly pesticides and petrochemical fertilizers. Yearly, over 2.6 billion pounds of pesticides are dumped on American food crops. Because sprays of pesticides and herbicides are used on so many commercially-grown fruits and vegetables, be sure to wash and scrub thoroughly with biodegradable soap.

Choose deep-colored, ripe, firm fruits and fresh, healthy vegetables. Use both the leaves and stems, as well as the body of the vegetable. They yield an abundance of organic minerals, even the tops of carrots contain phosphorus.

Fruit & Vegetable Health Power Drinks

Organic, raw, live fruit and vegetable juices can be purchased fresh from many health food stores or prepared at home with the wonderful juicers and blenders on the market. These health juices can be used full-strength or diluted with distilled water, consumed individually or blended as below. Try adding a dash of Bragg Liquid Aminos or Bragg Sprinkle (24 herbs & spices) to vegetable and tomato combinations for a delicious health drink.

When using fresh herbs in these drinks, use 1-2 leaves or a shake of Bragg Sprinkle (salt-free with 24 herbs & spices) and Bragg Sea Kelp. Both are delicious with vegetable juices.

Healthy, Powerful Juice and Blended Combinations:

- Beet, celery and alfalfa sprouts
- Cabbage, celery and apple
- Cabbage, cucumber, celery, tomato, spinach and basil
- Tomato, carrot and all greens
- Carrot, celery, watercress, garlic and wheatgrass
- Grapefruit, orange and lemon
- Beet, parsley, celery, carrot, mustard greens, and garlic
- Beet, celery, kelp and carrot
- Cucumber, carrot and parsley
- Watercress, cucumber, garlic, celery, carrot, kale and chard
- Asparagus, carrot and apple
- Carrot, celery, parsley, cabbage, onion and sweet basil
- Carrot, broccoli, lemon and cayenne
- Carrot, broccoli, celery, kale and rosemary
- Carrot, coconut and coconut milk
- Apple, carrot, celery and ginger
- Apple, pineapple and kiwi
- Apple, papaya and grapes
- Papaya, cranberries and apple
- Leafy greens, broccoli and apple
- Grape, blueberries and apple
- Watermelon (best alone)

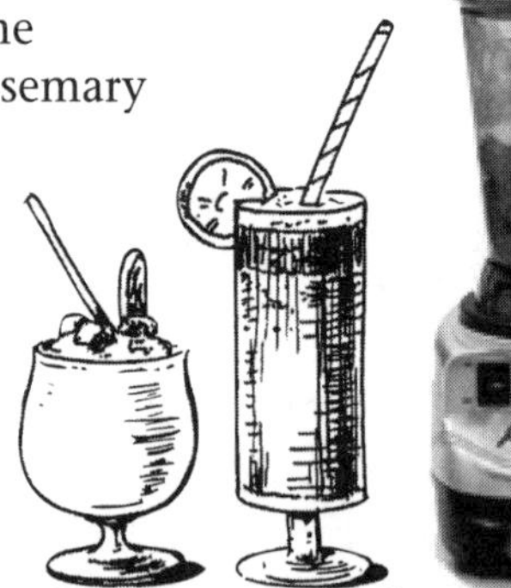

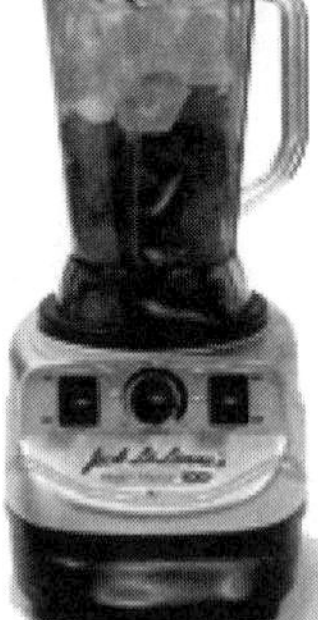

Ideal for Jack LaLanne HealthMaster 100. (see page 51)

Paul C. Bragg Introduced Juicing to America

Juicing has come a long way since my father imported the first hand operated vegetable-fruit juicer from Germany. Before, this juice was pressed by hand using cheesecloth. He introduced his new juice therapy idea, then pineapple juice, then later tomato juice, to the American public. These two juices were erroneously thought to be too acid. Now, these health beverages have become the favorites of millions. TV's famous *Juicemen* Jack LaLanne and Jay Kordich say Bragg was their early inspiration and health mentor! They both are ageless and are health inspirations to millions.

HEALTHY HERBAL TEAS

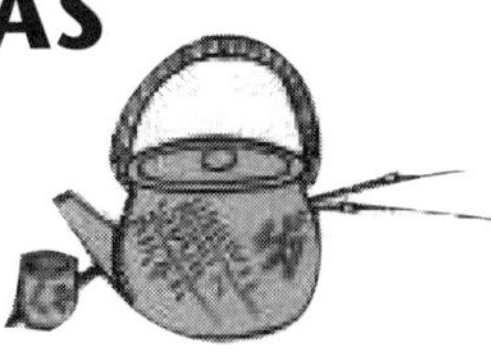

There is a wide variety of healthy, delicious herbal teas available in bulk and tea bags at health food stores. Brew as you would other teas, in glass or stainless steel.

HEALTHY FRUIT JUICE & POWER DRINKS

CAROB DELIGHT

1 cup rice milk
1½ tsps powdered carob
½ tsp soy milk powder
1 tsp raw honey
1 banana, mash
3 tsps shredded coconut

Put ingredients in blender or mix with hand beater. In a few minutes, you'll have a delicious drink, a meal in itself. Serves 1.

GRAPEFRUIT FOAM

Beat Egg Replacer equivalent to one egg. Add 2 teaspoons honey and 3 cups fresh grapefruit juice. Stir thoroughly and pour into glasses. Sprinkle with a dash of cinnamon or nutmeg. Serves 4.

MINT - LIME TINGLE

RF

18 fresh mint sprigs, chop
¾ cup distilled water
3 cups unsweetened fresh grape juice
¾ cup fresh lime juice
⅓ cup raw honey

Combine water and honey. Simmer 8 minutes. Pour over the chopped mint leaves. Cool; stir into combined fruit juices. Pour over shaved ice in glasses. Serve right away. Serves 4.

APRICOT AMBROSIA PUNCH

3 cups fresh apple juice
3 cups fresh orange juice
⅓ lb. fresh or unsulfured dried apricots
⅓ cup raw honey
⅔ cup fresh lemon juice

If dried apricots soak overnight until tender; then blend apricots and juice, add honey and fruit juices and blend well. Chill. Just before serving, pour over ice in punch bowl. Garnish with orange and lemon slices. Makes 12-14 punch-cup servings.

APPLE LEMONADE

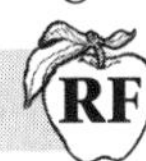

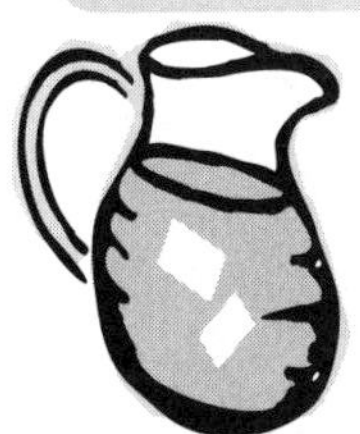

6 cups fresh apple juice
1⅛ cups fresh lemon juice
⅓ cup raw honey
fresh mint sprigs

Combine apple and lemon juice. Add honey and stir until the honey dissolves. Fill 5-6 glasses about ⅔ full with the apple lemonade. Add enough ice to fill the glasses. Place a sprig of fresh mint leaves in each glass. Serves 7.

PINEAPPLE MINT JULEP

8 fresh mint sprigs
½ cup fresh lemon juice
½ cup raw honey (or Stevia herb powder to taste)
3 cups unsweetened pineapple juice

Wash mint leaves, set aside 4 leaves for garnish. Bruise others with spoon to release flavor; cover with honey. Add lemon juice and let stand about 15 minutes. Add pineapple juice and blend. Pour over ice in pitcher or tall glasses. Garnish with remaining sprigs of mint. Makes 4 glasses.

FRUIT PUNCH

2 cups distilled water
1 cup fresh orange juice
¼ cup fresh lime juice
1 cup fresh pineapple juice
2 cups unsweetened fresh grape juice
1 cup fresh lemon juice
¼ cup raw honey (or Stevia to taste)
2 ripe bananas

Blend all ingredients thoroughly and chill. Serves 4-6.

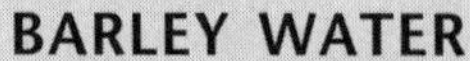

BARLEY WATER

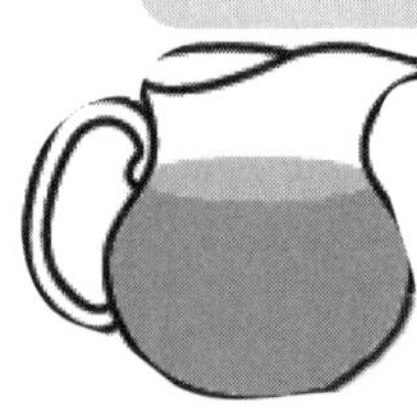

Wash ¼ cup natural barley and soak overnight. Drain. Add one quart distilled water and simmer until the barley is thoroughly done and about 1½ cups of liquid remains. Strain and serve plain, or add soy milk and season to taste with honey (or Stevia powder), pure vanilla, etc.

SPICED MINT TEA

2 cinnamon sticks
4 whole cloves
3 cups distilled water
¼ cup raw honey
½ cup lemon juice
4 whole allspice
3 bags mint tea or
3 Tbsps mint tea leaves
1 cup orange juice
½ cup grape juice

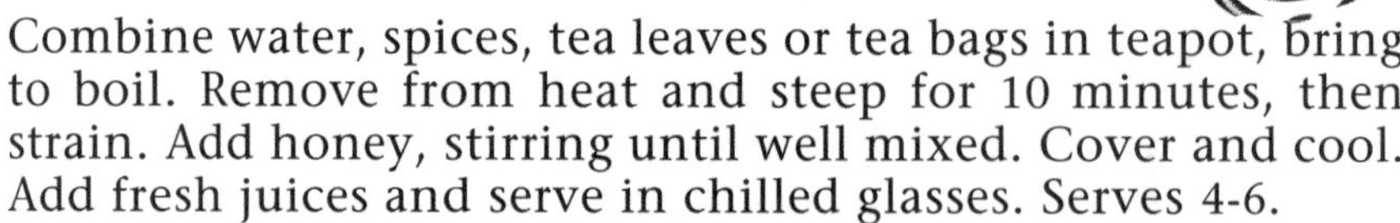

Combine water, spices, tea leaves or tea bags in teapot, bring to boil. Remove from heat and steep for 10 minutes, then strain. Add honey, stirring until well mixed. Cover and cool. Add fresh juices and serve in chilled glasses. Serves 4-6.

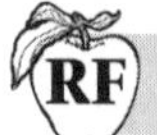

PROTEIN, PINEAPPLE, ALMOND MILK

1 cup raw almonds
2 bananas
1 Tbsp soy protein powder
2-4 cups fresh pineapple juice
Variation: Cashew or almond milk

Blend almonds and soy protein powder with small amount of pineapple juice and then add more pineapple juice to desired thickness. Follow same procedure for cashew or almond milk if desired. (see recipes page 41). Serves 4.

Studies on osteoporosis consistently conclude that vegetarians have stronger bones than meat-eaters. It is healthier and wise to avoid all meat and dairy products for optimum health!

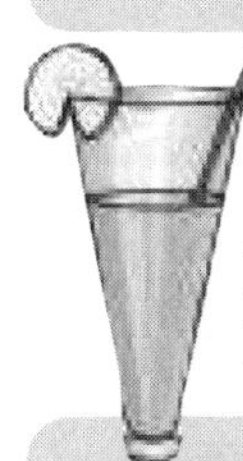

GRAPE COOLER

3 cups fresh orange juice
2 cups fresh grape juice
3 cups hot distilled water
1 cup fresh lemon juice
1 cup raw honey or herb Stevia powder to taste

Make syrup of honey and hot water; let cool. Add fruit juices. Pour over ice in pitcher or tall glasses. Serves 8-10.

BRAGG HEALTHY "ENERGY" SMOOTHIE

Prepare following in a blender. Add frozen juice cubes if desired colder. Mix 1½ to 2 cups of your choice of: fresh squeezed orange juice or grapefruit juice; carrot and greens juice; unsweetened pineapple, apple, cherry, cranberry, grape or other tropical fruit juices (papaya, passionfruit, kiwi); or just pure distilled water with:

2 tsps spirulina or green powder
1 Tbsp flax oil (or ground flax seeds)
½ tsp rice bran or oat bran
½ tsp lecithin granules
1-2 tsps Goji berries (dried)
2 Tbsps blueberries
½ tsp Vit C or Emergen-C powder
1 to 2 ripe bananas
1 tsp soy protein powder
1 tsp sunflower or chia seeds
1 tsp raw honey (optional)
2 dates or plum prunes, pitted
½ tsp Bragg Nutritional Yeast
⅓ cup soy yogurt or Silken tofu

Optional: four apricots (sundried, unsulphured) soaked in distilled water or unsweetened pineapple juice overnight. We soak enough to last for several days. Keep refrigerated. In summer you can add organic fresh fruit; peaches, papayas, blueberries, strawberries, all berries, and apricots instead of the bananas. In winter, add apples, kiwis, oranges, tangelos, persimmons or pears. If unavailable, try sugar free, frozen organic fruits. Serves 1-2.

BRAGG FAMOUS APPLE CIDER VINEGAR DRINK

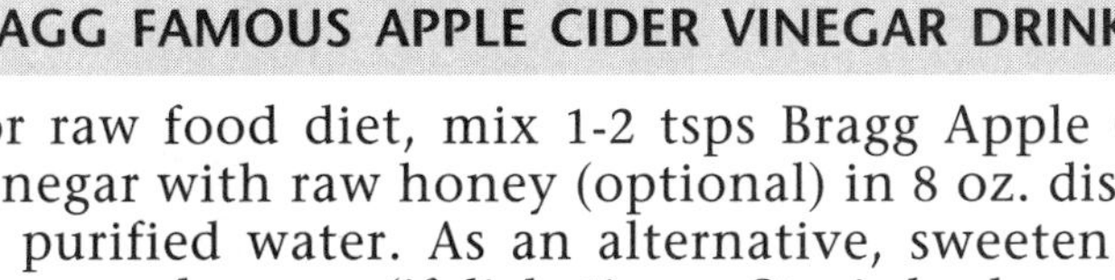

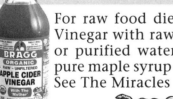

For raw food diet, mix 1-2 tsps Bragg Apple Cider Vinegar with raw honey (optional) in 8 oz. distilled or purified water. As an alternative, sweeten with pure maple syrup (if diabetic use Stevia herb powder). See The Miracles of Apple Cider Vinegar (page 202).

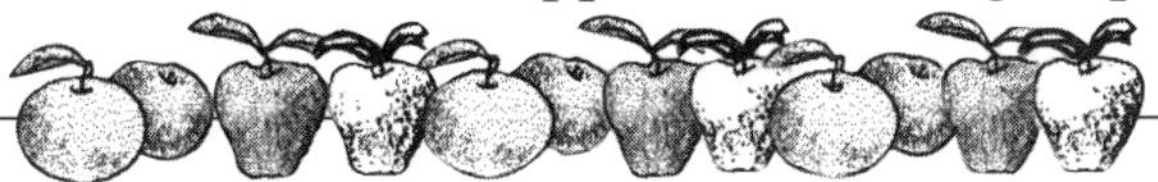

Potassium deficiency is a proven contributing cause of many illnesses, including: *Arthritis, kidney stones, atrial fibrillation, adrenal insufficiency, celiac disease, high blood pressure, coronary artery disease, ulcerative colitis, hypothyroidism, irritable bowel syndrome, Alzheimer's disease, multiple sclerosis, myasthenia gravis, Crohn's disease, lupus, atherosclerosis, diabetes and stroke.* – Linda Page, N.D., Ph.D., author *Healthy Healing* (visit her website: www.healthyhealing.com)

AMBROSIA SMOOTHIE

6 oz unsweetened pineapple juice (fresh squeezed when possible) or 1 cup fresh pineapple, chop
1 tsp Bragg Nutritional Yeast
2 bananas, ripe
1 Tbsp raw honey
1 tsp raw wheat germ
1 Tbsp soy powder

Blend all of the ingredients in blender and you have an excellent protein drink. You may blend in an ice cube to cool and pour into freezer-frosted glasses. Serves 1-2.

HI-PROTEIN SMOOTHIE

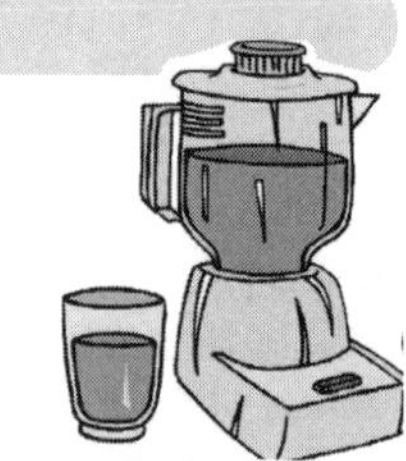

1 Tbsp soy powder
1 Tbsp flaxseed meal
1 Tbsp rice bran
⅓ pint plain soy yogurt
2 cups pineapple juice or fresh pineapple
1 Tbsp Bragg Yeast
2 Tbsps raw honey
1-2 ripe bananas
½ cup tofu
1 Tbsp tahini

Blend ingredients in blender until smooth. Serves 3-4.

PINEAPPLE - SESAME PROTEIN SMOOTHIE

3 cups unsweetened pineapple juice
½ cup sesame seeds or sesame butter
2 Tbsps soy powder
raw honey to taste

Place in blender: ¼ cup sesame seeds and 1 cup pineapple juice. Blend other ¼ cup of sesame seeds with second cup of pineapple juice. (*Optional:* use raw sesame butter or tahini.) Add more pineapple juice to mixture if needed. Add soy powder for more creamy texture. Add honey (or Stevia powder) to taste if desired. Serves 3-4.

GREEN POWER SMOOTHIES

Most Americans do not get enough raw greens in their diet. It's important to get ample raw greens, smoothies in your diet to achieve optimal nutrition and super health.

Green vegetables and fruits are packed with important nutrients and phytochemicals (see page 73). Dark green leafy vegetables are particularly nutrient rich. The National Cancer Institute (NCI) recommends making green vegetables an important part of your daily diet for the prevention of cancer. Green plant foods contain the important phytochemicals like chlorophyll, lutein and indoles. Chlorophyll (the blood of plants) is the green pigment which is responsible for the green color in green plants. Chlorophyll has anti-inflammatory, antioxidant, and wound-healing properties. It is referred to as "nature's purifier." Lutein is a powerful antioxidant found in green leafy vegetables that helps maintain good eye vision, protecting against cataracts and macular degeneration.

Indoles found in green plant foods help protect against breast cancer and prostate cancer. These are only a few of the thousands of health promoting phytochemicals (pg. 73) found in green plant foods and remember organic is best!

Many people find it difficult to eat enough green veggies in their daily diet. The easiest way to incorporate more raw greens into the diet is in the form of smoothies. Listed below are some great smoothies that will contribute green leafy vegetables and other green plant foods in your diet.

When making these Green Power Smoothies you will need to use a powerful blender. There are a few different powerful blenders on the market that we recommend. Our first recommendation is the Jack LaLanne HealthMaster 100 (*www.powerjuicer.com*). Also we recommend the VitaMix blender (*www.vitamix.com*), the K-Tec and Blendtec Home blenders (*www.blendtec.com*) for making these smoothies.

GREEN SPINACH - VEGGIE SMOOTHIE

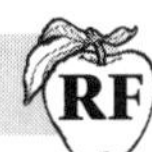

3 cups spinach
2 large tomatoes
½ cup fresh cilantro
1 lime, juice
½ green bell pepper
1 clove garlic, crush
2 cups distilled water
1 tsp raw honey or Stevia to taste

Blend all ingredients well. Makes about 1 quart.

GREEN KALE - VEGGIE SMOOTHIE

6 green kale leaves
¼ ripe avocado
1 lemon, juice
2 medium size tomatoes
1 tsp Bragg Liquid Aminos
2 green Romaine lettuce leaves
1 lime, juice
3 garlic cloves, crush
shake of Bragg Sprinkle
1½ cups distilled water

Blend all ingredients well. Makes about 1 quart.

GREEN ROMAINE AND WATERMELON SMOOTHIE

10 green Romaine lettuce leaves
7 cups cubed watermelon
¾ cup distilled water

Select the darkest green Romaine lettuce leaves and blend with the watermelon and distilled water. Makes about 1 quart.

GREEN PLANET SMOOTHIE

6 green kale leaves
1 green bell pepper
¼ cup fresh lime juice
shake of Bragg Sea Kelp
½ bunch parsley
1 ounce wheat grass juice
3 celery stalks, chop
1 tsp spirulina powder
4 apples, core, chop
1½ cup distilled water

Blend all ingredients well. Makes about 1 quart.

GREEN CITRUS DRINK

- 6 green Romaine lettuce leaves
- 3 celery stalks, chop
- 1-2 bananas (optional)
- ½ cup lime juice
- 4 kale leaves
- 1 cup green grapes
- 3 oranges, peeled
- 2 cups distilled water

Select darkest green leaves possible (Romaine, collards, kale, chard, etc.) and blend all ingredients. (You may add 1 to 2 ripe bananas if desired). Makes about 1 quart.

CRISP AND COOL GREEN DRINK

- 10 green Romaine lettuce leaves
- ½ medium honeydew melon, cubed
- 2 cups distilled water
- 2 cucumbers, peel, slice
- 2 celery stalks, chop
- 2-3 apples, core, chop

Select the darkest green Romaine lettuce leaves possible and blend all ingredients together. Makes about 1 quart.

VEGETARIAN SOURCES OF CALCIUM

FOOD	CALCIUM Content (mg)
Legumes (1cup, cooked)	
Black beans	103
Chick peas	78
Great Norther beans	121
Kidney beans	50
Lentils	37
Lima beans	52
Navy beans	128
Pinto beans	82
Vegetarian baked beans	128
Soyfoods	
Soybeans (1 cup, cooked)	175
Soymilk (1 cup)	250-300*
Soynuts	252
Tofu (1/2 cup)	120-350*
Tempeh (1/2 cup)	77
Fruits	
Dried figs (5)	258
Orange	56
Raisins (2/3 cup)	53

FOOD	CALCIUM Content (mg)
Vegetables (1/2 cup, cooked)	
Bok Choy	79
Broccoli	89
Collard greens	178
Kale	90
Mustard greens	75
Butternut squash	42
Sweet potato	35
Turnip greens	125
Nuts and Seeds (2 Tbsp)	
Almonds	50
Almond butter	86
Brazil nuts	50
Sesame seeds	176
Tahini	128
Grains	
Corn tortilla	53
Pita Bread (1 small pocket)	31
Other Foods	
Blackstrap molasses (1 Tbsp)	187

*Indicates a range of calcium found in different tofu products
Data from Bowes, *Church's Food Value of Portions Commonly Used.* 16th edition, by Pennington. Lippincott-Raven

Calcium is the major component of bones and is important for the smooth functioning of the muscles, including the heart, for blood clotting, and for nerve function. Calcium absorption is helped by adequate intake of vitamin D, zinc, and magnesium. Absorption of all the minerals, including calcium and zinc, is helped considerably by eating vitamin C-rich foods at the same time. – The Food Bible

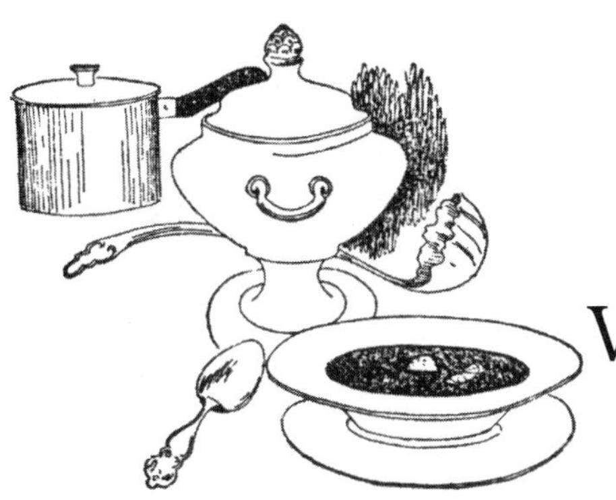

Chapter 5

Soups & Vitamin Broths

Some nutritionists look with respect on the tales of the "magic potions" of the Dark Ages: soups brewed with wild herbs and greens of the forest. Most agree now that the "magical broth" had practical and miracle curative properties, rather than supernatural charms.

Throughout history, Europe and Asia suffered from food shortages. Rather than roam the forest hunting for game and eating wild berries and herbs, Europeans crowded into small communities and concentrated efforts on wars and munitions instead of food. Death, rather than life, was paramount. Is it any wonder that the magician with his vitamin-rich herb pot, and the old crone with her love potions brewed from forest remedies, could seemingly work miracles? Of all the richness of nature's gifts to humanity, the living, growing foods that nurture our bodies are miracles in themselves!

The custom of having the soup pot on the back of the stove (into which all water left from cooking vegetables, as well as odds and ends of the vegetables themselves, were tossed) is a healthy practice in nutritional cookery. Far too many people destroy their foods. First, they take carrots, scrape all the vitamin-rich skin off; toss them in large quantities of boiling water; boil the life out of them; and throw all the water, into which the vitamins and minerals have escaped, down the drainpipe. Millions feed their sink nature's richest gifts and keep the dead, lifeless remainder to eat!

Save those beet tops, extra spinach leaves, green lettuce leaves that you think are too dark to serve on the table, tomato skins, skin from any vegetable you feel you absolutely must peel – all the little odds and ends and leftovers that you would normally throw away – toss them into the soup pot. I call it my "vitamin pot." Above all, save the precious liquids that remain in a pot after cooking. You will find no more delicious soup in the world than the rich soup made of pot liquids and mixtures of vegetables that you would ordinarily discard. That, above all, is your basic soup recipe. Here are some delicious, healthy soup recipes you and your family will enjoy!

BRAGG LIQUID AMINOS – CONSOMMÉ

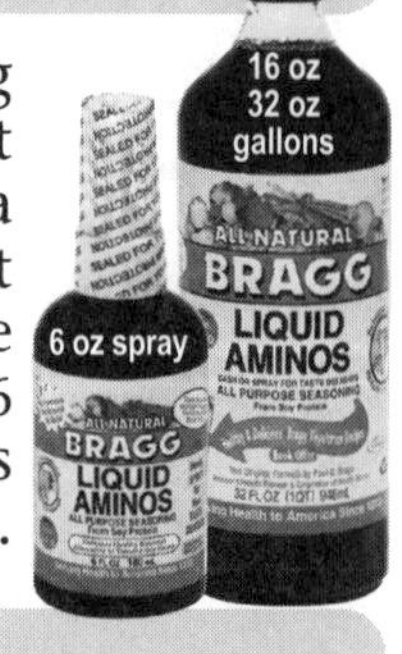

A delicious consommé can be made by adding Bragg Liquid Aminos (1-2 tsps per cup) to hot distilled water. Seasonings may be added for extra flavor. Bragg Liquid Aminos give an excellent flavor to broth and soups when used as base stock. It is the healthiest of broths. It contains 16 essential amino acids from soy. Sip this delicious consommé as is, or add it to flavor other soups.

ROYAL SOUP

3¾ cups potatoes, dice
1½ cups fresh or frozen peas
1½ cups asparagus stalks, chop
3 Tbsps Bragg Organic Olive Oil
1½ qts boiling distilled water
½ tsp Bragg Liquid Aminos
4½ Tbsps chives, chop
¼ tsp thyme
shake of Bragg Sprinkle (24 herbs & spices) and Bragg Sea Kelp

Cook potatoes in boiling water for 15 minutes until tender. Drain, reserving liquid; press potatoes through a strainer and add to saved potato liquid. Add peas and chopped asparagus. Simmer 10-15 minutes or until tender. Add chives, olive oil, Bragg Aminos, Bragg Sprinkle and Sea Kelp. Serves about 6.

SPRING BROTH OR SOUP

1 cup celery, finely chop
1 cup parsley, chop
1 cup zucchini, grate
1 tsp Bragg Liquid Aminos
1 cup raw spinach, chop
2 qts distilled water
1 cup carrots, grate
1 cup beets, grate
½ tsp Bragg Sprinkle (24 herbs & spices)

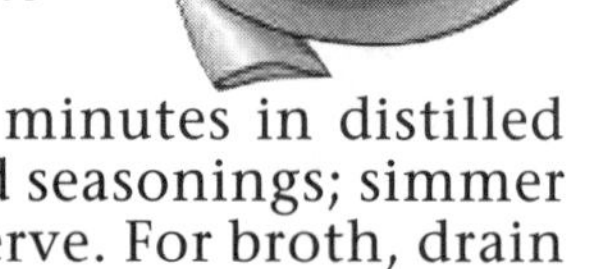

Simmer celery, beets and carrots for 15 minutes in distilled water. Add spinach, parsley, zucchini and seasonings; simmer ten more minutes. For soup, blend and serve. For broth, drain vegetables and add Bragg Aminos. Serves 6-8.

BROCCOLI SOUP

1 Tbsp Bragg Organic Olive Oil
1½ cups vegetable stock (page 10)
1 tsp Bragg Liquid Aminos
1 Tbsp Sesame Tahini
½ tsp sweet basil
1 Tbsp whole-grain flour
1 cup soy milk
2 cups broccoli florets
½ cup soft tofu
a dash of grated nutmeg

Heat olive oil. Stir in flour and sweet basil. Add stock and bring to a boil. Add broccoli florets (save stems for another vegetable dish) and simmer 5-8 minutes. Mix tahini and tofu in blender. Add cooked broccoli mixture, soy milk, Bragg Aminos and nutmeg. (*Optional*: Bragg Sprinkle, 24 herbs & spices, will add more herbal flavors.) Process at low speed, then medium until smooth. Serve hot. Serves 4.

BASIC CREAMED SOUP RECIPE

2 to 2½ Tbsps onion, mince
2 Tbsps whole-grain flour
1 Tbsp Bragg Liquid Aminos
pinch cayenne pepper (optional)
1 Tbsp watercress, garnish
2 Tbsps Bragg Olive Oil
1½ cups silken tofu
Bragg Sprinkle (to taste)
1 cup vegetable stock
pinch of paprika
2 cups raw or cooked veggies of choice, chop

Sauté onion in olive oil. Place in double boiler; blend with flour until smooth. Add liquids. Cook until slightly thickened and smooth. Add cooked or raw blended vegetables, herbs, tofu and Sprinkle. Garnish with paprika and watercress. Serves 4.

CREAMED SPINACH SOUP

Use the Basic Creamed Soup Recipe (above) and add to it 1 cup of chopped raw or cooked spinach and blend. Use ¼ teaspoon chervil or Bragg Sprinkle for herb flavoring.*

CREAMED CELERY SOUP

Use the Basic Creamed Soup Recipe (above), and add 1 cup finely chopped raw or cooked celery. *Optional:* add 1 teaspoon chopped mint for herb flavoring.*

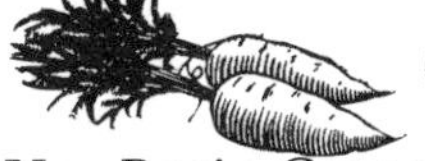

CREAMED CARROT SOUP

Use Basic Creamed Soup Recipe (above), and add 1 cup finely chopped raw or blended cooked carrots. Use 1 tablespoon freshly chopped parsley and Bragg Sprinkle for herb flavoring.*

CREAMED BROCCOLI SOUP

To Basic Creamed Soup Recipe, add 1⅓ cups chopped raw or blended cooked broccoli. Garnish with soy Parmesan cheese.*

CREAMED CORN SOUP

To Basic Creamed Soup Recipe, add 1¼ cups fresh raw or canned corn kernels. Blend. Garnish with chopped parsley.*

CREAMED PEA SOUP

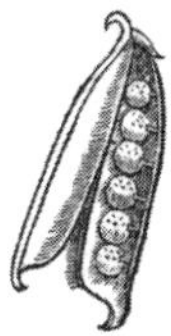

To Basic Creamed Soup Recipe, add 1 cup fresh raw or canned cooked or blended peas. Use ¼ teaspoon dried sweet basil, shake of Bragg Sprinkle and 1 tablespoon finely chopped fresh mint for herb flavoring.*

******All creamed soup recipes can be sprinkled with pine nuts or sunflower seeds for added health and protein benefits.*

CREAM OF TOMATO SOUP

2 cups soy milk
4 Tbsps Bragg Organic Olive Oil
2 Tbsps potato or whole-grain flour
2 cups fresh or can tomatoes
shake of Bragg Sprinkle & Kelp
2 tsps red onion, mince
pinch of celery seed
2 cloves garlic, crush
¼ tsp basil
shake Bragg Yeast Flakes

Pureé or blend tomatoes. Cook 10 minutes with onions, herbs and seasonings. Thicken to paste by adding blended flour and olive oil, then re-cook. Heat soy milk to scalding. Be sure tomato mixture is same temperature as soy milk before adding, and then add to soy milk very slowly. Serve at once. Serves 4.

CAUTION: If heated soy milk and heated tomato mixture are not the same temperature or are not combined slowly enough, the soy milk could curdle.

CREAMED WATERCRESS SOUP

To Basic Creamed Soup Recipe (page 55), add small bunch finely chopped watercress. Substitute vegetable juice for stock. Cook watercress 5 minutes before adding.

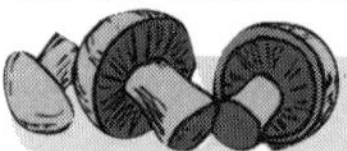

CREAM OF MUSHROOM SOUP

½ lb fresh mushrooms, of your choice, slice
2 Tbsps celery, mince
shake of Bragg Sprinkle
shake of Bragg Kelp
4 Tbsps Bragg Organic Olive Oil
2 Tbsps onion, mince
3 cups vegetable stock (page 10)
1 cup soy milk
2 Tbsps whole-grain flour

Wash and slice the mushrooms. Sauté onion, celery and mushrooms in 1 tablespoon olive oil until tender. Blend and add vegetable stock. In a separate pot, blend flour and remaining oil. Add soy milk and seasonings, stirring until thick and smooth. Add to mushroom purée and vegetable stock mixture. Simmer 3-5 minutes and serve. Serves 4.

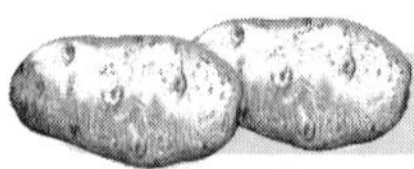

CREAM OF POTATO SOUP

1 Tbsp Bragg Organic Olive Oil
1 carrot, chop (optional)
3 medium-sized potatoes, chop
3 celery stalks, chop
1 red onion, chop
2 cups soy milk
½ tsp Bragg Sprinkle
Bragg Liquid Aminos, to taste

Chop vegetables, cook until tender. Add Bragg Olive Oil, Bragg Aminos, Sprinkle and soy milk. Blend and serve. Serves 2.

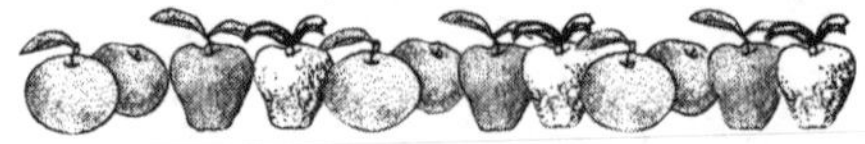

Amino acids are needed for building every part of the body, including bones, blood, hair, skin, nails and glands, and are Mother Nature's and God's secret to a long, healthy, vital life. – Paul C. Bragg, ND, PhD., Originator of Health Stores

---

Amino acid are the very soup of life. – H.J. Hoegerman, M.D., (Bragg Aminos Fan)

VEGGIE SOUP

1½ cups potatoes, chop
½ cup leeks, chop
shake of Bragg Sprinkle
2 cloves garlic, mash
½ cup organic brown rice
1 cup condensed tomato soup
2 Tbsps Bragg Olive Oil
1 cup onion, chop
1 cup celery, chop
1 cup carrots, chop
1 cup peas or green beans
1⅓ qt cold distilled water
½ cup whole-grain macaroni
1 Tbsp Bragg Liquid Aminos

Put all vegetables, macaroni (or pasta of your choice), rice and seasonings in large heavy soup pot with tight fitting lid. Cover. Cook until vegetables are tender. Serves 4-6.

CORN CHOWDER

1 small red onion, slice
1 Tbsp raw honey
3 cups potatoes, dice
1 cup soy milk
1 Tbsp Bragg Organic Olive Oil
1½ cups corn kernels
1 cup fresh or can tomatoes
1 tsp Bragg Liquid Aminos
shake of Bragg Sprinkle (24 herbs & spices) and Bragg Yeast Flakes

Add the onion to the olive oil and slowly sauté for five minutes without browning. Add vegetables to 1 qt. boiling distilled water; cook until tender. Slowly add soy milk, Bragg Aminos, Sprinkle and honey. Serve hot. Serves 4.

AVOCADO SOUPS - HOT OR COLD

Avocado soups are great favorites in the tropics. The avocado is used frequently and generously in all kinds of soups. It is generally diced into small cubes and added just before serving.

AVOCADO - TOMATO SOUP

Dilute tomato juice with small amount of Bragg Organic Olive Oil. Add desired amount of diced avocado just before serving.

BLACK OLIVE SOUP

4½ cups soy milk
2¼ Tbsps whole-grain flour
shake of Bragg Sprinkle
1½ cups black olives, pitted
1½ Tbsps onion, grate
3 Tbsps Bragg Organic Olive Oil
½ cup cooked celery, dice
1 tsp Bragg Liquid Aminos

Sauté onion in 1 tablespoon olive oil. Combine soy milk and onion. Blend in blender. Mix flour in 2 tablespoons olive oil, Bragg Aminos and Sprinkle. Mix with celery and olives. Cook for 10 minutes on low heat. Serves 6.

Eating a diet rich in plant foods, in the form of fruits, vegetables, and whole-grain cereals, probably remains the best option for reducing the risk of colon cancer, and for more greater health protection. – The Lancet, May 3, 2003

To feel safe and warm on a cold night, all you really need is soup. – Laurie Colwin

TURNIP - CARROT SOUP

6 white turnips, slice
4 carrots, slice
2 cups distilled water
2 Tbsps Bragg Organic Olive Oil
½ cup organic brown rice
4 cups vegetable stock (page 10)
Bragg Sprinkle (24 herbs & spices), to taste

Put sliced turnips, carrots, brown rice, seasonings, stock and water in heavy soup pot with olive oil. Cover, cook for 30 minutes. Garnish with Bragg Nutritional Yeast Flakes. Serves 4.

CINCINNATI'S FAMOUS SPLIT PEA SOUP

2 cups dried peas, (soak overnight)
2 cups celery, chop
3 Tbsps Bragg Olive Oil
shake of Bragg Sprinkle
2 qts distilled water
1 cup red onions, chop
1 cup parsley, chop
2 leeks, slice thin (optional)
1 tsp Bragg Liquid Aminos

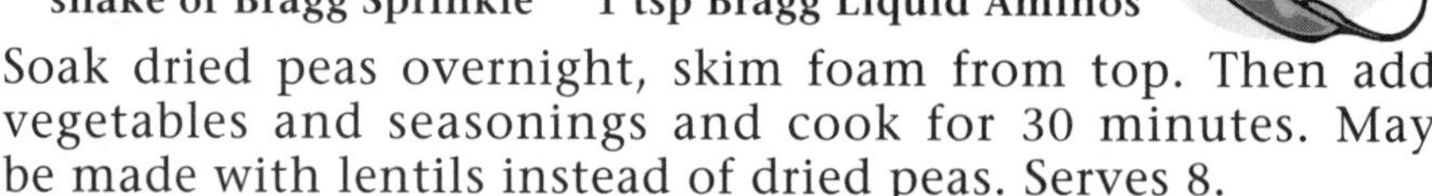

Soak dried peas overnight, skim foam from top. Then add vegetables and seasonings and cook for 30 minutes. May be made with lentils instead of dried peas. Serves 8.

SOYBEAN SOUP

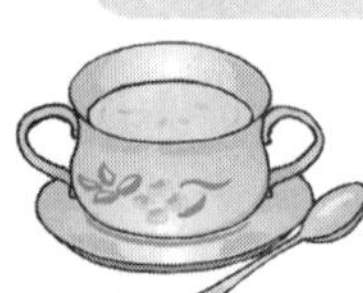

1 cup soybeans, soak
4 cups distilled cold water
1 Tbsp Bragg Olive Oil
1 Tbsp whole-grain flour
1 tsp Bragg Liquid Aminos
¼ cup celery, dice
½ small onion, slice
pinch mustard powder
shake of Bragg Sprinkle

Soak soybeans overnight. Drain and rinse. Add water and cook for 2 hours or until tender. Purée in blender. Sauté sliced onions and celery in olive oil. Add whole-grain flour, Bragg Aminos, seasonings, Sprinkle, and soybean purée. Reheat and serve. Serves 4.

BLACK SOYBEAN SOUP

1 pt black soybeans, soak overnight
6-8 cups cold distilled water
1 tsp lemon rind, finely chop
1 Tbsp Bragg Liquid Aminos
2½ Tbsps Bragg Olive Oil
⅛ tsp peppercorns, freshly ground
1 medium onion, mince
3 celery stalks, chop
2 Tbsps potato flour
¼ cup parsley, chop
⅛ cup fresh lemon juice
¼ tsp mustard powder

Sauté onion in olive oil until golden brown; add water, beans, lemon juice, lemon rind, celery and parsley, then cook until beans are tender (about 4 hours). Add more water if necessary. Blend. Add potato flour, Bragg Aminos and seasonings. Mix well. Simmer for 15 minutes before serving. Serves 4.

Just before serving soups, veggies, and potatoes, sprinkle on top some Bragg Nutritional Yeast Flakes. They are so delicious and great for you!

Only I can change my life. No one can do it for me. – Carol Burnett, Actress

CHESTNUT SOUP

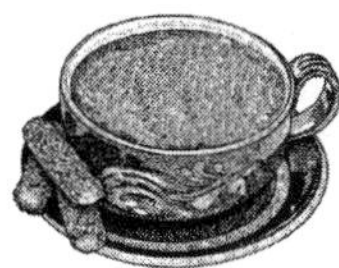

3 cups chestnuts, blanch
1 small red onion, mince
3 cups soy milk
½ tsp Bragg Liquid Aminos
chopped parsley (garnish)
4½ cups distilled water
shake of Bragg Sea Kelp
⅓ tsp Bragg Sprinkle
3 Tbsps whole-grain flour
pinch of celery seed
3 Tbsps Bragg Organic Olive Oil

To shell and blanch chestnuts: first wash and discard those that float. Let dry. Now with a sharp knife, make a cross on both sides of the shell. Place in a baking dish with 1 teaspoon olive oil and bake in hot oven (450°F) for ten minutes. Cool, and remove shell and the brown skin with a knife. Cook chestnuts in water until tender, then press through a sieve and add soy milk. Sauté onion in olive oil until tender, but not brown. Blend in whole-grain flour, seasonings. Now add the soy milk and chestnut mixture gradually, stirring constantly. Cook gently for 5 minutes. Garnish with parsley and sprinkle with Bragg Nutritional Yeast Flakes. Serves 6-8.

SWEET POTATO SOUP

3 steamed sweet potatoes
4 cups soy milk or silken tofu
1 tsp Bragg Organic Olive Oil
Bragg Sprinkle to taste

Blend cooked sweet potatoes (with skin), add soy milk or silken tofu. Add Bragg Olive Oil and Sprinkle. Reheat to warm. (This recipe is good for all types of potatoes.) Serves 4.

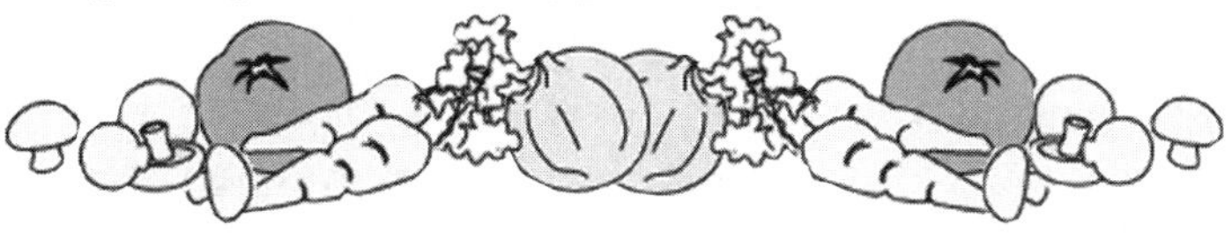

At least 50% of all U.S. children are allergic to milk, many undiagnosed. Dairy products are the leading cause of food allergy, often revealed by constipation, diarrhea, and fatigue. Many cases of asthma and sinus infections are reported to be relieved and even eliminated by cutting out dairy!
– Frank Oski, M.D., Chief of Pediatrics at John Hopkins Medical School

---

Vegetarian diets offer disease protection benefits because of their lower saturated fat, no cholesterol, no animal protein content and often higher concentrations of folate (which reduces serum homocysteine levels), antioxidants such as vitamin C and E, carotenoids, and phytochemicals.
– Journal of the American Dietetic Association, 1995

Researchers have discovered that the more healthy habits an individual practices, the longer they live and the healthier they are!
– Elizabeth Vierck, *Health Smart*

If you step back, look at the data, the optimum amount of red meat you eat should be zero. – Dr. William Castelli, famous Medical Director
see web: FraminghamHeartStudy.org

WARM OR CHILLED RED CURRANT SOUP

½ cup barley
½ cup raw honey
1⅓ qts red currants
½ tsp cinnamon powder
⅔ cup distilled water
¼ tsp Bragg Liquid Aminos

Soak barley overnight in distilled water. Wash and stem currants and add honey, water and cinnamon powder. Cook currants over low heat for 15 minutes. Drain and put through a coarse sieve. Add soaked barley with ½ cup water and Bragg Aminos; simmer until barley is soft and liquid thickened. Blend currants and barley. Serve soup warm or chilled. Serves 4-6.

GOLDEN SOUP

1 sweet onion, chop
2 large ripe tomatoes, chop
1½ qts vegetable stock (page 10)
3 Tbsps Bragg Organic Olive Oil
1 tsp Bragg Liquid Aminos
½ tsp Bragg Sprinkle
½ cup soy Parmesan cheese
2 cloves garlic, slice

Cook the onion and garlic in olive oil until golden. Add the tomatoes to vegetable stock and cook for 15 minutes. Add Sprinkle and Bragg Aminos. Simmer very slowly for 10 minutes. Pass soup through a sieve, return to soup pot and reheat. Put heaping tablespoon grated Parmesan cheese in soup bowls, ladle soup over it and serve. Serves 4-6.

ZUCCHINI SOUP

1 pound zucchini (5 medium), wash and slice
⅛ tsp basil
½ Tbsp Bragg Liquid Aminos
2 cloves garlic, mash
½ cup soy milk
1 cup distilled water
1 bay leaf
½ cup parsley, chop
½ tsp Bragg Sprinkle
½ cup soy yogurt
½ cup soy Parmesan cheese

Place the zucchini, herbs, Sprinkle, garlic, and water in a covered saucepan and simmer gently until tender. Add Bragg Aminos. Stir in soy milk and heat, do not boil. Serve topped with soy yogurt or grated soy parmesan cheese. Serves 4.

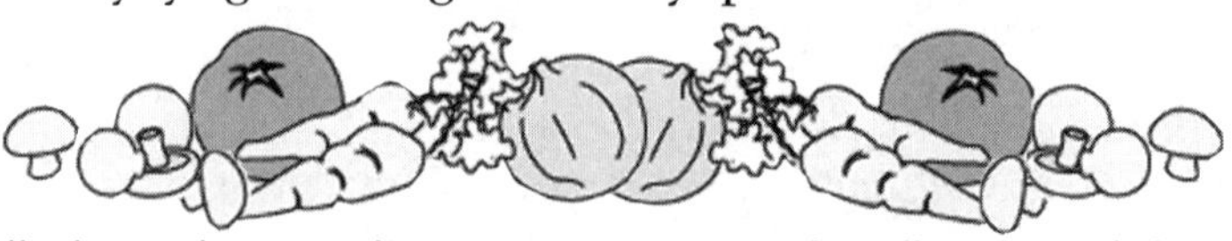

Well-planned vegan diets are appropriate for all stages of the life cycle. Including during pregnancy and lactation. Appropriately planned vegan and the lacto-ovo-vegetarian diets satisfy nutrient needs of infants, children, and adolescents and promote healthy, normal growth.
– Journal of the American Dietetic Association, November 1997

Vegetarians are healthier and have lower rates of heart disease and high blood pressure, colon cancer, osteoporosis, lung cancer, breast cancer, kidney stones, gallstones and diabetes. – American Dietetic Association

SUNFLOWER SEED SOUP

¾ cup carrots, grate
1 large red onion, finely chop
2 Tbsps Bragg Organic Olive Oil
3 medium sized tomatoes
1 tsp raw honey
1½ cups distilled water
1 Tbsp Bragg Liquid Aminos
½ cup sunflower seed meal*
shake of Bragg Sprinkle (24 herbs & spices)

Skin tomatoes, if desired (see page 105) and blend in food processor until smooth. Slowly heat olive oil in saucepan, sauté carrots and onions over low heat, 3 minutes. Add water, cover and cook until vegetables are tender. To tomato mixture add cooked vegetables including water and blend in food processor until smooth. Pour mixture back into saucepan, add Bragg Aminos, Sprinkle, honey and sunflower seed meal. Reheat to below simmer point, stirring constantly. For more nutrition, garnish with soy yogurt, finely chopped green onions with stems, or avocado slices. Serves 4.

SOYBEAN AND VEGETABLE STEW

4 potatoes, thinly slice
2 large red onions, slice
2 celery stalks, dice
1 green pepper, slice
4 Tbsps Bragg Olive Oil
2½ cups cooked soybeans
4 large tomatoes, slice
Spray of Bragg Liquid Aminos
½ tsp Bragg Sprinkle
3 cups of distilled water
dash of cayenne pepper
shake of Bragg Kelp

In a heavy skillet sauté olive oil, potatoes (with skins), onions, celery and green pepper 5 minutes. Spray of Bragg Aminos, add Sprinkle, Kelp and cayenne over vegetables. To 3 cups water add vegetable mixture, soybeans and tomatoes. Cover, cook slowly for 20 minutes or until tender. Serves 6.

VEGETABLE BARLEY SOUP

1 cup red onions, chop
1 cup celery, chop
1 cup fresh parsley, mince
1 cup mushrooms, slice
1 cup carrots, dice
½ cup unpearled barley
2 cloves garlic, mash
2 cups yellow squash, dice
2 cups cauliflower florets
2 tomatoes
1 Tbsp Bragg Liquid Aminos
2 qts distilled water
½ tsp Bragg Sprinkle
3 Tbsps Bragg Olive Oil

Soak barley for one hour. In large soup kettle sauté onions, celery and garlic in oil for 5 minutes. Add mushrooms and continue to sauté. Add water, barley and other ingredients. Cook for 45 minutes until done. Serve in soup bowls and garnish with sunflower and sesame seed meal*. This garnish tastes delicious and fortifies the soup with protein. Serves 6-8.

**Sunflower seed and nut meals can be purchased at health stores, or better to make your own in blender or grain or electric coffee grinder.*

BRAGG LENTIL SOUP

1½ cups lentils, wash
1 qt distilled water
1 Tbsp Bragg Liquid Aminos
1 cup parsley, chop
1 cup carrots, chop
1 cup bell peppers, chop
1 cup celery, chop
3 tomatoes
2 cloves garlic, mash
1 cup onions, chop
½ tsp Bragg Sprinkle (24 herbs & spices)

Combine ingredients; simmer covered for 30 minutes, until done. You may add other vegetables, rice, etc. Serves 6-8.

BARLEY, TOMATO AND BEAN SOUP

½ cup barley
3¾ cups vegetable broth
1 red onion, chop
2 celery stalks, thinly slice including tops
2 carrots, dice
2 - 15 oz cans cannellini beans, drain and rinse
4 tomatoes, chop
½ tsp Bragg Sprinkle
pinch of black pepper
shake of Bragg Sea Kelp

Combine the barley, vegetable broth, onion, celery, carrot and seasonings in a large soup pot. Simmer until the barley is tender, about 25 minutes. Add the remaining ingredients and simmer an additional 20 minutes. Serves 6.

CREAMY TOMATO AND POTATO SOUP

2 red onions, chop
2 celery stalks, chop
6 russet potatoes, unpeeled, dice
2 - 15 oz cans crushed tomatoes
1 cup distilled water
1 Tbsp Bragg Organic Olive Oil
3 Tbsps whole-grain pastry flour
2½ cups soy milk
1 Tbsp raw honey
1 tsp Bragg Sprinkle
2 tsps Bragg Liquid Aminos
¼ tsp black pepper
pinch of cayenne powder
shake of Bragg Sea Kelp

Combine onions, celery, potato and tomatoes in a large pot. Add water, then bring to a simmer. Cover and cook 15 minutes. Heat olive oil in a saucepan, then whisk in flour to form a thick paste. Stir constantly over low heat for 3 minutes, then whisk in soy or rice milk. Cook over medium heat, stirring constantly for 5 minutes. Combine with tomato mixture. Add honey, Sprinkle, Kelp, Bragg Aminos, black pepper and cayenne to taste. Heat over a low flame until hot and steamy. Serves 6-8.

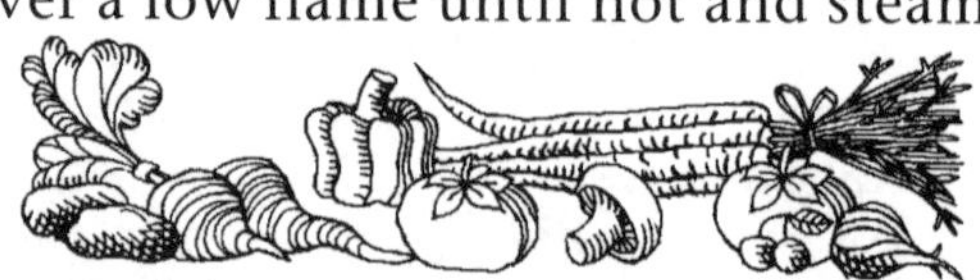

I live on good, hearty soup, not on fine words. – Moliere

Good soup is one of the prime ingredients of good living. For soup can do more to lift the spirits and stimulate the appetite than any other one dish. – Louis P. DeGouy, The Soup Book, 1949

An old-fashioned vegetable soup, is a more powerful anti-carcinogen than any known medicine. – James Duke, Ph.D., USDA Herbal Medicine Expert

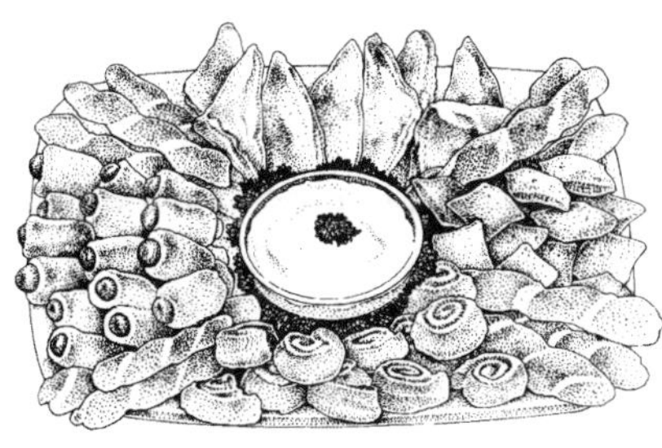

Chapter 6

Canapés ~ Healthy Appetizers

"Appetizers" are a misnomer. Contrary to popular belief, they dull the appetite rather than stimulate it. The very best health appetizer for a meal is a small plate of fresh sliced fruit, or fruit juice, vegetable juice, or a nutritious salad. For a gala occasion, the so-called appetizers, or canapés, are nice to serve with fruit punch or vegetable juice cocktails, and they can be prepared to be both healthy and appetizing.

Canapés should never be substantial. They should be small, spicy tidbits of distinctive flavor to pique the activity of the gastric juices. If they are to be served just prior to a meal, the soup course of the meal should be omitted. Always start your dinner meal with a healthy salad, then follow with soup if desired.

Delicious health canapés can be made without the usual smoked, pickled or processed meats or fish. Most of the canapé tidbits to follow may be served on small squares of dry, toasted whole-grain bread or crackers. We suggest replacing the cheeses and fatty, dairy based spreads in your favorite canapé recipes with health, non-dairy alternatives. Soup, immediately following the canapés, can cause an excessively rapid and essentially false sense of satisfaction, which dulls the appetite.

ASPARAGUS TIPS

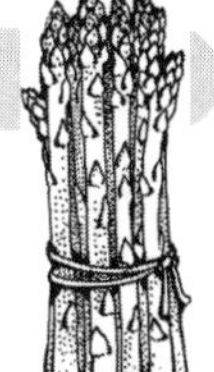

Lightly baste 3-inches of asparagus tips in Bragg Olive Oil, then roll in granulated soy Parmesan cheese and heat briefly under broiler. Insert toothpicks and serve.

SOY CHEESE CAPERS

Spread small toasted squares of whole grain bread with Cheese Sauce (page 161) or place slices of soy cheese atop squares. Dot with 2 or 3 capers. Place under broiler for a few moments.

ARTICHOKE HEARTS

Stuff artichoke hearts with a mixture of soy cheese and whole-grain bread crumbs. Sprinkle with Bragg Liquid Aminos and celery, poppy or mustard seed. Place under broiler for a few moments until brown. Cut in quarters, place on toothpick, and serve on a bed of lettuce or cabbage.

TOFU KNOBBY BALLS

Blend or mix well-drained firm tofu with green and red bell pepper, watercress, cilantro and shake of Bragg Sprinkle (24 herbs & spices). Mix mashed avocado or Tofunaise (page 139) to hold the balls together. Form into small balls. Roll in poppy or sesame seeds, insert toothpick in each one and serve on a bed of lettuce. Spray with Bragg Aminos.

SNAPPY CHEESE BALLS

Using soft spicy soy cheeses, cut and form into balls or cubes. Roll in celery or mustard seed. Place small leaf of watercress or mint on top of each ball or cube and insert a toothpick. Serve on a bed of lettuce or in a hollowed out cantaloupe shell.

STUFFED CELERY

2 Tbsps soy cheese
2 lbs firm tofu, well-drained
¼ tsp Bragg Liquid Aminos
celery stalks

Mash soy cheese, tofu and Bragg Aminos and blend thoroughly. Spread mixture on celery stalks. Sprinkle top of cheese with celery, caraway, sesame or anise seeds. (Do not combine seeds; use only one for flavoring.)

SPREAD VARIATIONS FOR CELERY AND VEGETABLES

1. Organic (non-hydrogenated) peanut or nut butter with minced apple.
2. Mash avocado, add pinch of minced chives and shake of Bragg Sprinkle (24 herbs & spices).
3. Any soy cheese blend with minced chives, parsley and a dash of Bragg Sprinkle (24 herbs & spices) to taste.
4. Blend tofu or soy cheese with mustard and minced onion.

AVOCADO PASTE

Blend avocado, minced chives and a spray of Bragg Aminos and shake of Bragg Sprinkle with lemon juice, mustard powder, sesame or caraway seeds.

Vegetarians consume more antioxidants than meat-eaters. Antioxidants reduce the risk for cancer, heart disease, cataracts and possibly arthritis. Dietary antioxidants include vitamins E and C, and carotenoids as well as many other phytochemicals (page 73). Most vegetarians consume over 100% more vitamin E and vitamin C and total antioxidants than meat-eaters.

Serving appetizers shows your guests that you care about their enjoyment with starting the main meal off with some light, healthy delicacies.

PEANUT BUTTER OR TAHINI SESAME BALLS

1 cup soy powder
½ cup raw honey
2 Tbsps boiling distilled water
1 cup uncooked rolled oats
¾ cup toasted sesame seeds
1 tsp pure vanilla extract
1 cup organic Tahini or non-hydrogenated, creamy peanut butter

Combine all ingredients except sesame seeds and form into balls. Roll balls with generous amounts of sesame seeds. These are delicious without baking or you can bake at 200°F for 10 minutes.

SPROUTS - BEANS APPETIZER

3 cups sprouted alfalfa seeds, mung beans and lentils
1 lb cooked kidney or garbanzo beans, drain
1 lb cooked fresh or canned yellow beans, drain
1 lb cooked fresh green beans
½ cup Bragg Apple Cider Vinegar
1 Tbsp Bragg Liquid Aminos
1 cup red onion, chop
⅓ cup raw honey
3 cloves garlic, crush
½ cup Bragg Organic Olive Oil
shake of Bragg Sprinkle

Put sprouts and beans in bowl. Mix and purée remaining ingredients in blender. Pour purée over beans and sprouts, toss well, cover and marinate for one hour before serving.

HI-PROTEIN CEREAL MIX SNACK

MIX LIGHTLY IN A BOWL:
3 qts raw oatmeal
1 cup natural cornmeal
½ cup raw wheat germ
½ cup soy flour
½ cup unsweetened coconut flakes
¾ cup sunflower meal or any other nut meal
1 cup nuts, chop such as peanuts, walnuts or pecans
½ cup seeds such as pumpkin, sesame or sunflower
¾ cup unsulphured raisins, or currants, chop

THEN MIX WITH DRY INGREDIENTS:
1½ cups distilled water
⅔ cup raw honey
1⅓ cups sesame seed oil

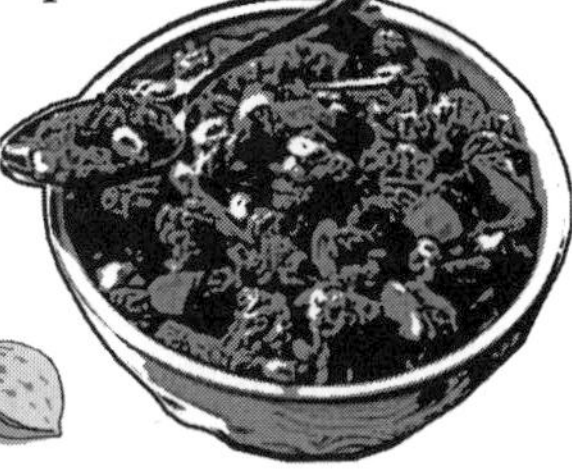

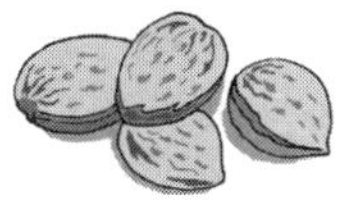

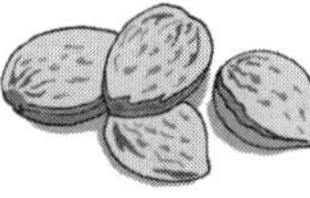

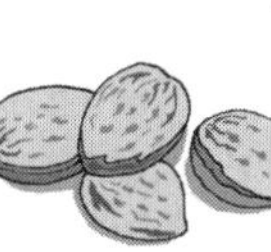

As a single footstep will not make a path on the earth, so a single thought will not make a pathway in the mind. To make a deep physical path, we walk again and again. To make a deep mental path, we must think over and over the kind of thoughts we wish to dominate our lives. – Henry David Thoreau

---

You simply will not be the same person two months from now after consciously giving thanks each day for the abundance that exists in your life. And you will have set in motion an ancient spiritual law: the more you have and are grateful for, the more will be given to you. – Sarah Ban Breathnach

---

Nothing can bring you peace but yourself and God. – Ralph Waldo Emerson

ROASTED MUSHROOM - ONION - WALNUT CAVIAR

1 lb mushrooms, of choice
3 medium garlic cloves, peel
1 Tbsp Bragg Apple Cider Vinegar
1 red onion, coarsely chop
¾ cup walnut pieces
2 Tbsps Bragg Olive Oil
shake of Bragg Sprinkle
1 tsp Bragg Liquid Aminos

Preheat oven to 450°F. Trim stems off mushrooms and cut caps into 1-inch pieces. Smaller mushrooms may be halved or left whole. In large baking pan combine mushrooms, onions, and garlic cloves. Drizzle with olive oil and toss to coat well. Distribute evenly in pan, then roast undisturbed for 10 minutes, stir well, redistributing evenly, and roast for 10 more minutes. Sprinkle walnuts over mushrooms and onions, add Sprinkle (24 herbs & spices) and roast for 5 minutes. Remove from oven and let cool for a few minutes. In food processor, combine all ingredients. Run motor until coarse paste is formed, scraping down sides as necessary. Serve on dry whole grain toast, pitas or crackers.

COUSCOUS PACKETS

½ cup distilled water
⅓ cup couscous
2 Tbsps raisins or currants
pinch curry powder
1 tsp Bragg Olive Oil
2 Tbsps toasted pine nuts
6 lettuce or large spinach leaves, wash and dry

In a small bowl, soften currants in warm distilled water. Stir in couscous, olive oil, and curry powder. Let sit for 10 minutes. Stir in pine nuts. Fill each spinach leaf with about 1 Tbsp of couscous and fold over sides to form a packet. Secure packets with toothpicks, if desired. Serves 4-6.

CHERRY TOMATO BRUSCHETTA

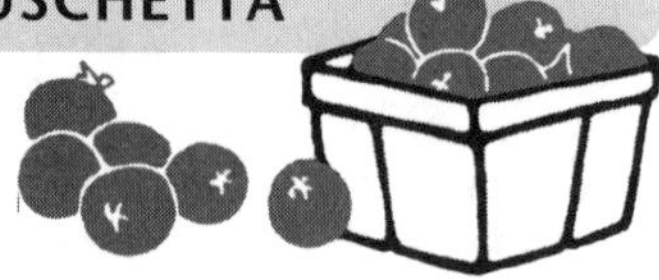

1 slender whole-grain baguette
⅓ cup hummus (page 69)
8 cherry tomatoes
Bragg Organic Olive Oil

Preheat broiler. Cut 2 inch slices from baguette and place on a baking sheet. Lightly oil both sides with olive oil. Watching carefully, toast the slices under broiler. They will be done in a few seconds. Turn to toast both sides. Remove from oven and place on serving dish. Halve cherry tomatoes and place on baking sheet, cut side down. Lightly oil. Broil until skins wrinkle and brown lightly, 1-3 minutes. Remove from broiler. Top each toasted sliced baguette with a teaspoon of hummus and a tomato half. Serves 4.

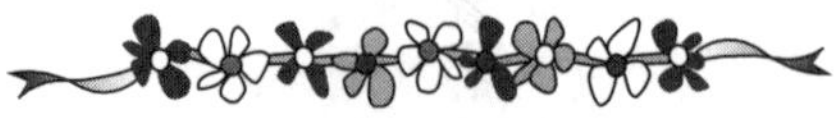

It's difficult to think anything but pleasant thoughts while eating a delicious homegrown tomato. – Lewis Grizzard, American writer and humorist

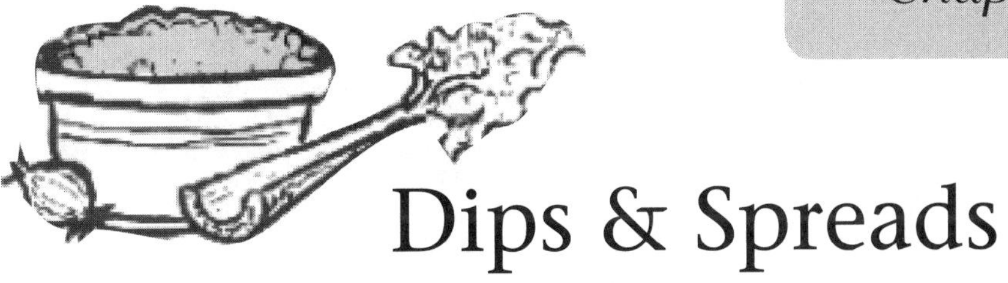

Chapter 7

Dips & Spreads

Dips and spreads are great for appetizers and party fare. Many tend to be high in fat content and loaded with calories. Here are some to try that are healthy, tasty and low in fat.

PATÉ OF SEEDS

RF

1 cup raw pumpkin seeds
1 medium red onion, chop
½ cup basil, chop
1 cup raw sunflower seeds
1 tsp Bragg Liquid Aminos
shake of Bragg Sprinkle

Soak pumpkin and sunflower seeds for 6-12 hours. This gives them the desired taste and texture. It also starts the sprouting process, which improves the nutritional value of the seeds and aids digestion. Drain, rinse thoroughly, and drain again. Put the soaked seeds and all the remaining ingredients in a food processor fitted with a metal blade. Process until smooth. Mound the paté in the center of a serving dish, cover, and refrigerate for at least 1 hour before serving. This paté will keep up to 2 days in the refrigerator. Makes 2 cups.

MUSHROOM - WALNUT PATÉ

1 Tbsp Bragg Organic Olive Oil
½ lb mushrooms, slice
½ lb firm tofu, crumble
2 Tbsps Bragg Liquid Aminos
1 red onion, finely chop
2 cups walnuts, toast
½ tsp Bragg Sprinkle
2 tsps Bragg Nutritional Yeast Flakes

Cook the onions in olive oil in a large frying pan over medium heat, stirring, until translucent (about 6 minutes). Add mushrooms, cover and cook for 3 minutes. Uncover and cook, stirring occasionally, until mushrooms have wilted, about 5 minutes. Then process in a blender and add remaining ingredients and process until smooth. Place in serving bowl, cover and refrigerate for at least 1 hour before serving. The paté keeps up to one day in the refrigerator. Makes 3 cups.

CARROT HUMMUS

2 cups cooked carrots
⅓ cup tahini
15 oz can chickpeas, drain and reserve liquid
2 cloves garlic
pita bread triangles
⅓ cup fresh lemon juice
Bragg Liquid Aminos to taste

In a food processor or blender, purée carrots, chickpeas, tahini, garlic and lemon juice until smooth. Add reserved liquid from chickpeas as needed to make a thick purée. Makes 2 cups.

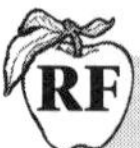

CASHEW DIP AND TOPPING

This recipe can be used as a dip for vegetables, or as a topping on vegetables, salads, pasta and pizza.

½ cup raw cashews
¼ cup lemon juice
¼ tsp Bragg Liquid Aminos
¼ tsp garlic powder
2 oz canned pimientos
1 Tbsp Bragg Nutritional Yeast Flakes
½ tsp Bragg Sprinkle
1½ cups distilled water

Place all ingredients in blender and process until very smooth. You can vary nut choices. Makes 2 cups.

BABA GHANOUSH DIP

4 medium eggplants
1 cup tahini
1 lb carrots, shred
4 cloves garlic, press
½ tsp Bragg Sprinkle
½ cup Bragg Organic Olive Oil
½ cup fresh squeezed lemon juice
½ tsp Bragg Liquid Aminos
1 red onion, mince
Serve with crackers or heated pita

Bake eggplants at 350°F until soft, about 45 minutes to 1 hour. Pierce the skin with a fork before baking to prevent exploding. Scoop the meat from the skin and place in mixing bowl, adding Sprinkle and remaining ingredients; mix well. Chill. Serve with crackers or heated pita bread. Yields 2 cups.

PINTO BEAN DIP

2 cups cooked pinto beans
2 cloves garlic, press
½ Tbsp Bragg Liquid Aminos
2 red onions, mince
1 chili pepper, mince
1 tomato, chop
½ tsp Bragg Sprinkle (24 herbs & spices)

Mash beans in large bowl with drizzle of olive oil. Add all other ingredients and place in a blender and purée until smooth. Serve with whole-grain crackers or pita bread. Makes 2½ cups.

EGGPLANT DIP

1 large globe eggplant
⅓ cup silken soft tofu
⅓ cup dry whole-grain bread crumbs
2 Tbsps lemon juice
1 tsp garlic, mince
¼ tsp red pepper sauce
3 Tbsps parsley, mince
½ tsp Bragg Sprinkle (24 herbs & spices)

Pierce eggplant in several places with a fork and place it on a baking sheet. Broil about 6-inches from the heat until blackened on all sides. Remove from oven and set aside to cool. When the eggplant is cool enough to handle, cut it open and spoon the flesh into a large bowl. Mash it with a fork, breaking up any long strands. Stir in bread crumbs, silken tofu, lemon juice, garlic, Sprinkle and red pepper sauce. Spread on decorative plate. Sprinkle with parsley. Chill completely. Serve with thin rounds of crisp raw vegetables, such as zucchini, jicama, celery, carrots, turnips, sweet potatoes. Delicious on heated pita bread. Makes 2 cups.

CUCUMBER DIP

2 large cucumbers
½ cup red onion, finely dice
2 Tbsps Bragg Organic Apple Cider Vinegar
2 cloves garlic, crush
1 lb fresh firm tofu
2 Tbsps cilantro, mince
shakes of Bragg Sprinkle
½ tsp Bragg Liquid Aminos

Peel, seed and mince cucumbers and place in a mixing bowl with the onion. In blender, combine tofu, apple cider vinegar, garlic, Bragg Aminos, and Sprinkle. Blend until smooth, then pour over cucumbers and mix well. Transfer to serving dish and chill 2-3 hours. Garnish with fresh cilantro and serve. Makes 2 cups.

HUMMUS*

2 cups cooked garbanzo beans
1 tsp Bragg Liquid Aminos
shakes of Bragg Sprinkle
juice of 1 lemon
1 cup tahini
2 cloves garlic, chop

In blender, place cooked garbanzos with enough liquid to keep wet, about the consistency of peanut butter. Add tahini, garlic, lemon juice, Sprinkle and Bragg Aminos. Blend well and chill for 1 hour before serving. This makes nutritious pita sandwich spreads and tasty dips. This combination is important in a vegetarian diet since it supplies a substantial amount of vegetable protein. Makes 2 cups.

BEAN SPREAD*

Combine cooked beans of your choice with chopped onion, minced parsley, tofunaise (page 139). Blend into a spread for dips, sandwiches or stuffings. When making sandwiches, prepare open face with a lettuce leaf or cabbage leaf on top.

NUT BUTTER AND VEGETABLE SPREAD*

Combine grated or ground raw carrots, celery, and onions with nut butter of choice. Season to taste.

******Hummus, Bean Spread, Nut Butter and Vegetable Spreads are delicious and nutritious. Perfect for sandwiches, pitas, spreads, dips, appetizers and toppings for salads and vegetables.*

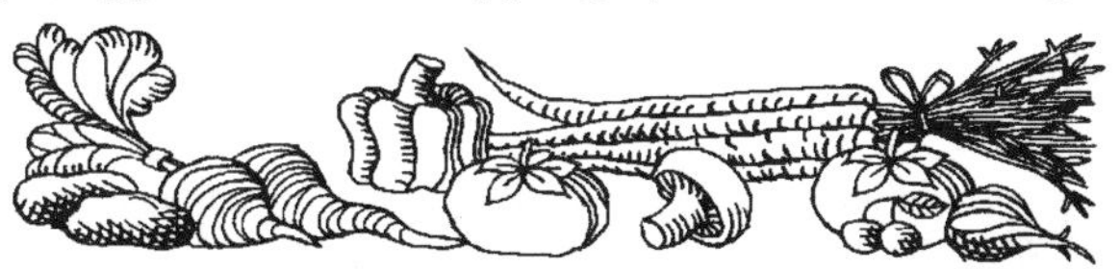

Let food be your medicine and medicine be your food. – Hippocrates, 400 B.C.

Healthy foods, when broken down during the digestive process, provide the ingredients your cells need to grow, replenish & repair.– Adele Puhn, M.S., C.N.S.

ROSEMARY AND WHITE BEAN SPREAD

1 Tbsp Bragg Organic Olive Oil
$1\frac{1}{3}$ Tbsps Bragg Apple Cider Vinegar
2-15 oz cans white beans, drain and rinse
2 cloves garlic, mince
1 cup red onion, chop
1 tsp dried rosemary, chop
$\frac{1}{4}$ tsp crushed red pepper
pinch of paprika, to garnish
$\frac{1}{3}$ tsp Bragg Sprinkle

Heat olive oil over medium heat. Cook and stir onions, garlic and rosemary until soft. Blend with remaining ingredients in a food processor until smooth. Transfer to baking dish. Garnish with paprika and bake at 350°F for 25 minutes. Makes 2 cups.

PEANUT OR ALMOND BUTTER - YEAST SPREAD

$\frac{1}{2}$ cup creamy peanut or almond butter
2 Tbsps Bragg Olive Oil
$\frac{1}{2}$ cup Bragg Nutritional Yeast Flakes

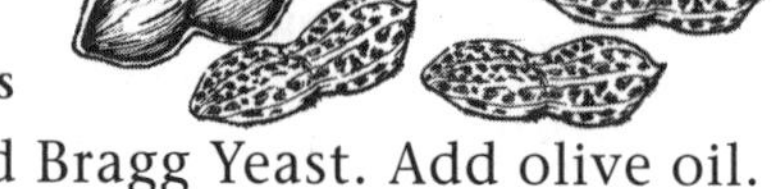

Combine nut butter of choice and Bragg Yeast. Add olive oil. Mix until smooth. Store covered in refrigerator. Makes 1 cup.

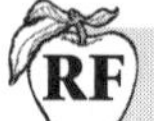

ALMOND SPREAD

2 cups raw almonds
1 Tbsp orange rind
2 cups wheat germ
2 Tbsps raw honey or stevia to taste
2 Tbsps Bragg Organic Olive Oil
$1\frac{1}{4}$ cups Bragg Apple Cider Vinegar

Grind almonds. Try pinch of stevia powder instead of honey. Add remaining ingredients. Blend until smooth. Makes 2 cups.

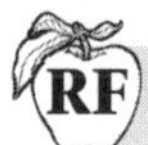

DATE SPREAD

Grind 1 cup pitted dates and 4 tablespoons nuts of choice. Blend using food processor. Add enough fresh orange juice to make the mixture spreadable. A squeeze of fresh lemon juice reduces sweet taste if desired. Makes 1 cup.

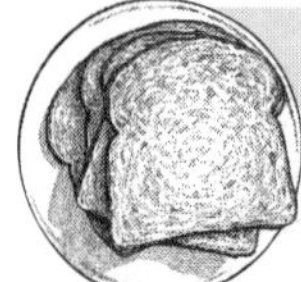

SOY - NUT SANDWICH SPREAD

2 cups cooked soybeans, mash
1 cup cashews, finely ground
1 tsp Bragg Liquid Aminos
1 cup avocado (optional)
2 tsps lemon juice
$\frac{1}{2}$ tsp Bragg Sprinkle

Blend ingredients thoroughly, place in container, refrigerate. Use as sandwich spread, topping or appetizer dip. Makes 3 cups.

Scientific research shows that peanuts can improve your health and prevent disease. Peanuts provide benefits to everyone. – www.peanut-institute.org

---

Fast Foods, processed meats and sugared foods up weight and medical bills!

Although we think we are one and we act as if we are one, human beings are not natural carnivores. When we kill animals to eat them, they end up killing us because their flesh, which contains cholesterol and saturated fat, was never intended for human beings, who are natural herbivores.
– William Clifford Roberts, M.D., Editor In Chief, American Journal of Cardiology

Chapter 8

Vegetables

Vegetables Make for a Healthy Menu

Vegetables and fruit, both raw or lightly cooked, are among the "curative" foods, and should represent at least three-fifths of the diet. These foods not only contribute vitamins and minerals to the diet, but add the fiber required for proper body functioning, in addition to helping maintain the alkaline reserve of the body. They add variety, color, tasty flavor and texture to your meals.

For some people vegetables are an unappetizing, uninteresting food – sad loss! The customary method of over-cooking garden-picture vegetables and serving them straight from a pool of surplus cooking water is certainly an unappetizing way to serve nature's gifts. Any cook with ingenuity can prepare a vegetable to be a beautiful delicacy. Properly prepared vegetables, raw or cooked, combined with delightful herb seasoning will enhance flavors and conserve vitamins, minerals, and food value. It is not necessary to prepare them with rich sauces or heavy spices. They can be standard items of fine food, exquisitely flavored and served in entirely new ways designed to excite the palate and nourish the body.

Cooking with herbs is a delightful and healthy experience. Herbs enhance the flavor of vegetables. The chapter on cooking with herbs and this vegetable section should be used interchangeably. Vegetables can become healthy delicacies rather than boring foods to be regarded with distaste.

Buying Organic Vegetables for Your Family

It is often very difficult to buy vegetables for a family of two or even four people without running the risk of having leftovers. Of all foods, vegetables have the least food value after they have been cooked and then stored. Vegetables are meant to be eaten as soon as possible after cooking, to obtain the utmost of their vitamin and mineral content. Avoid saving cooked vegetables for a second meal or a second day. Instead buy wisely and cook carefully to avoid waste or leftovers.

New research shows that cruciferous vegetables like Brussels sprouts, broccoli, bok choy, kale, cabbage, cauliflower, collard greens, radishes, rutabagas, turnips, etc. offers health protection against colon cancer.

How to Select Healthy, Fresh Vegetables

Although canning has become almost an exact science, fresh vegetables still outrank canned foods in all possible aspects of flavor and vitamin/mineral content. Buy all the fresh, organic vegetables possible, when they are in season. You will find many in the market year round, as modern scientific agriculture has extended the season of many previously limited vegetables. Some vegetables, when out of season, may lack freshness and flavor. Frozen foods have overcome this handicap. Learn to buy your vegetables when they are fresh, firm and ripe. Avoid moldy, withered, bruised, over-soft, over-hard or colorless-looking vegetables. They not only lack flavor, but contain less of the vitamin and mineral content.

There are five classifications of vegetables, and each should be selected with attention to its freshness and quality (please note that we recommend eating organically grown produce):

• *Root Vegetables*

Beets, carrots, turnips, potatoes, etc., should be firm, not withered. They should never have sprouts. Root vegetables like potatoes and turnips should not be green.

• *Stem Vegetables*

Asparagus, bean sprouts, celery, etc. should be crisp, fresh and have good color.

• *Leaf and Flower Vegetables*

Spinach, chard, kale, bok choy, lettuce, etc., should be deep green in color, crisp, fresh and, if in head form (cabbage, head lettuce, etc.), solid and firm.

• *Fruit Vegetables*

Represented by the squash family: eggplant, okra and tomato. They should be fresh, firm and deep in color.

• *Seed Vegetables*

Corn, peas, beans and other legumes should be firm and vibrant in color.

• *The Stem, Leaf & Fruit Vegetables*

Easily distinguishable as vegetables grown above the ground; usually lower in starch content than the root vegetables; the smaller the root vegetable, the less starch content. If you are counting your calories or are on a low-carbohydrate or restricted-carbohydrate diet, select small carrots, beets and turnips as they are more suitable. Not only do smaller-sized root vegetables provide lower starch content for the diet, but they are more flavorful. For general purposes, medium-sized vegetables are usually preferred.

Nature's Miracle Phytochemicals Help Prevent Cancer:

Make sure to get your daily dose of these naturally occurring, cancer-fighting super foods – phytonutrients that are abundant in apples, tomatoes, onions, garlic, beans, legumes, soybeans, cabbage, cauliflower, broccoli, citrus fruits, etc. The champions with the highest count of phytonutrients go to apples and tomatoes.

Class	Food Sources	Action
PHYTOESTROGENS ISOFLAVINS	*Soy products, flaxseed, seeds & nuts, yams alfalfa & red clover sprouts, licorice root (not candy)*	*May block some cancers, & aids in menopausal symptoms and helps improve the memory*
PHYTOSTEROLS	*Plant oils, corn, soy, sesame, safflower, wheat, pumpkin*	*Blocks hormonal role in cancers, inhibits uptake of cholesterol from diet*
SAPONINS	*Yams, beets, beans, cabbage, nuts, soybeans*	*May prevent cancer cells from multiplying*
TERPENES	*Carrots, winter squash sweet potatoes, yams apples, cantaloupes*	*Antioxidants – protects DNA from free radical-induced damage*
	Tomatoes & its sauces, tomato-based products	*Helps block UVA & UVB & may help protect against cancers, prostate, etc.*
	Spinach, kale, beet & turnip greens, cabbage	*Protects eyes from macular degeneration*
	Red chile peppers	*Keeps carcinogens from binding to DNA*
QUERCETIN (& FLAVANOIDS)	*Apples especially the skins, red onions & be sure that green tea has no caffeine*	*Strong cancer fighter, protects heart & arteries. Reduces pain, allergy & asthma symptoms*
	Citrus fruits (flavonoids)	*Promotes protective enzymes*
PHENOLS	*Apples, fennel, parsley, carrots, alfalfa, cabbage*	*Prevents blood clotting & may have anticancer properties*
	Cinnamon	*Promotes healthy blood sugar and glucose metabolism*
	Citrus fruits, broccoli, cabbage, cucumbers, green peppers, tomatoes	*Antioxidants – flavonoids block membrane receptor sites for certain hormones*
	Apples, grape seeds	*Strong antioxidants; fights germs & bacteria, strengthens immune system, veins & capillaries*
	Grapes, especially skins	*Antioxidant, antimutagen; promotes detoxification. Acts as carcinogen inhibitors*
	Yellow & green squash	*Antihepatoxic, antitumor*
SULFUR COMPOUNDS	*Onions & garlic, (fresh is always best) Red onions (our favorite) also contain Quercetin*	*Promotes liver enzymes, inhibits cholesterol synthesis, reduces triglycerides, lowers blood pressure, improves immune response, fights infections, germs & parasites*

Serving Sizes Chart for Vegetables

Fresh Vegetables	for 2 People	for 4 People
Asparagus	1¼ lbs	2½ lbs
Beets (including beet tops)	1¼ lbs	2½ lbs
Broccoli	1¼ lbs	2½ lbs
Brussels sprouts	¾ lb	1½ lbs
Cabbage	¾ lb	1½ lbs
Carrots	½ lb	1 lb
Cauliflower	1 small head	1 large head
Corn of the Cob	2 to 4 ears	8 ears
Greens (kale, spinach, etc.)	1¼ lbs	2½ lbs
Lima Beans	1¼ lbs un-shelled	2½ lbs unshelled
Onions	1 lb	2 lb
Parsnips	1 lb	2 lb
Peas	1¼ lbs un-shelled	2½ lbs unshelled
Potatoes (white & sweet)	1 lb	2 lbs
Squash (almost any kind)	1 lb	2 lbs
Green Beans	¾ lb	1½ lbs
Turnips	1¼ lbs	2½ lbs
Zucchini	¾ lb	1½ lbs

How to Store Vegetables Before Preparation

To retain their mineral and vitamin content vegetables should be cooked soon after buying or picking. If it's impossible to cook them soon, store in refrigerator or a cool place. Greens and other crisp vegetables should be thoroughly washed and dried, placed in Evert-Fresh Green Bags (*www.evertfresh.com*), and stored in refrigerator. For salad vegetables, if necessary to store for any length of time, do not wash them until just before using. For certain vegetables, like winter squash, eggplant, onion and potatoes, store at room temperature, displayed spread out, (wired hanging baskets) away from direct sun.

How to Clean Vegetables Before Cooking

There may be hazards in using commercially grown vegetables, unless they are properly cleaned. This is because many sprays are used in truck gardening. It is also possible to obtain vegetables carrying infectious forms of bacteria because of irrigation with unsanitary water in some areas. For these reasons, it is absolutely essential to wash all vegetables.

To clean fresh produce: 1) Rinse under cold running water. For extra protection add ¼ cup white vinegar to ¾ cup water, (we use *white vinegar* for cleaning only). Don't use soap or detergents. It is important to rinse food even if you are going to peel it. 2) Use a scrub brush to remove additional dirt and bacteria. 3) Cut out bruised or damaged areas; bacteria can thrive there. 4) Final rinse, then dry with clean cloth or paper towel. See web – washing fruits & veggies: *www.nutrition.about.com*.

Use scrub brush to remove dark spots. In most cases, they should not be scraped. Do not remove their skins as the richest portion of their food content lies just beneath the skin covering. When you peel potatoes, carrots and other vegetables, you waste a nutritious part of their food value. It's best to steam, roast or bake vegetables in their skins.

Healthy Cooking of Vegetables

Vegetables should always be prepared with the least amount of water to retain health nutrients, distilled or reverse osmosis waters are purest and best to use. We prefer steaming (use steamer basket), baking and woks because they conserve more vitamins and minerals. The small convection ovens are ideal for healthy baking.

Below are some suggestions for waterless cooking using little or no water:

Steaming: Any quality stainless steel, enamel, glass or iron pan with a tight-fitting cover is preferable. You may use a steamer basket that fits in most pans. We prefer to use steamers, but more water can be used and the remaining liquids are delicious served with the vegetables in shallow soup bowls and any excess saved for other uses such as vegetable stock (see page 10). For a tasty delight, try a spray of Bragg Liquid Aminos and dash of Bragg Sprinkle over steamed veggies.

The pan used should be sized to suit the amount of vegetables you are preparing. If vegetables are cut or sliced in small pieces and the container is filled to the brim, very little water is required. Sliced carrots or beets steamed this way usually require only a cup of water. Cover tightly and cook over medium heat for 8-12 minutes.

Baking: Casserole cookery may be applied to this health method by slicing, dicing or chopping root vegetables and the succulent vegetables. This fast method uses about a ½ cup of distilled water and 1 Tablespoon of Bragg Organic Olive Oil or sesame oil, fresh sliced garlic, Bragg Liquid Aminos and Bragg Sprinkle. Bake in a moderate oven, about 350°F. Cooking time varies depending on type of vegetable.

Stir Frying: Wok & light stir-frying are popular methods for preparing veggies and main entrées. Woks originated in Asian cooking, and have been used for centuries. We enjoy this fast, easy, almost waterless method of preparing our foods.

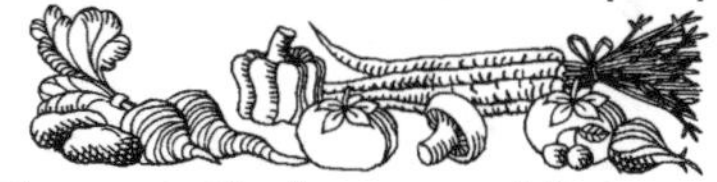

We must use time creatively . . . and forever realize that the time is always ripe to do right. – Martin Luther King, Jr.

Some Important Points to Remember When Cooking Vegetables:

1. Do not remove the lid while the vegetable is cooking. When lid is removed while cooking, essential vitamins and minerals are lost. You also allow water in the vegetables (or, "self-cooking liquids-vapors") to escape.
2. Low heat should be used whenever possible. Vegetables should be cooked for as little time as possible, just enough to tenderize them.
3. Vegetables taste best lightly cooked, almost raw.
4. Vegetables may be prepared in a variety of ways, including broiling, roasting, sautéing, baking, boiling, steaming, and in wok for stir frys.
5. Don't allow vegetables to stand in water before cooking, as the minerals dissolve and are lost in the water.
6. Cut, trim or prepare the vegetables just before cooking to prevent loss of vitamin C and nutrients.

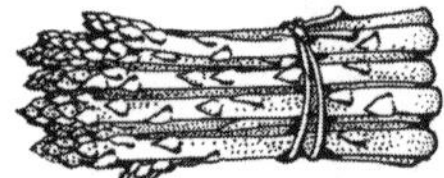

ASPARAGUS

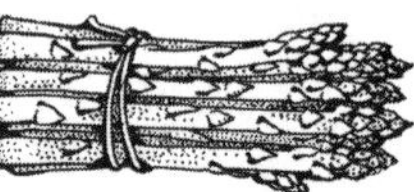

Asparagus, with its delicate flavor, is an early spring vegetable. It's high in minerals and vitamins. Select medium to large, crisp green stalks. Wash thoroughly, cut off lower white, coarse stalk 1-2" if needed. Cook in steamer basket with ample water 10 minutes or until tender. Also tender raw asparagus is delicious. Serve with Bragg Ginger & Sesame or Braggberry Dressing (see page 304). 2½ pounds of asparagus serves 4-6.

BAKED ASPARAGUS

2 lbs asparagus
¼ cup Bragg Organic Olive Oil
1 cup whole-grain bread crumbs
Egg Replacer equal to 1 egg
½ tsp Bragg Liquid Aminos
shake of Bragg Sprinkle

Cut and wash asparagus and roll in bread crumbs. Dip in Egg Replacer with Bragg Aminos and Sprinkle, then roll again in bread crumbs. Pour olive oil in baking dish, arrange asparagus. Bake at 350°F until tender. Also raw and steamed is delicious. Serves 4.

ASPARAGUS ON WHOLE GRAIN TOAST

Cut coarse white ends off asparagus stalks. Steam until tender. Serve on toast with Bragg Olive Oil or Bragg Ginger Dressing.

Asparagus is a nutrient-dense food which is high in folic acid and is a good source of potassium, fiber, vitamin B6, vitamins A and C, and thiamin. Asparagus has no fat, no cholesterol and is low in sodium.

ROASTED ASPARAGUS WITH TAPENADE

2 lbs asparagus, trim
Bragg Liquid Aminos to taste
¼ cup Bragg Organic Olive Oil
¼ cup olive tapenade (page 35)
Bragg Sprinkle (24 herbs & spices), to taste

Place asparagus in single layer in heavy roasting pan in 475°F oven. Pour oil over asparagus and turn spears to coat. Lightly spray with Bragg Aminos. Roast asparagus for 15 minutes, turning at least once. Dot with tapenade and season with Sprinkle.

COLD ASPARAGUS WITH SESAME SEEDS

1 lb asparagus
1 Tbsp sesame seeds
1 Tbsp raw honey
½ tsp Bragg Liquid Aminos
2 Tbsps Bragg Apple Cider Vinegar
1 Tbsp Bragg Organic Olive Oil

Cut off tough ends of asparagus, and cut them on the diagonal into ½-inch slices. Place into steamer basket, steam for 10 minutes or until tender (test with fork). Pat dry. Toast sesame seeds in heavy skillet over medium heat for 2-3 minutes, stirring constantly. Mix vinegar, Bragg Aminos, honey and olive oil in bowl. Add asparagus and 2 teaspoons of the sesame seeds. Toss to mix. Refrigerate 1-3 hours, toss occasionally. Garnish with remaining sesame seeds and sprinkle of Bragg Nutritional Yeast Flakes before serving.

ARTICHOKES

Artichokes have important nutritional value! A medium sized artichoke delivers 2 grams of protein, 10 mg of vitamin C, plus healthy dose of most minerals. Globe artichokes contain more protein than most vegetables. It is excellent for low-calorie diets as they contain only 25 calories and zero fat. *We grow artichokes and asparagus in our vegetable garden – PB.*

Do not confuse the globe artichoke with the Jerusalem. The globe are a green, clustered-bud type; the Jerusalem is a root vegetable like a small potato – both are delicious baked.

ARTICHOKES WITH GARLIC & HERBS

4 artichokes
3 Tbsps fresh squeezed lemon juice
¼ cup Bragg Organic Olive Oil
4 cloves garlic, slice
1 tsp Bragg Liquid Aminos
⅓ tsp Bragg Sprinkle

Wash artichokes thoroughly. Cut one inch off the tops. Remove stems. Place sliced garlic between the leaves of the artichokes. Mix Sprinkle, olive oil, Bragg Aminos and lemon juice and sprinkle over artichokes. Stand artichokes on end in a saucepan using steamer basket. Steam for 30 minutes or until tender. Serve hot or cold, whole or halved, with tofunaise (pg. 139). Serves 4-8.

Artichokes have strong choleretic activity – increases excretion of cholesterol and decrease manufacture of cholesterol in the liver. – elements4health.com.

STEAMED ARTICHOKES

4 artichokes
4 garlic cloves, slice
dried bread crumbs (optional)
1 tsp Bragg Liquid Aminos
Bragg Organic Olive Oil
¼ cup Bragg Apple Cider Vinegar (added to water for steaming)
⅓ tsp Bragg Sprinkle
⅓ tsp Bragg Sea Kelp
Tofunaise (page 139)

Wash artichokes thoroughly. Cut 1-inch off tips of leaves to prevent the sharp thorns from pricking. Slice garlic and put in between leaves and add dried bread crumbs (optional). Add Sprinkle and Sea Kelp among inner leaves. Place artichokes in steamer basket, steam with vinegar-water for 30 minutes until tender. Drain, serve with tofunaise, Braggberry Dressing or warm Olive Oil and garlic. To eat, dip bottom part of leaves in sauce and scrape with teeth. Remove and discard inner fibers from inside heart. Cut heart into small pieces and dip in sauce. Serves 4.

SCALLOPED GLOBE ARTICHOKES

6 cooked artichokes
1 cup soy milk
1 tsp Bragg Liquid Aminos
1½ Tbsps fresh squeezed lemon juice
1 cup dry whole-grain bread crumbs
Egg Replacer equal to 2 eggs
shake of Bragg Sprinkle (24 herbs & spices)

Scrape edible portion from cooked artichoke leaves, remove fibers and dice heart. Mix artichoke scrapings, whole-grain bread crumbs, Egg Replacer, soy milk, lemon juice, Bragg Aminos and Sprinkle. Place in oiled baking dish. Bake in moderate oven (375°F) about 15 minutes. Serves 6.

ARTICHOKES SAUTÉED WITH MUSTARD & CHIVES

24 baby artichokes, tops trimmed
7 Tbsps Bragg Organic Olive Oil
1 Tbsp lemon juice
2 Tbsps chives, finely sliced
½ cup almonds, chopped
2 Tbsps Dijon-style mustard
¼ cup parsley, chopped
⅓ tsp Bragg Sprinkle

Saute almonds in 1 Tbsp of olive oil until golden; reserve. Quarter baby artichokes lengthwise. Saute artichokes in 4 Tbsps of olive oil, 10-15 minutes or until tender. Add mustard and lemon juice, saute 1 minute longer. Toss with almonds, parsley, chives and remaining 2 Tbsps olive oil and Bragg Sprinkle. Serves 6.

Diets High in Vegetables & Fruits Protect Against Cancer

- *A diet high in vegetables and fruits helps reduce the risk of cancer.*
- *Diets rich in beta-carotene (the plant form of vitamin A) and vitamin C helps reduce the risk of certain cancers.*
- *Reducing fat in the diet helps reduce cancer risk, and helps in weight control, and helps reduce the risk of heart attacks and strokes.*
- *Diets high in fiber-rich foods (such as blueberries, raspberries and apples and broccoli) helps reduce the risk of colon and rectal cancers.*
- *Vegetables from cabbage family helps reduce risk of colon cancer.*

National Cancer Institute • www.cancer.gov

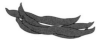

GREEN BEANS

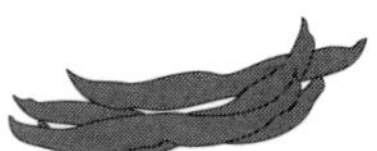

One pound of green beans serves 4. Tender, young raw beans are also delicious. Gently snap tip ends off. If the beans snap easily, they are young, fresh beans. Wash thoroughly, remove the ends; cut lengthwise or crosswise into thin pieces, or leave whole if desired. Steam in a small amount of water until tender. Green beans can be used in the following recipes:

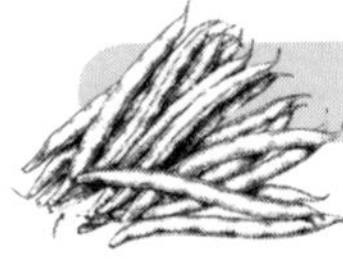

GREEN BEANS WITH HERBS

2 lbs green beans
3 Tbsps Bragg Olive Oil
½ tsp Bragg Sprinkle
2 cloves garlic, slice
pinch of soy Parmesan cheese
½ tsp Bragg Liquid Aminos

Cut washed beans to desired length. Steam or cook with small amount of water over low heat. Lightly sauté garlic in olive oil in wok or pan. Add cooked beans, Sprinkle and Bragg Aminos. Sauté 2 minutes and sprinkle with soy parmesan cheese. Serves 4-6.

GREEN BEANS WITH MINT

3 cups green beans, slice
3 Tbsps Bragg Olive Oil
½ tsp Bragg Liquid Aminos
¼ cup mint, chop
sweet basil, fresh
shake of Bragg Sprinkle

Combine ingredients, sauté in wok 15 minutes. Serves 4-6.

GREEN BEANS WITH MUSHROOMS

3 cups green beans, slice
1½ Tbsps Bragg Organic Olive Oil
3 garlic cloves, mince
1 cup mushrooms, slice
½ tsp Bragg Liquid Aminos
Braggberry Marinade
shake of Bragg Sprinkle (24 herbs & spices)

Sauté green beans, garlic and mushrooms in wok or pan with olive oil for 15 minutes or until tender. Add Sprinkle and Bragg Aminos. Garnish with Braggberry Marinade. Serves 4-6.

SPANISH SNAP BEANS

2 medium red onions, slice
1 green bell pepper, dice with seeds
2 cups fresh or canned tomatoes
2 tsps Bragg Organic Olive Oil
2 lbs cooked snap beans,
cut beans into one-inch pieces
1 cup distilled water
shake of Bragg Sprinkle
2 garlic cloves, slice
2 Tbsps whole-grain flour
a dash of sesame oil
1 tsp Bragg Liquid Aminos

Combine tomatoes, onions, bell pepper, Sprinkle, garlic, water and Bragg Aminos. Simmer for 10 minutes. Blend olive oil with a dash of sesame oil for flavor with the whole-grain flour; stir into tomato mixture. Stirring frequently. Cook until thick and smooth. Add cooked beans and heat for 5 minutes. Serves 4-6.

The most healthful calcium sources are green leafy vegetables and legumes, or "greens and beans" for short. Broccoli, Brussel sprouts, collards, mustard greens, kale (which is the highest in calcium) and other greens are loaded with absorbable calcium and host of other nutrients and phytochemicals.

LIMA BEANS

All lima beans, legumes, etc. are very high in protein. They are the healthy "life builders" of the body's blood, muscle and tissue. For this reason, they can be used as a vegetable, as well as a protein, substituting for meat, eggs and other animal proteins.

BAKED LIMA BEANS

3 cups cooked lima beans
2 Tbsps arrowroot flour
1 tsp Bragg Liquid Aminos
½ cup whole-grain bread crumbs
3 Tbsps Bragg Olive Oil
½ tsp Bragg Sprinkle
1 cup soy milk
Egg Replacer equal to 2 eggs

Add arrowroot flour to olive oil. Add soy milk gradually, stir over low heat until thick. Purée (cooked) lima beans in blender, add to sauce. Add Bragg Aminos, Sprinkle and Egg Replacer. Place in oiled casserole dish, cover with bread crumbs and olive oil. Bake 15 minutes in 350°F oven. Serves 4.

BABY LIMAS MARJORAM

3 cups cooked baby limas
2 Tbsps parsley, chop
3 garlic cloves, chop
2 large tomatoes, dice
½ tsp Bragg Liquid Aminos
⅓ tsp marjoram
1 small red onion, chop
2 Tbsps Bragg Organic Olive Oil
shake of Bragg Sprinkle
shake of Bragg Kelp

Combine garlic and onion with olive oil and sauté in wok or pan for 2-3 minutes. Add diced tomato and remaining ingredients. Cook 5-10 minutes until done, stirring frequently. Serves 3-6.

BAKED BEANS BASIC RECIPE

(This can be used for kidney beans, pink beans, navy beans, etc., all garden peas or any variety of similar legumes.)

1 quart dried beans
2 Tbsps brown rice syrup
1 cup unsulfured molasses
½ cup Bragg Organic Olive Oil
½ tsp Bragg Sprinkle
1 tsp Bragg Liquid Aminos

Cover beans with cold distilled water and soak overnight (to reduce cooking time). Drain and rinse. Cover beans with distilled water again, place in bean pot, crockpot or iron kettle. Heat slowly. Add other ingredients. Keep below boiling and always keep enough water to cover the beans. When skin begins to burst, cover the bean pot and bake 1½ hours in 350°F oven until done. You can also prepare beans in a crockpot overnight on low. Serves 6-8.

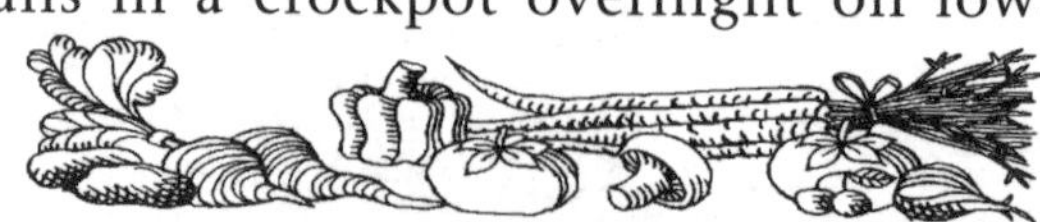

One cup cooked beans provides between 9 to 13 grams of healthy fiber.

SOYBEANS

The soybean is a rich source of protein and other nutrients. It also makes a delightful addition to healthy meals. They have an ancient heritage, having been used for thousands of years in Asian cuisine. Only in recent years have Americans and Europeans become aware of the soybean possibilities as a meat and dairy substitute and its great value as a healthy food staple.

Add Soybeans to Your Diet

Soybeans are used in thousands of products and are now the second-largest cash crop in the United States, topped only by corn. The FDA has recently ruled that soy products with at least 6.5 grams of soy per serving can carry this label: "Twenty-five grams of soy protein a day, as part of a diet low in saturated fat and cholesterol, may reduce the risk of heart disease." In fact, soybeans contain more protein and iron than beef, more calcium than milk and more lecithin than eggs. Soybean protein also has all of the essential amino acids, making it the only plant protein equal to animals products in these essential nutrients. Plus, a good source of B vitamins, potassium, zinc and other minerals.

Soy can aid those who are lactose-intolerant. There is a wide-range of soy products to choose from such as yogurts, cheeses and even soy ice cream. Adding soy to your meals can be delicious and great for your health.

Try Bragg's Natural Liquid Aminos which is made from soybean protein (certified non-GMO); it adds zest to meals – a healthy alternative to salt, Tamari and traditional soy sauce.

CHOLESTEROL COUNT OF COMMON FOODS

Food from Animal		Food from Plant	
Cholesterol Count	**(mg)**	**Cholesterol Count**	**(mg)**
Brain, 3 oz.	1,749	All beans	0
Liver, chicken, 1 cup	883	All fruits	0
Liver, beef, 3 oz.	331	All grains	0
Kidney, beef, 3 oz.	329	All legumes	0
Butter, 1 pat	250	All nuts	0
Egg, whole,	213	All seeds	0
Cream cheese, 8 oz.	120	All vegetables	0
Ice cream, 1 ½ cups	88	All vegetable oils	0
Lamb, 3 oz..	78		
Beef, sirloin steak, 3 oz..	77		
Pork, 3 oz..	77		
Chicken breast, 3 oz.	73		
Chicken leg, 2 oz.	48		

Sources:
1. J. Pennington, Food Values of Portions Commonly Used
2. Family and Consumer Services, University of Georgia

How to Make Sprouts
Soybeans, Sunflower, Alfalfa, Lentil, Mung Beans, etc.

Sprouts are a nutritional food that can be used in many recipes. In the life of a plant, sprouting is the moment of the greatest vitality and energy of the plant. When a seed sprouts, it activates many metabolic systems. It begins the synthesis of many different enzymes. Some vitamins increase during sprouting by up to 500%! Sprouting significantly increases protein bio-availability by 30% and more. The protein in sprouts are among the most digestible of all proteins found in foods.

The sprouts of these beans and seeds are used as a salad vegetable to replace salad greens, and in sandwiches to replace lettuce. Sprouts are a healthy, attractive garnish and a highly nutritional addition to dishes of all kinds.

It's important to have organic beans and seeds and not over one year old for sprouting. Seeds for sprouting can be found at your local health food store. With viable beans and seeds obtained for sprouting, you can create a vegetable in any climate, winter or summer, that is fresh, matures quickly (a few days), does not require soil cultivation or variations of sunshine, and has high healthy nutritional value!

Sprouts are very tender. To hold crispness when adding to hot mixtures, it is best to add just before serving.

Excellent Method for Sprouting Beans and Seeds

from the U.S. Department of Agriculture

Soybeans, mung beans and other seeds can be sprouted in a large glass jar, flower pot, a sink strainer or any container that you can drain from the top or bottom and can be covered with cheesecloth or mesh. Be sure the container is large enough, because the beans or seeds may swell from six to ten times their original bulk as they sprout:

- Soak overnight.
- The next morning, put them in the container, cover it, with cheesecloth and leave it in a warm place.
- Rinse with lukewarm water at least three or four times each day during the sprouting period.
- In 4-6 days, the sprouts will be 2 to 3 inches long.
- Then sprouts should be loosely placed spread out in container, refrigerated or stored in cool place until served.

Note: See Salad Section for recipe on Sprouted Soybean Salad (pg. 23).

It's bizarre that the vegetable and fruit produce managers are more important to my children's health than the pediatrician. – Meryl Streep

SOY MILK

Soy milk is a liquid resembling cow's milk that is made from soybeans. Today's soy milks are nutritionally close to cow's milk, but healthier because they don't contain cholesterol and saturated fat (see website: *www.notmilk.com*). Soy can be used in any recipe calling for cow's milk with the same proportions. However, soy milk curdles when boiled, so it's best to add to a recipe as the final ingredient. There are several ways of making organic soy milk. Here's a simple, practical recipe:

Soak soy beans overnight. Measure out 3 times amount of liquid in proportion to soaked soy beans you have prepared; grind beans, slowly adding some of this liquid as you go, proportioning liquid so that all of it is used up by the time you have ground all the beans. Add vanilla bean to pulpy mass and simmer slowly 1 hour. Strain through cheese cloth or strainer.

SOY CHEESE

To prepare soy cheese, allow soy milk to curdle, just as you would cow's milk. Set the soy milk in a warm place, and when it has soured and thickened, cut into sections and bring to a boil in a saucepan. Then strain through cheese cloth. The remaining cheese can be seasoned with Bragg Aminos, onions, chopped chives, or Bragg Sprinkle (24 herbs & spices).

SOYBEAN CASSEROLE

4 cups soybeans
1 cup celery, chop
½ cup carrots, chop
½ cup red onions, chop
1 green pepper, chop
2½ cups fresh tomatoes
1 cup raw walnuts, chop
1 can tomato sauce
6 fresh mushrooms
3 Tbsps whole-grain bread crumbs
1 tsp Bragg Liquid Aminos
2 Tbsps molasses
3 Tbsps raw honey
2 Tbsps Bragg Organic Olive Oil
2 Tbsps parsley, chop
1½ Tbsps fresh grated ginger
½ tsp Bragg Sprinkle
2 cloves garlic, press

Soak soybeans overnight. Next day cook for 30 minutes. Add all other ingredients and mix well. Bake in oiled casserole dish in 350°F oven for 45 minutes. Serves 6-8.

Soybeans and other foods rich in omega-3 fatty acids all help to maintain a healthy heart, among other benefits. – Alternative Medicine Magazine

BAKED SOYBEAN CROQUETTES

- 2 Tbsps onion, mince
- 1 garlic clove, mince
- 1½ cups celery, dice
- 1½ tsps Bragg Liquid Aminos
- 1 cup tomato purée
- 2 Tbsps Bragg Organic Olive Oil
- 5 Tbsps whole-grain flour
- 3 cups soybean pulp*
- shake of Bragg Sprinkle
- raw wheat germ
- Egg Replacer equal to 1 egg
- 2 Tbsps distilled water

Add minced onion, garlic, celery, Sprinkle and Bragg Aminos to tomato purée, bring to a boil. Mix flour and olive oil together and slowly add to boiled tomato purée mixture. Cook to thick paste. Cool and add soybean pulp. Shape into croquettes. Add water to Egg Replacer. Roll croquettes in wheat germ, then in Egg Replacer and again in wheat germ. Place them on oiled baking sheet. Bake at 400°F for 20 minutes. Serves 6.

**Soybean pulp is prepared by pressing cooked soybeans through a coarse sieve or by grinding them in a food grinder or blender.*

SOYBEAN SPROUTS CASSEROLE

- 3 cups sprouted soybeans
- ½ cup whole-grain bread crumbs
- 3 Tbsps Bragg Organic Olive Oil
- 2 Tbsps soybean flour
- Egg Replacer equal to 2 eggs
- 2 red onions, chop
- ¾ cup celery, dice
- 1 cup soy milk
- ½ cup soy Parmesan cheese
- 1 tsp Bragg Liquid Aminos
- shake of Bragg Sprinkle (24 herbs & spices)

Lightly sauté onions and celery in olive oil, adding sprouts last. Add this to Egg Replacer, soy milk, flour, bread crumbs, Sprinkle and Bragg Aminos. Pour mixture into oiled casserole and top with grated soy Parmesan cheese. Bake in 350°F oven 5-8 minutes or until delicately brown. Serves 4-6.

SOYBEAN SPROUTS WITH ONIONS & MUSHROOMS

- ½ cup green onion tops, finely chop
- 1 Tbsp Bragg Liquid Aminos
- 3 Tbsps Bragg Organic Olive Oil
- 3 cups sprouted soybeans
- 1 cup mushrooms, slice
- ⅓ tsp Bragg Sprinkle

Sauté onion tops, soybean sprouts and mushrooms lightly in olive oil. Shake Bragg Aminos and Sprinkle over mixture and allow to simmer a few minutes before serving. Serves 5.

COOKING DRIED SOYBEANS

Soak organic soybeans overnight. In the morning, drain and wash again. Drain and add boiling water three times the original amount of soybeans (example: 1 cup dry beans to 3 cups of water). Simmer at least two hours, or overnight in a crockpot. Soybeans will not cook into a soft, mushy mass. They will remain firm and hold their shape better than other dry beans.

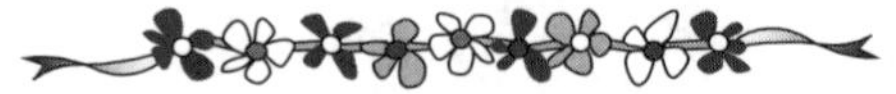

Soybeans have abundant heart healthy lecithin. – Prevention Magazine

GREEN SOYBEANS

Allow soybean pods to stand ten minutes in boiling water. Drain and shell beans. For each cup of shelled beans, add ½ cup of boiling water. Bring to a boil and cook until beans are tender (10-15 minutes). Drain and season as desired.

SAUTÉED SOYBEAN SPROUTS AND ONIONS

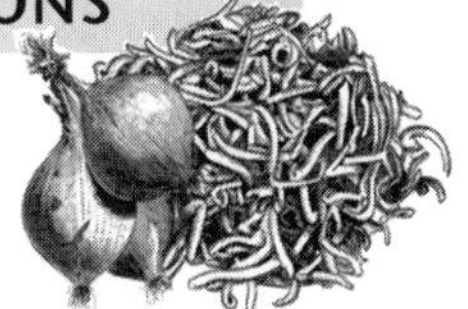

1 pound soybean sprouts
4 Tbsps Bragg Olive Oil
2 tsps Bragg Liquid Aminos
1 cup vegetable stock
2 red onions, chop
1½ Tbsps potato flour
4 Tbsps distilled water
½ tsp Bragg Sprinkle

Lightly sauté sprouts and onions in olive oil. Add vegetable stock, Sprinkle and Bragg Aminos. Thicken with potato flour (or rice flour) and water made into paste and serve hot. Serves 4.

SOYBEAN PATTIES WITH TOMATO SAUCE

1 cup soybeans, soak overnight
2 Tbsps Bragg Nutritional Yeast
pinch of poultry seasoning
1 Tbsp Bragg Liquid Aminos
1 Tbsp Bragg Organic Olive Oil
½ cup distilled water
¼ tsp onion powder
pinch of garlic powder
½ tsp Bragg Sprinkle
⅔ cup organic rolled oats

Grind soybeans in a food processor. Combine remaining ingredients, with the exception of the rolled oats, and chop fine in the food processor. Then add the oats and mix thoroughly. Let ingredients stand for 10 minutes to absorb all of the moisture. Form into patties on well-oiled baking pan. Bake in 350°F oven for 10 minutes or until browned. Turn, cover and bake 10 more minutes. Reduce heat to 325°F and cook additional 10 minutes. Serve with tomato sauce (page 111 or 163). Serves 4.

SOYBEAN STUFFED PEPPERS

½ cup fresh tomatoes, chop
1 tsp Bragg Liquid Aminos
2 cups soybean pulp*
whole-grain bread crumbs
3-4 green peppers
shake of Bragg Kelp
½ cup celery, dice
1 tsp red onion, mince

Remove seeds and inner partitions from green peppers. Parboil peppers 3 minutes. At same time simmer celery in another pan containing ¼ cup of distilled water. Add in soybean pulp, tomatoes, onions and Bragg Aminos. Stir until combined. Sprinkle inside of peppers with Kelp seasoning. Fill with soybean mixture. Cover tops with whole-grain bread crumbs. Place in an oiled pan and bake in 400°F oven for 30 minutes or until the peppers are soft. Serves 3-4.

**Soybean pulp is prepared by pressing cooked soybeans through a coarse sieve or by grinding them in a food grinder or blender.*

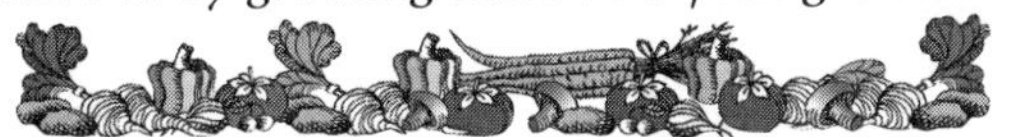

SOYBEAN LOAF

2 cups soybeans
1 cup whole-grain bread crumbs
¼ cup uncooked whole-grain cereal
1 cup raw carrots, finely grate
2 Tbsps Bragg Organic Olive Oil
1 red onion, chop
1 bunch spinach, chop
½ tsp Bragg Sprinkle
2 garlic cloves, mash
1 tsp Bragg Liquid Aminos

Soak beans overnight, skim off foam and grind in blender. Cover with soaking water, and cook in double boiler for approximately 1 hour. Add remainder of ingredients to cooked soybeans and pour into a loaf or ring pan. Bake 30 minutes in 350°F oven or until lightly browned.

BEETS

Beets are one of the most nutritional and economical vegetables. Both root and leaves are an excellent source of vitamins and minerals. For delicious beets, steam them in their skins for 20 minutes, serve sliced. We also love beets raw, grated in our salads or sliced as a garnish for dips.

BAKED BEETS - WHOLE, SLICED OR GRATED

Select medium-sized, tender beets. Remove tops. Wash but do not peel. Bake whole, sliced or grated. If grated, fill casserole very full; sprinkle with a small amount of water. Cover tightly and bake in a 350°F oven. Grated beets will bake within ten minutes of being thoroughly heated; whole and sliced beets, 20-40 minutes in a casserole dish. Remove cover, season with Bragg Olive Oil and Bragg Sprinkle.

JULIENNE BEETS, BAKED

Remove tops from six beets and save them to cook as greens. Wash medium-sized beets (do not peel) and cut into julienne strips. Put in baking dish or casserole. Add ½ cup boiling water. Bake at 350°F for 30-45 minutes with a tight-fitting cover. Remove from the oven, add one teaspoon of fresh lemon or lime juice, one tablespoon of Bragg Organic Olive Oil and a dash of Bragg Aminos. Serves 4.

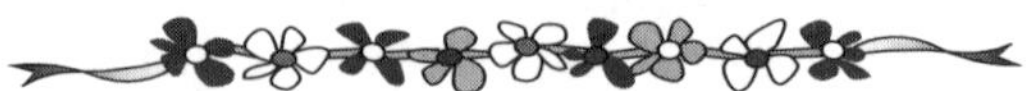

Read labels carefully! Beware of store-bought, processed foods such as canned soups, salty chips, frozen dinners, etc., which account for more than three-fourths of high salt intake most people eat, causing many health problems.

One cannot think well, love well, sleep well,
if one has not dined well. – Virginia Woolf

How good it is to be well-fed, healthy and kind, all at the same time.
– Henry Heimlich, vegetarian physician, inventor of Heimlich Maneuver

BEETS EN ORANGE

¾ cup freshly squeezed orange juice
1¼ tsps grated organic orange rind
2 Tbsps Bragg Organic Olive Oil
2 Tbsps potato flour or arrowroot flour
3¼ cups cooked beets, slice
¾ cup distilled water
2 tsps raw honey

Stir potato or arrowroot flour into olive oil; add water slowly. Add orange rind, orange juice and honey. Cook until smooth and thick. While stirring, add cooked sliced beets and cook 3-5 minutes. Serves 4-6.

LEMON BEETS, PICKLED

10 small beets
½ cup distilled water
2 Tbsps raw honey
1 cup lemon juice
1 Tbsp pickling spices
1 Tbsp Bragg Apple Cider Vinegar

Mix lemon juice and vinegar with water, bring to a boil and cook for 10 minutes with pickling spices tied in a muslin cooking bag. Cool. Sweeten with two tablespoons of honey, or to taste. Cook small beets with skins until tender; plunge into cold water and slice. Cover with seasoning mixture in a bowl and allow to marinate overnight or longer. Store in refrigerator.

BEET GREENS

Tender beet greens and stems are delicious. If you have a vegetable garden, you can eat beet greens as you thin your beets. Select beets with care when you buy them at stores, so that they have tender green tops. Wash thoroughly and steam or cook covered, in a ½ cup distilled water for 5 minutes or until tender. Season with dash or spray of Bragg Aminos, Bragg Organic Olive Oil, Bragg Sprinkle and Bragg Apple Cider Vinegar. Serve in bowl with liquid left.

BROCCOLI

The rich green broccoli florets, leaves and stem have a delicate flavor cooked or raw. Delicious rich source of vitamins, minerals and other nutrients.

BROCCOLI WITH SOY CHEESE

1 lb broccoli, break apart
½ cup soy cheese, grate
1 tsp Bragg Liquid Aminos
2 Tbsps Bragg Organic Olive Oil
2 cloves garlic, slice
½ cup whole-grain bread crumbs

Wash broccoli thoroughly, removing tough end parts of the stem. Steam 10 minutes until tender. Place in casserole dish, add Bragg Aminos, bread crumbs and top with soy cheese. Brown garlic slowly in olive oil and pour oil over broccoli, and bake in 350°F oven for 10 minutes. Serves 4.

CABBAGE

Eat Plenty of Raw Cabbage – Miracle Cleanser & Healer

Cabbage (raw) has amazing properties. It stimulates the immune system, kills bacteria and viruses, heals ulcers, and according to Dr. James Balch in *Prescription for Dietary Wellness*, your chances of contracting colon cancer can be reduced by up to 60% by eating raw cabbage weekly. Dr. Saxon-Graham states that those who never consumed cabbage were three times more likely to develop colon cancer. A Japanese Study shows people who ate raw cabbage had the lowest fatality rate from any cancer. Therapeutic benefits have also been attributed to raw cabbage in relation to scurvy, gout, rheumatism (arthritis), eye diseases, asthma, pyorrhea, and gangrene. We add raw cabbage to salads and even make sandwiches wrapped in cabbage leaves instead of bread. These cabbage wraps are so delicious!

GREEN CABBAGE

When cooking cabbage, remove tough or bruised outer leaves (save for soup stock). But not too many because outside leaves contain more vitamins and food value. Remove tough end stalk. Slice finely, put in oiled baking dish, cover with whole-grain bread crumbs and ¼ cup Bragg Organic Olive Oil. Add 3 tablespoons soy milk or water, short bake until tender. Brown a few minutes under broiler. Spray with Bragg Aminos and dash of Bragg Vinegar and serve.

RED CABBAGE

2 lbs red cabbage, slice
½ tsp nutmeg
½ cup distilled water
2 large apples, core, chop
2 Tbsps Bragg Olive Oil
⅛ tsp Bragg Liquid Aminos
2 Tbsps raw honey
½ cup lemon juice

Slice cabbage; mix together with apples, lemon juice, nutmeg, honey, oil, Bragg Aminos and water. Cook until tender.

CARROTS

Carrots are a valuable source of vitamin A. When cooking carrots, as with all vegetables, use the smallest possible amount of water. For flavor enhancement, when serving carrots in a sauce, be sure to include the cooking water in the sauce, making it part of the liquid content.

CARAMELIZED CARROTS

2½ lbs carrots, cut in sticks or slices
2 Tbsps Bragg Organic Olive Oil
shake of Bragg Sprinkle (24 herbs & spices)
2 Tbsps raw honey
3 Tbsps distilled water

Place cut carrots in oiled casserole dish; add dash of Sprinkle, water and honey. Top with olive oil. Cover tightly and bake at 400°F for about 15 minutes or until tender. Serves 6.

CARROTS AND CELERY

3 cups carrots, thinly slice
¼ tsp Bragg Sprinkle
2 Tbsps Bragg Organic Olive Oil
2 cups green celery, chop thin
½ tsp Bragg Liquid Aminos
2½ Tbsps parsley, finely chop

Add the smallest amount of boiling water possible to the carrots and celery in a saucepan. Add Bragg Sprinkle and Bragg Aminos. Cover tightly and simmer for 10 minutes or until tender; toss with parsley and olive oil. Serves 6-8.

SPICED CARROTS CASSEROLE

15 baby carrots
2 Tbsps raw honey
1 cup boiling distilled water
¼ cup Bragg Organic Olive Oil
¼ tsp cinnamon
½ tsp ginger, fresh grate

Wash, brush carrots (don't scrape or pare), place in casserole. Now blend olive oil, honey, cinnamon and ginger together, add water, mix well and pour over carrots, cover tightly and bake at 350°F for 20 minutes or until tender. Serve in bowls with liquid, garnish with Bragg Nutritional Yeast. Serves 4-6.

GLAZED CARROTS WITH HONEY

6 carrots, ½ inch slices
1 Tbsp raw honey
1 Tbsp Bragg Organic Olive Oil
1 Tbsp organic orange rind, grate

Wash carrots thoroughly, slice into ½-inch thick rounds; cook in steamer basket until tender about 10 minutes in distilled water. Blend the raw honey, olive oil and orange rind in a saucepan. Bring to a boil, add steamed carrots with liquids and continue to simmer for 5 more minutes to glaze. Serves 4.

CARROTS WITH TURNIPS

4 carrots, slice
2 cloves garlic, mince
2 small red onions, chop
⅓ tsp Bragg Liquid Aminos
3 Tbsps soy cheese, grate
2 turnips, slice
3 Tbsps Bragg Olive Oil
½ tsp Bragg Sprinkle
2 Tbsps parsley, chop
½ cup distilled water

Wash carrots and turnips thoroughly, then slice. Place oil in a wok or pan with chopped onions and minced garlic. Cook slowly for 3 minutes. Add carrots and turnips, then Sprinkle, Bragg Aminos and water. Cook very slowly. When carrots and turnips are almost tender, add soy cheese and parsley. For delicious option add torn chard leaves last minute. Serves 4.

Carrots are rich in beta-carotene, dietary fiber, antioxidants, and minerals.

Make sure to get your daily dose of the naturally-occurring, cancer fighting biological substances that are abundant in onion, garlic, beans, legumes, soybeans, cabbage, cauliflower, broccoli, citrus fruits, etc. (page 73). The winner tomato, which contains the largest amount of the miracle phytochemicals!

CARROTS WITH PARSLEY

1 bunch young carrots, slice
1 Tbsp parsley, chop
2 Tbsps Bragg Organic Olive Oil
1 Tbsp raw honey

Wash the carrots and slice in rounds. Add a small amount of distilled water and cook in a covered pan until tender. Allow the cooking water to evaporate rather than draining it from the carrots by covering the pan and increasing the heat. Watch carefully to see that the carrots don't burn. When practically dry, add the olive oil, honey and parsley. Serves 3-5.

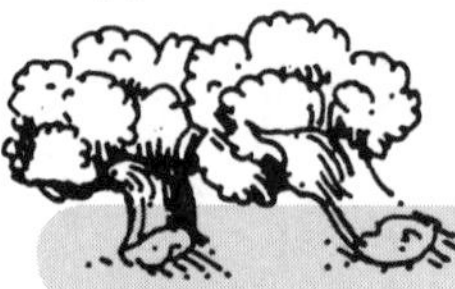

CAULIFLOWER

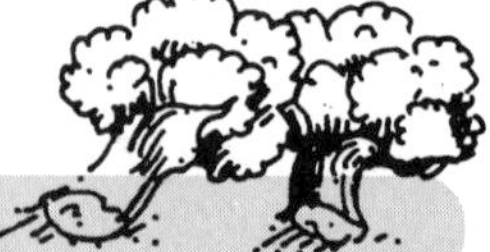

BAKED CAULIFLOWER

Remove florets from cauliflower head, and slice leaves and stems – it's all edible. Wash thoroughly. Prepare as follows:

½ cup whole-grain bread crumbs
1 cup soy milk or distilled water
3 Tbsps Bragg Organic Olive Oil
2 cloves garlic
shake of Bragg Sprinkle
½ cup grated soy cheese
3 cups cauliflower florets, leaves and stems

Brown garlic in oil. Place cauliflower florets in a baking dish. Cover with garlic-seasoned oil, Sprinkle, bread crumbs and soy milk or water. Bake in a 350°F oven for 30 minutes until tender. Cauliflower can be browned under the broiler before serving. Just before putting under broiler, top with grated soy cheese. Serves 4.

ROASTED CAULIFLOWER

1 head cauliflower, broken into florets
3 Tbsps Bragg Organic Olive Oil
½ tsp Bragg Liquid Aminos
shake of Bragg Sprinkle
shake of Bragg Kelp
parsley, chop

On large baking sheet, toss cauliflower florets with olive oil, Bragg Aminos, Kelp and Sprinkle. Bake at 350°F until tender and lightly brown, about 20 minutes. Place in bowl. Garnish with Braggberry or Bragg Ginger Dressing and parsley. Serves 4.

Various Types of Vegetarian Diets

- **Vegan** – Diet based on plant foods only. No animal products. No flesh foods, and no eggs and no dairy products of any kind.
- **Lacto Vegetarian:** No meat, fish or poultry, no eggs, but does include dairy.
- **Lacto-ovo Vegetarian:** No meat, fish or poultry, but does include milk & eggs.

Most vegetarians consume adequate protein and no animal protein. Most meat-eaters consume a diet that is 14% to 18% protein, lacto-ovo vegetarians consume a diet comprising of 12% to 14% protein, and vegan diets are only 10% to 12% protein. Excess animal protein is linked to higher risk for osteoporosis, kidney disease, heart disease and premature ageing. Research also indicates that animal protein raises blood cholesterol levels, while vegetable protein sources as beans and soy reduces blood cholesterol levels. For more info see Vegetarian Protein % Chart (page 138).

CELERY

Celery contains vitamin C and other nutrients that promote health, including *phalides*, which helps lower cholesterol. We love raw celery and add it to most all salads.

BRAISED CELERY

2 large red onions, slice
4 Tbsps Bragg Organic Olive Oil
shake of Bragg Sprinkle
4 cups finely cut celery
¼ cup distilled water
2 garlic cloves, mince

Place onions in baking dish. Brown celery in olive oil. Combine with onions, garlic, water and Sprinkle. Cook 5 minutes, then bake in 325°F oven for 15 minutes. Serves 6-8.

CELERY ROOT AND WILD RICE

⅓ cup wild rice
1⅓ cups distilled water

Cook rice in distilled water for 20 to 30 minutes. Do not stir. Drain off most of the water and steam until fluffy.

½ cup vegetable stock
1 celery root, thin slices
Egg Replacer equal to 1 egg
3 Tbsps red onion, chop
⅓ cup Bragg Olive Oil
spray of Bragg Liquid Aminos

Now mix and pour in oiled casserole dish with rice and bake in 350°F oven 30 minutes, or until celery root is tender. Serves 4.

CORN

Corn is best cooked soon after picking. For retaining flavor, steaming is best, usually takes 3 to 6 minutes. (We also love raw corn!) Serve with spray of Bragg Aminos and Olive Oil, then shake Bragg Sprinkle, Kelp and Bragg Nutritional Yeast Flakes over each ear of organic corn.

EGGPLANT

The eggplant, perhaps more than any other vegetable, lends itself to a variety of preparations. Almost any seasoning and herb within the boundary of the imagination can be put to use by the inventive cook with this delightful vegetable.

Eggplant, skin and all, can be prepared as an entrée, as a meat substitute, or as an accompanying vegetable. It can be boiled, baked, broiled or prepared in so many delicious ways that it can be the "luxury dish" of any meal.

Only a few of the hundreds of eggplant recipes can be included, but a good cook can successfully experiment with this versatile vegetable. Enjoy garden fun, grow eggplants.

The more natural food you eat, the more you'll enjoy radiant health and be able to promote the higher life of love and brotherhood. – Patricia Bragg, ND, PhD.

EGGPLANT AND OKRA

1 eggplant, un-peeled, chop
½ tsp Bragg Liquid Aminos
1 tsp Bragg Olive Oil
2 large tomatoes, dice
1 Tbsp bell pepper, chop
2 cups okra, slice
soy Parmesan cheese
2 cloves garlic, slice
⅓ cup chives or green onion tops
shake of Bragg Sprinkle

Sauté all of the ingredients except soy cheese, together in wok or pan for about 10-12 minutes, or until tender. Sprinkle with soy Parmesan cheese before serving. Serves 4-6.

EGGPLANT WITH HERBS AND SOY CHEESE

2 eggplants, slice
2 Tbsps Bragg Organic Olive Oil
2 cloves garlic, slice
1 cup tomato juice
½ cup chives or green onion tops, chop
¼ tsp rosemary
¼ tsp marjoram
¼ tsp Bragg Sprinkle
2 tsps lemon juice
1 Tbsp parsley, chop
½ cup grated soy cheese

Place sliced eggplant in oiled casserole dish. Pour about 1 cup of boiling water over it. Allow to bake in 325°F oven while mixing sauce containing all other ingredients, except soy cheese. Pour the sauce over eggplant, cover and allow to bake about 20 more minutes. When done, sprinkle with soy cheese and allow to lightly brown under broiler. Serves 4-6.

STUFFED BAKED EGGPLANT

1 large, firm eggplant
2 tsps grated soy cheese
½ tsp Bragg Liquid Aminos
1 Tbsp Bragg Organic Olive Oil
1 cup whole-grain bread crumbs
2 tomatoes, chop
1 green pepper, mince
1 cup celery, finely cut
2 Tbsps red onion, mince
shake of Bragg Sprinkle

Cut eggplant in half, remove pulp, leaving thick layer in hulls. Cut pulp into bits, mix with all ingredients. Fill eggplant hulls, place in baking casserole with one cup distilled water in bottom. Cover and bake 30 minutes or until done at 325°F. Serves 4.

EGGPLANT CASSEROLE

1 large eggplant
½ tsp Bragg Liquid Aminos
1 clove garlic, mince
shake of Bragg Sprinkle
¼ tsp sweet basil
4 Tbsps Bragg Organic Olive Oil
2 medium onions, chop
3 large tomatoes, chop
1 cup grated soy cheese

Slice eggplant in six slices without peeling; brush with olive oil. Broil until partly tender, turning once. Sauté onion and garlic in remaining oil; add tomatoes, Bragg Aminos and seasonings. Simmer until thickened, stirring often. Arrange eggplant slices, soy cheese and sauce in layers in oiled casserole dish, bake in 325°F oven for about 20 minutes. Serves 4-6.

GREEN LEAVES
NATURE'S CHOICE VEGETABLES

All green leafy vegetables: spinach, Swiss chard, kale, mustard greens, beet tops, turnip tops, etc. can be prepared (cooked or raw) to delight any taste. They are all rich in nature's colors, chlorophyll, vitamins and minerals. They are an excellent source of fiber, color and visual appeal. All greens adapt themselves to the same basic recipes. The recipes below can be used interchangeably with any of the green, leafy vegetables. The cooking time will vary. Mustard greens take longer to cook than spinach leaves, for instance, but all can be cooked by following the simple basic recipe pattern "cooked until tender".

PREPARATION OF GREEN LEAFY VEGETABLES

All green, leafy vegetables, particularly spinach and Swiss chard, tend to have sand and soil on the surface. Wash thoroughly. They should be rinsed in several cold water baths, or until sand and soil are removed. To cook, place in a saucepan with small amount of water, plus using water left on leaves from the washing. Cover, steam until tender. All green, leafy vegetables should be cooked only minutes at low temperature in steamer pan. Season and serve greens with liquid in bowls.

BASIC GREENS RECIPE NO. 1

2 lbs greens of choice
shake of Bragg Sprinkle
¼ tsp Bragg Liquid Aminos
1 small onion, mince
dash of nutmeg
2 Tbsps Bragg Organic Olive Oil

Steam greens and add olive oil, minced onion, nutmeg, Sprinkle and Bragg Aminos. Serve greens and liquid in bowls. Serves 4.

BASIC GREENS RECIPE NO. 2

2 cups cooked greens of choice
1 Tbsp pimento, chop
5 Tbsps Bragg Organic Olive Oil
½ tsp Bragg Liquid Aminos
2 Tbsps green pepper, chop
2 Tbsps onion, finely chop
2 Tbsps lemon juice
2 cloves garlic, mashed
shake of Bragg Sprinkle (24 herbs & spices)

Sauté green pepper, pimento, Sprinkle, garlic and onion in olive oil. Add cooked greens. Thoroughly heat, then add lemon juice and Bragg Aminos and serve in bowls. Serves 3.

Vegetables and fruits are endowed with naturally occurring pigments called flavonoids, which, among many other health benefits, may be a natural weapon in the weight-loss dept. See page 73 for list of food sources.

A laugh is just like sunshine. It freshens all the day. – Heart Warmers

BASIC GREENS RECIPE NO. 3

2 lbs steamed greens of choice
4 Tbsps Bragg Organic Olive Oil
1 Tbsp chives, chop
¼ tsp Bragg Liquid Aminos
2 cloves garlic, mince
1 tsp chervil
¼ tsp nutmeg
shake of Bragg Sprinkle

Steam the greens. Sauté garlic in olive oil, browning slightly. Place greens and liquid in saucepan, add Sprinkle, chervil and chives. Pour garlic and oil mixture over greens; stir in nutmeg and Bragg Aminos. Serve greens and liquid in bowls. Serves 4.

BASIC GREENS RECIPE NO. 4

2 lbs steamed greens
¼ tsp Bragg Liquid Aminos
2 Tbsps fresh squeezed lemon juice
2 cloves garlic, chop
4 Tbsps Bragg Organic Olive Oil

Brown garlic in olive oil, add lemon juice and Bragg Aminos. Remove garlic and pour the garlic flavored oil over steamed greens before serving. Serve greens and liquids in bowl. Serves 4.

BASIC GREENS RECIPE NO. 5

2 lbs greens
¼ cup green onions, chop
1 Tbsp Bragg Organic Olive Oil
½ cup parsley, chop
¼ tsp Bragg Liquid Aminos
½ tsp Bragg Sprinkle

Steam greens, parsley and onions for 3 minutes. Place greens and some liquid in oiled casserole, add Sprinkle, Bragg Aminos (*optional:* tofu) and bake at 325°F for 10 minutes. Serves 4.

BASIC GREENS RECIPE NO. 6

2 lbs greens
2 cloves garlic, crush
4 Tbsps Bragg Organic Olive Oil
⅓ tsp Bragg Liquid Aminos
½ cup Bragg Liquid Aminos consommé (page 54)

Steam greens. Prepare sauce by crushing garlic and add to consommé and olive oil. Heat sauce thoroughly and pour over greens before serving. Season with Bragg Aminos and Bragg Nutritional Yeast. Serves 4.

KALE

Kale is a highly nutritious, healthy vegetable, with powerful antioxidant properties and is anti-inflammatory. Kale is very high in beta carotene, vitamin K, A, and C and is rich in calcium.

KALE AND SOFT TOFU

4 cups kale, cut large
1 tsp lemon juice
¼ tsp sweet anise
1 Tbsp Bragg Organic Olive Oil
1 tsp raw honey
1 cup soft tofu, crumble

Place kale in saucepan. Add next four ingredients. Heat thoroughly, then reduce heat and stir in soft tofu. Serves 6.

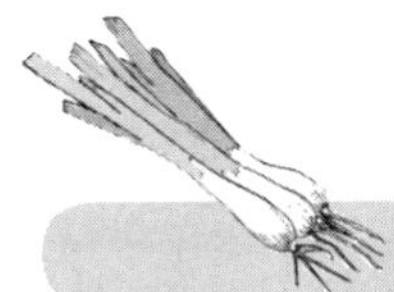

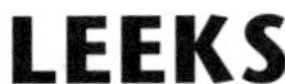

LEEKS

LEEKS AU GRATIN

1 bunch leeks, thinly slice
½ tsp Bragg Liquid Aminos
shake of Bragg Sprinkle
½ cup soy Parmesan cheese, grate

Wash and slice leeks. Steam for 15 minutes until tender. Drain. Arrange in oiled baking dish and add Sprinkle, Bragg Aminos and grated soy Parmesan cheese. Heat under broiler until cheese is golden brown. Serves 4.

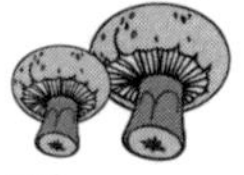

MUSHROOMS

The popular button mushroom is the most widely used and is readily available, fresh or canned. Asian mushrooms are high in protein, and have great health benefits: shiitake, reishi, oyster, portobello, porcini, chanterelle, crimini, etc., are available dried and fresh in many wholefood supermarkets, health stores and Asian markets. Mushrooms are a delicious addition to vegetables, soups, pastas and casseroles. They can also be used as an entrée. Experiment with different types of mushrooms in the following recipes.

BROILED BUTTON MUSHROOMS

8 large button mushrooms, fresh
2 Tbsps Bragg Organic Olive Oil
dash of Bragg Liquid Aminos
whole grain toast or lettuce

Wash mushrooms and remove stem (save stems for soups). Place mushrooms, cap side down in an oiled pan. Broil for three minutes, about 3 inches below flame. Turn over mushrooms and broil on the other side three more minutes. Put olive oil and Bragg Aminos in each cap; broil until warm in center. Serve on whole-grain toast or a bed of shredded lettuce. Serves 2-4.

AVOCADO AND MUSHROOMS

10 mushrooms, slice
2 Tbsps Bragg Organic Olive Oil
1 ripe avocado, dice
sliced pimento, fresh or canned
parsley, chop
1 tsp Bragg Liquid Aminos
corn tortilla, pita bread or whole-grain toast
soy Parmesan cheese and Bragg Nutritional Yeast

Wash mushrooms, slice and sauté with olive oil in wok or pan until tender (7-8 minutes). Add diced avocado, pimento and Bragg Aminos. Serve on warmed corn tortilla, pita bread, or whole-grain toast. Garnish with chopped parsley, Parmesan soy cheese and Bragg Nutritional Yeast Flakes and top with Braggberry Dressing. Serves 4.

Studies show both beta-carotene and vitamin C, found abundantly in fruits and vegetables, play vital roles in preventing heart disease and cancers.

MUSHROOM DELIGHT SANDWICH

Place following on slice of 100% whole-grain toasted bread: sliced mushrooms, sliced red onion, soy cheddar cheese and sliced tomatoes. Broil 5 minutes. Serve open face with alfalfa sprouts, lettuce leaves, Braggberry or Ginger & Sesame Dressing over top.

MUSHROOM - BROWN RICE BAKE

2 cups brown rice, cook
2 red onions, chop
½ tsp Bragg Sprinkle
1 Tbsp Bragg Liquid Aminos
1½ cups mushrooms, fresh
4 oz soy cheddar cheese, grate
Egg Replacer equal to 2 eggs
Bragg Organic Olive Oil
1 tsp Bragg Nutritional Yeast Flakes, garnish before serving

Wash and cook rice in boiling water until tender. Wash and roughly chop mushrooms. Sauté mushrooms and red onions in olive oil and Bragg Aminos for 10 minutes, then mix in Egg Replacer with grated soy cheese, Sprinkle, onions, mushrooms and rice. Place in oiled baking dish. Bake in 400°F oven for 15 minutes. Garnish with Bragg Nutritional Yeast. Serves 4.

STUFFED MUSHROOMS BAKE

14 large mushrooms
½ cup raw wheat germ
2 Tbsps onions, mince
3 garlic cloves, mince
3 Tbsps sunflower seeds, chop
1 Tbsp Bragg Liquid Aminos
2 Tbsps soy cheddar cheese, grate
⅓ cup Bragg Organic Olive Oil
¼ cup sunflower seeds, chop or whole (for topping)

Remove mushroom stems and finely chop. Add remaining ingredients and mix well. Top mushroom caps with this mixture and sprinkle with chopped or whole sunflower seeds. Lightly broil in pie tin until caps are tender. Serves 4.

MUSHROOM STUFFING FOR BAKED POTATO

2 large russet potatoes
½ cup mushrooms, finely chop
½ cup green onions, finely chop
1 Tbsp Bragg Organic Olive, per potato
⅓ tsp Bragg Sprinkle
⅓ cup soy cheese
shake Bragg Sprinkle (24 herbs & spices)

Before baking, scrub potatoes thoroughly so that skins can be eaten. Many important nutrients, particularly proteins, are contained in the skins. Bake potatoes for 1 hour at 400°F.

After baked, cut in half and scoop out the inside, leaving ¼ inch of the potato against the skin. In a mixing bowl, mash potatoes thoroughly and add mushrooms, green onions, soy cheese and 1 Tbsp olive oil per potato. Return mixture into potato shells, season with Bragg Sprinkle (24 herbs & spices) and bake 15 minutes or until soy cheese has melted. Serves 2-4.

Mushrooms are a rich source of Vitamin D, riboflavin, niacin and selenium.
– Dr. Winston Craig, Andrews University, Berrien Springs, Michigan

MUSHROOM - SOYBEAN PATTIES

1 cup mushrooms, chop
1½ cups cooked soybeans
Egg Replacer equal to 2 eggs
½ cup onions, finely chop
½ cup powdered soy milk
½ cup raw wheat germ
¼ cup crumbled soft tofu
1 Tbsp Bragg Liquid Aminos
shake of Bragg Sprinkle
½ cup sesame seeds

Mash soybeans to fine pulp in blender or mixing bowl. Add all other ingredients, mix well. If mixture is too dry, add small amounts of hot water until it can be shaped into patties. Dry mixture for about 15 minutes; then sauté patties in olive oil a few minutes, until both sides are brown. Serves 4-6.

PROTEIN MUSHROOM LOAF

2 cups mushrooms, finely chop
⅓ cup red onions, chop
⅓ cup green peppers, chop
½ cup tomatoes, diced
Egg Replacer equal to 2 eggs
2 cups whole-grain bread crumbs
½ cup soy cheese, grate
1 Tbsp Bragg Liquid Aminos
⅓ cup sunflower seeds, chop
⅓ cup walnuts, chop
2 cloves garlic, mash
½ tsp Bragg Sprinkle

Mix all ingredients together. Bake in oiled loaf pan 30 minutes in 375°F oven. Top with sauce (see pages 161-164). Serves 6.

BROWN RICE - MUSHROOM LOAF

2 cups cooked brown rice
1 cup mushrooms, chop
Egg Replacer equal to 2 eggs
½ tsp Bragg Sprinkle
½ cup red onions, mince
⅓ cup sunflower seeds, chop
½ cup soy cheese, grate
1 tsp Bragg Liquid Aminos

Combine all ingredients. Season as desired and pack in oiled casserole dish. Bake for 30 minutes in 375°F oven. Serves 4.

BUCKWHEAT GROATS WITH MUSHROOMS

1 cup buckwheat groats or kasha
Egg Replacer equal to 2 eggs
1 cup mushrooms, slice
1 tsp Bragg Liquid Aminos
2 cups distilled water
2 Tbsps Bragg Olive Oil
shake of Bragg Sprinkle
1 clove garlic, press

Beat the Egg Replacer and add to groats. Mix thoroughly coating the grains. In a heavy skillet, slowly brown mixture in olive oil. Add sliced mushrooms and garlic. Bring water to a boil and add the mixture together with the Bragg Aminos and Sprinkle. Mix well. Cover and cook very slowly, on low heat until all the liquid is absorbed and the kasha is light and fluffy. Serves 4.

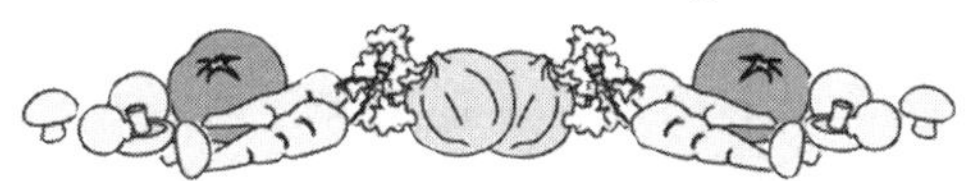

Plant based diets are low in fat and high in healthy fiber and other substances such as antioxidants, which are proving to be important in preventing cancer. – Cornell University Study

SAUTÉED MUSHROOMS ON WHOLE GRAIN TOAST

Wash mushrooms thoroughly. Separate large from the small, cutting large mushrooms down center of stem. Sauté in heavy skillet, using generous amount of Bragg Organic Olive Oil and the following: mushrooms, chopped garlic (optional), 1 tsp Bragg Aminos, ½ tsp Bragg Sprinkle and ½ tsp lemon juice. Gently stir with wooden spoon, until done. Arrange generous amount on toasted whole grain bread, topping with the sauce from the sautéed mixture.

MUSHROOM BURGERS

1 small onion, finely chop
Egg Replacer equal to 1 egg
Bragg Organic Olive Oil
2 cups mushrooms, finely chop
1 tsp Bragg Liquid Aminos
1 cup whole-grain bread crumbs

Mix all ingredients well and form into small burgers. Sauté in olive oil, turning until brown on both sides. Serves 4-6.

MUSHROOM - LENTIL BURGERS

1 cup mushrooms, finely chop
3 Tbsps Bragg Organic Olive Oil
1 cup whole-grain bread crumbs
1 clove garlic, press (optional)
½ cup parsley, finely chop
shake of Bragg Sprinkle
½ cup red onion, chop
2 cups cooked lentils
1 Tbsp Bragg Liquid Aminos
shake of Bragg Kelp

Mash lentils lightly. Add remainder of ingredients, except bread crumbs and olive oil. Form the mixture into patties. Coat or roll in finely ground whole-grain bread crumbs or potato flour. Heat the olive oil in a skillet and lightly sauté the patties on both sides until brown. Serves 4-6.

OKRA

Okra has the peculiar property of being a gentle, slippery bulk, which makes it excellent for those whose diets cannot tolerate roughage. Because of its blandness, it should be combined with either vegetables of decided flavor or a herbal seasoning. Okra is perfect for soups, especially with potatoes.

TOMATO OKRA

1 lb okra, slice
1 red onion, chop
2 cups tomatoes, chop
½ tsp Bragg Liquid Aminos
1 Tbsp Bragg Organic Olive Oil
½ tsp Bragg Sprinkle

Cook okra in olive oil until tender; add tomatoes, onions, Bragg Aminos and Sprinkle (24 herbs & spices). Simmer until done. This recipe is also delicious with 1 teaspoon sweet basil added at end of cooking. Serve in small bowls. Serves 2-4.

Mushrooms are the only source of Vitamin D in the produce aisle.
– visit informative web: *www.mushroominfo.com*

OKRA SPECIALTY

2 cups okra, thinly slice
2 large tomatoes, chop
2 cloves garlic, mince
1 large red onion, slice
1 tsp Bragg Liquid Aminos
shake of Bragg Sprinkle

Cut and mix ingredients. Add enough distilled water to steam until tender. Serve in shallow bowls with liquid. Serves 4.

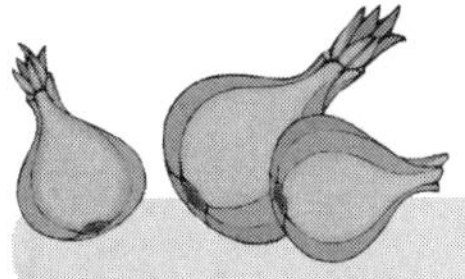

ONIONS

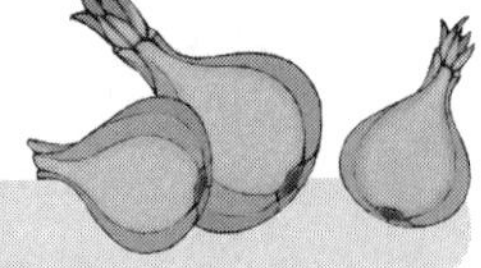

ONIONS AND TOFU

2 cups red onions, slice
1 package firm tofu, slice
1 Tbsp Bragg Organic Olive Oil
shake of Bragg Sprinkle
1 tsp Bragg Liquid Aminos
shake of Bragg Kelp

In wok, lightly sauté onions, tofu, Bragg Aminos, Kelp and Sprinkle in olive oil for 4-6 minutes. Cover, let steam 10 minutes or until onions are slightly brown. Serves 4-6.

WHOLE ONIONS WITH SOY CHEESE

6 medium-sized onions
¼ tsp Bragg Liquid Aminos
¾ cup soy cheese, grate
¼ tsp Bragg Sprinkle

Peel outer skins, slice even onion tops. Steam 15 minutes. Place up in oiled casserole. Season with Sprinkle and Bragg Aminos. Cover onions with grated soy cheese (croutons optional). Bake at 375°F for few minutes until warmed through. Serves 4.

NUTTED ONION CUPS

6 large red onions
½ cup walnuts, chop
¼ cup celery, dice
shake of Bragg Sprinkle
1 clove garlic, mince
¼ cup Bragg Olive Oil
¼ cup parsley, mince
1 Tbsp Bragg Liquid Aminos
¼ cup soy Parmesan cheese, grate
1 cup dry whole-grain bread crumbs

Peel outer skin and cut thin slice from onion tops. Center onions upright in steamer basket in saucepan in which they fit snugly, add water and cover pot. Steam 15 minutes or until onions are tender, cool and scoop out centers. Chop centers and set aside.

Meanwhile, heat olive oil in heavy skillet and cook celery and scooped out onion in remaining oil until celery is tender. Add Sprinkle, garlic, parsley and dried bread crumbs. Mix well and remove from heat. Stir in chopped nuts, soy cheese and Bragg Aminos. Spoon mixture into onion cups. Arrange in oiled baking dish and bake in 325°F oven for 15 minutes. Serves 6.

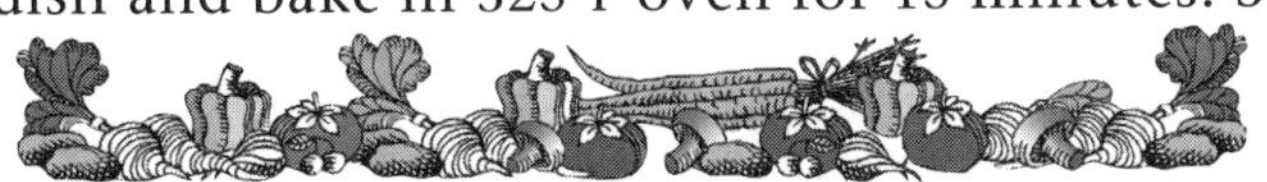

Onions are a good source of vitamin C, potassium, dietary fiber and folic acid. They contain calcium, iron and are high in protein. Onions are low in sodium and contain no fat. – National Onion Association, www.onions-usa.org

We prefer red onions, they are our favorite – raw and cooked. – PB

PARSNIPS

Due to improper cooking, the parsnip has gained a negative reputation. Traditionally parsnips have been prepared with sweeteners, but the sugar content of parsnips is higher than most vegetables and, for this reason, does not require excessive amounts of added sweetener. We prefer these methods given here:

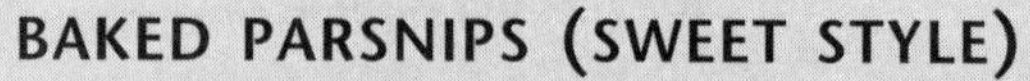

BAKED PARSNIPS (SWEET STYLE)

3 cups cooked parsnips, slice
⅓ cup raw honey
¼ cup Bragg Organic Olive Oil

Place sliced, cooked parsnips in oiled casserole dish and drizzle with honey. Bake at 400°F for 15 minutes. Serves 6.

PARSNIP PATTIES

6-8 parsnips, thin slice
1 red onion, mince
2 Tbsps Bragg Organic Olive Oil
whole-grain dry bread crumbs
¼ tsp Bragg Sprinkle (24 herbs & spices)

Wash and cut young parsnips into thin slices. Steam in small amount of purified water until tender. Mash and add Sprinkle, olive oil and small amount of very finely minced onion. Mix well; shape into small patties. Dip and roll in whole-grain bread crumbs; place on baking sheet and bake at 350°F oven for 20 minutes. Serves 6.

PEAS

Peas, like beans, have high protein content and are a good source of dietary fiber. I love raw peas in salads. – PB

PEAS BASQUE

2 lbs tender young peas
4 leaves Romaine lettuce
1 Tbsp Bragg Organic Olive Oil
shake of Bragg Sprinkle

Place olive oil in saucepan, add peas, Sprinkle and cover with lettuce leaves that have been rinsed in cold water. Cook over low heat until peas are tender. Serves 4-6.

PEAS EN CASSEROLE

4 small red onions, dice
1 cup hot distilled water
4 cups fresh, can or frozen peas
½ tsp mint, chop
2 Tbsps Bragg Organic Olive Oil
½ tsp Bragg Sprinkle

Place all ingredients in casserole dish. Cover, cook in 350°F oven 20 minutes. Serve in bowls and top each serving with shake of Braggberry Dressing and Nutritional Yeast. Serves 5-6.

Peas are a good source of vitamin A, C, folate, thiamine, iron and phosphorus, rich in protein and fiber and low in fat. No matter what season, freshly frozen organic garden peas are available throughout the year. – www.Peas.org

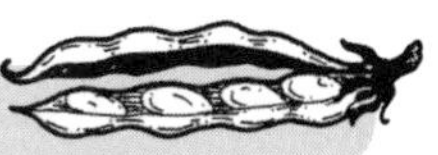

PEAS IN ONION SAUCE

2 lbs peas, shelled
2 Tbsps Bragg Organic Olive Oil
1 red onion, finely chop
shake of Bragg Sprinkle

Cook peas until tender, about 5 minutes, in a small amount of water. Sauté chopped onion in olive oil, then add cooked peas and Sprinkle, heat slowly in a covered pan. Serves 4.

PEAS & CARROTS WITH 24 HERBS & SPICES

2 cups peas, shelled
½ tsp of Bragg Sprinkle
1 cup carrots, large grate
1 tsp Bragg Organic Olive Oil

Cook peas, carrots and Sprinkle (24 herbs & spices) in small amount of water until tender. Add olive oil and serve. Serves 2.

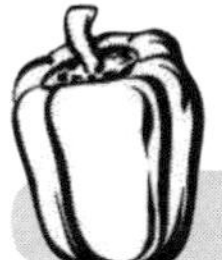

PEPPERS

SAUERKRAUT - STUFFED PEPPERS

3 medium-sized bell peppers
½ tsp Bragg Liquid Aminos
1 red onion, slice thin
½ cup whole-grain bread crumbs
½ cup sauerkraut
¼ tsp Bragg Sprinkle

After removing seeds and partitions, parboil peppers for 5 minutes. Mix Bragg Aminos, onion, sauerkraut and Sprinkle and fill empty peppers. Place in oiled baking dish, top with whole-grain bread crumbs, and pour half-inch of water into pan. Bake at 350°F for 30 minutes. Serve hot. Serves 3.

SPINACH WITH PEPPERS

1½ Tbsps bell pepper, mince
1½ Tbsps red onion, mince
½ Tbsp pimento, mince
1 Tbsp lemon juice
2 cups cooked spinach, mince
3 Tbsps Bragg Organic Olive Oil
½ tsp Bragg Liquid Aminos
½ tsp Bragg Sprinkle

Sauté green pepper, pimento and onion in olive oil 10 minutes. Add spinach, lemon juice, Sprinkle and Bragg Aminos. Serves 3.

POTATOES

Potatoes are low in fiber, which makes them practical for people on soft food diets. They are easily digested and assimilated. Potato skins are highly nutritious and should be eaten with the rest of the potato. Baking is one of the best ways to prepare potatoes.

POTATOES AU GRATIN

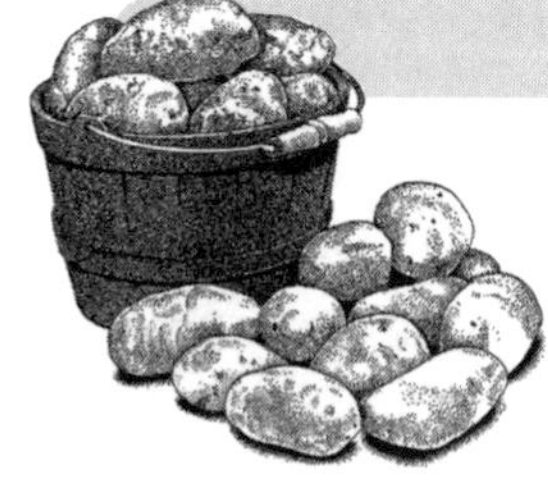

Thinly slice 6 medium russet potatoes and four red onions. Alternately arrange in layers in oiled baking dish, season with Bragg Sprinkle and Bragg Aminos, and top with a layer of grated soy cheese. Bake in a 350°F oven for 30 minutes until done. Serves 4-6.

POTATOES STUFFED WITH SOY CHEESE

3 large potatoes
¼ lb soy cheese, grate
Seasonings of your choice

Scrub and dry potatoes. Use apple corer to remove center of each potato. Fill each center cavity with soy cheese and seasonings of choice. Plug ends with pieces of remaining potato. Bake at 400°F until tender, 30-45 minutes. Serves 3.

ZESTY POTATO CASSEROLE

2 cups raw potatoes, slice
2 Tbsps Bragg Olive Oil
½ tsp Bragg Sprinkle
¼ cup parsley, chop
1 clove garlic, slice
1 cup can or fresh tomatoes
¼ cup distilled water
1 cup soy Parmesan cheese, grate

Alternate layers of potatoes and tomatoes in casserole dish. Combine olive oil, water, Sprinkle, garlic and parsley. Pour over potatoes and tomatoes. Cover, bake 375°F 30 minutes, until tender. Top with Parmesan cheese, Bragg Nutritional Yeast. Serves 3.

HEALTH-BAKED FRENCH FRIES

5 large white potatoes
Spray of Bragg Liquid Aminos
5 Tbsps Bragg Organic Olive Oil
shake of Bragg Sprinkle

Cut potatoes lengthwise into long strips. Arrange in baking pan so they don't overlap. Pour olive oil and shake Sprinkle over them. Bake 450°F for 30 minutes or until tender, turning occasionally. Before serving spray with Bragg Aminos and top with Bragg Nutritional Yeast Flakes. Serves 4.

STUFFED BAKED POTATOES

Bake three large russet potatoes at 400°F for one hour. When done, cut in half, scoop out up to ¼ inch of the skin. Place the scooped out portion into a mixing bowl and add:

3 Tbsps Bragg Organic Olive Oil
½ cup green onions, finely chop
1 cup soy cheese, grate
shake Bragg Sprinkle & Aminos

Spoon the mashed mixture into half potato shells; add Sprinkle and spray of Bragg Aminos. Heat in 375°F oven for 10 minutes to allow cheese to melt. Top with Bragg Nutritional Yeast. Serves 6.

Vegetarians have the best, healthiest diet. They have the lowest rates of coronary disease of any group in the U.S.! Some people scoff at vegetarians, but they have a fraction of our heart attack rate and only 40% of our cancer rate. They out-live other men and women who eat meat.
– William Castelli, M.D., world famous heart disease researcher

---

To our minds the greatest mistake a person can make is to remain ignorant when surrounded every day of his life, by the knowledge he needs to grow and be healthy, happy and successful. It's all there. We need only to observe, read, learn and apply. – Paul C. Bragg, ND, PhD., Originator Health Stores

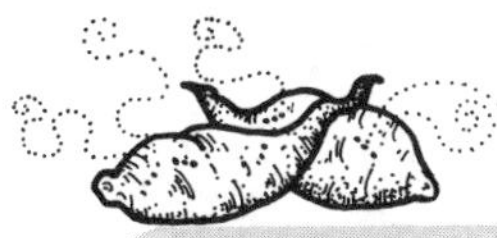

SWEET POTATOES

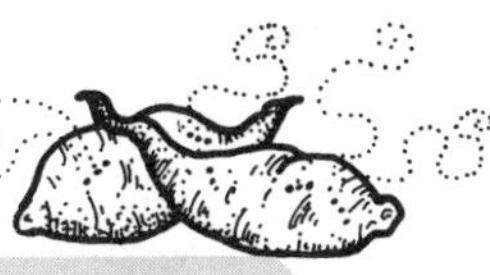

MAPLE - CANDIED SWEET POTATOES

3 medium sweet potatoes
½ Tbsp Bragg Organic Olive Oil
¼ cup distilled water
¼ cup 100% pure maple syrup
½ cup unsweetened apple juice

Steam potatoes in jackets 20 minutes. Then put 1 inch slices into baking dish. Heat remaining ingredients to boiling, pour sauce over potatoes, bake 300°F for 15 minutes. Serves 4.

SWEETS IN BAKED APPLES

2 Tbsps Bragg Organic Olive Oil
2 Tbsps raw honey
3 large apples
2 Tbsps raisins
2 medium cooked yams (or sweet potatoes), mash

Cut a slice from top of each apple, and core. Scoop out inside of apples. Scallop edge with a sharp knife, as desired. Combine olive oil, mashed sweet potatoes, honey and raisins. Mix well. Fill apple shells. Place in baking dish (covered optimal) with small amount of water. Bake at 375°F for 20-30 minutes. Serves 3.

SAUERKRAUT

HAWAIIAN SAUERKRAUT*

½ pound sauerkraut, with juice
½ pound red cabbage, shred
2 Tbsps Bragg Organic Olive Oil
1 cup fresh/can pineapple, dice
1 tsp fresh ginger, grate
½ tsp Bragg Liquid Aminos

Sauerkraut comes in its own juice. Shred red cabbage and simmer all ingredients except Bragg Aminos and olive oil for 15 minutes. Cool, add olive oil and Bragg Aminos. Serve hot or cold. Delicious side dish or salad topping. Serves 4-6.

SQUASH

BAKED ACORN SQUASH

3 acorn squash
⅓ cup raw honey
⅓ cup Bragg Organic Olive Oil

Cut three acorn squash in half lengthwise. Remove seeds. Brush lightly with olive oil. Lay halves flat side-down in a baking pan with ½ cup distilled water in bottom. Bake 30 minutes at 350°F. Turn face up; brush with mixture of ⅓ cup honey and ⅓ cup olive oil. Bake 10 minutes until tender and golden, brushing frequently with honey/oil mixture. Serves 6.

**The Bragg* Health Sauerkraut Recipe Book *was first published in the 1950's. Soon it will be available as a Bragg e-book on demand. Check web:* www.bragg.com

ZUCCHINI WITH HERBS

1 lb zucchini, cut thin rounds
1 cup distilled boiling water
2 Tbsps parsley, chop
5 tomatoes, chop
1 Tbsp Bragg Liquid Aminos
soy Parmesan cheese, grate
2 cloves garlic, chop
shake of Bragg Sprinkle
1 tsp sweet basil
1 red onion, chop
2 Tbsps Bragg Olive Oil
shake Bragg Nutritional Yeast

Wash, cut zucchini in thin rounds. In wok sauté onion, garlic in olive oil until slightly brown. Add zucchini and seasonings with cup boiling water, cook 10 minutes. Add tomatoes, cook few minutes more. Serve in bowls, top with parsley, soy Parmesan cheese and Bragg Nutritional Yeast. Serves 8.

SQUASH AND LIMA BEANS

3 cups lima beans, fresh or frozen
2 cups boiling distilled water
4 cups squash or zucchini, slice
1 tsp Bragg Liquid Aminos
1 cup red onion, mince
shake of Bragg Kelp
3 Tbsps whole-grain flour
¼ tsp paprika
3 Tbsps Bragg Olive Oil
½ tsp Bragg Sprinkle

Combine lima beans, Bragg Aminos, seasonings and boiling water in pan, cover. Bring to boil, cook until tender. Add thinly sliced squash. Continue cooking (covered) for 10 more minutes until tender, stirring occasionally. Drain, reserve liquid. Meanwhile, heat olive oil in wok; add onions and sauté until tender. Blend in remaining ingredients. Measure one cup of reserved liquid; add to onion mixture and cook until thickened, stirring constantly. Pour over squash and beans. Heat and serve in bowls. Serves 6-8.

SQUASH SURPRISE

1½ lbs summer squash or zucchini
2 large tomatoes, chop
½ tsp Bragg Liquid Aminos
pinch dill seeds
1 red onion, chop
shake of Bragg Sprinkle

Cut and mix ingredients. Cook 10 minutes until tender. *Variation:* Add torn chard, kale, or greens of choice. Serve in bowls with liquids. Serves 6.

BROILED STUFFED SQUASH

4 large summer squash
½ cup soy cheese, crumble
⅓ cup raw wheat germ or small dry whole-grain bread crumbs
1 Tbsp Bragg Liquid Aminos
1 clove garlic, press
1 tsp Bragg Olive Oil
shake of Bragg Sprinkle

Cut off stem end of squash. Blanch in boiling water for 4 minutes. Drain and scoop out inside, leaving shells whole. Combine squash pulp, olive oil, garlic, Bragg Aminos, Sprinkle and wheat germ or small dry whole-grain bread crumbs with soy cheese. Fill shells with mixture and place in shallow baking pan. Broil 5 minutes to melt soy cheese. Serves 4-6.

TOMATOES

Tomatoes are rich in Vitamin C, phytochemicals and other nutrients. (See Phytochemical Chart on page 73.) They are one of the highest forms of miracle phytochemicals and are a sturdy vegetable, in spite of their delicate delicious flavor and perishability. They are one of our most adaptable vegetables and can be used as a main dish when properly seasoned, or combined with small amounts of other vegetables, pastas or dishes as a flavor enhancement.

BAKED TOMATOES

Pick firm, medium-sized tomatoes. Cut out a small piece of tomato where stem meets tomato. Lay close together in a baking pan. Put small amount of Bragg Organic Olive Oil and dash of Bragg Aminos and Sprinkle in each cavity. You may also stuff tomatoes by scooping out half of the insides and fill with dry whole-grain bread crumbs, crumbled tofu or soy cheese. Bake at 350°F until done.

BROILED TOMATOES

1 tomato for each serving
whole-grain bread crumbs
Bragg Organic Olive Oil
Spray of Bragg Liquid Aminos

Wash ripe tomatoes, halve crosswise, brush olive oil on top, then on top sprinkle dry or toasted whole-grain bread crumbs. Place face-up under broiler 8 minutes or until lightly browned. Spray on Bragg Aminos and Bragg Nutritional Yeast.

TOMATOES CREOLE

3 green bell peppers, chop
1 red onion, mince
1 tsp Bragg Liquid Aminos
2 Tbsps Bragg Olive Oil
6 large tomatoes
2 garlic cloves, mince
shake of Bragg Sprinkle
shake of Bragg Sea Kelp

Cut green bell peppers into medium-sized pieces; quarter the tomatoes. Put minced onion, garlic and oil in wok or pan, and sauté for 5 minutes. Add tomatoes, bell peppers, Bragg Aminos, Bragg Kelp and Sprinkle. Mix well, cook slowly until bell peppers are tender. Serves 4-6.

HOW TO SKIN TOMATOES IF DESIRED

Bring a large pot of water to boil and then turn off heat. Meanwhile, fill a pan with cold water. Using a large serving spoon, place one tomato at a time into the boiled water. After one minute, remove the tomato from the boiled water and put into cold water. After one minute remove tomato from cold water, then pull off skins. The skins will easily pull away from the tomato. *But we prefer the skins. – PB*

ONION TOMATO BAKE

15 spring onions and green tops
1 Tbsp grated soy Parmesan cheese
½ cup whole-grain bread crumbs
2 Tbsps Bragg Organic Olive Oil
6 ripe tomatoes
1 tsp Bragg Liquid Aminos
1 Tbsp raw honey
shake of Bragg Sprinkle

Chop the green spring onions and tops into small circlets. Cut tomatoes into small sections; combine onions, tomatoes, Bragg Aminos, Sprinkle and honey in oiled casserole dish. Sprinkle with whole-grain bread crumbs and top with oil. Bake about 20 minutes at 350°F. Garnish with grated soy Parmesan cheese and Bragg Nutritional Yeast. Serves 4-6.

SPINACH STUFFED TOMATO

6 large ripe tomatoes, halve
2 Tbsps Bragg Organic Olive Oil
1 tsp Bragg Liquid Aminos
Soy Parmesan cheese, grated
2 cups cooked spinach
½ red onion, finely chop
shake of Bragg Sprinkle (24 herbs & spices)

Prepare tomatoes for stuffing by scooping out half of insides. Carefully wash spinach and stems, drain. Lightly steam without added water. The small amount of water left on the leaves from washing is enough to cook spinach in its own juice. Cook 2-3 minutes, until tender. Combine cooked spinach with olive oil, finely chopped onion, Bragg Aminos and Sprinkle. Stuff tomato shells, place in oiled casserole dish, bake 10-15 minutes at 350°F. At the last minute sprinkle with grated soy Parmesan cheese. Serves 6.

CORNBREAD STUFFED TOMATOES

6 large tomatoes
½ cup green or red bell pepper, finely chop
2 Tbsps Bragg Organic Olive Oil
1 tsp Bragg Liquid Aminos
⅓ tsp Bragg Sprinkle
2 Tbsps parsley, mince
2 cups cornbread, coarsely crumble
2 cloves garlic, press
Soy Parmesan cheese, grated

Cut thin slice from stem end of each tomato. Gently spoon out seeds and most of tomato pulp, leaving firm shells. Chop ½ cup of cut-out tomato pulp and set aside. Turn tomatoes upside down to drain. Saute pepper in olive oil until tender, but not brown. Add Bragg Aminos, Sprinkle, garlic, parsley, cornbread, chopped tomatoes. Mix lightly, then stuff loosely into the tomato shells. Place in oiled shallow baking dish. Bake at 350°F for 15 minutes. At last minute sprinkle with grated soy Parmesan cheese. Serves 6.

Anyone who stops learning is old, whether 20 or 80. Anyone who keeps learning stays youthful. The greatest thing in life is to keep your mind young. – Henry Ford

---

Paul Bragg before putting his head on his pillow each night said he had to learn something new before going to sleep. Good youthful habit to follow.

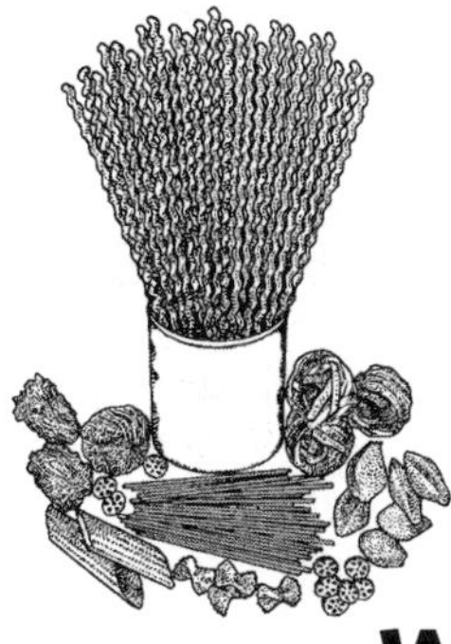

Chapter 9

Patricia's Favorite Vegetarian Recipes

WHOLE GRAIN PASTA

Pasta is an easy dish to prepare. It meets the needs of a cook who has little time and wants to make healthy meals. Sauces can be prepared ahead and frozen while pasta can be made fresh in minutes. Pasta is available in fresh or dried varieties. Be sure to read the labels; buy pasta made with whole, organically-grown grains! Avoid all bleached grains.

Nutritionists world-wide proclaim the health benefits of the Mediterranean diet. It is low in the bad fats and has good nutrition, rich in healthy fats (olive oil). It's moderate in protein, rich in vitamins and healthy carbohydrates. Remember, to retain nutritional value, pasta should not be overcooked.

PASTA WITH BASIL (PESTO) SAUCE

1 lb pasta
36 basil leaves
3 cloves garlic
½ cup pine nuts
1 tsp Bragg Liquid Aminos
½ cup Bragg Organic Olive Oil
1 cup hard soy cheese, grate
⅓ tsp Bragg Sprinkle

To make sauce, wash and thoroughly dry basil leaves. Place clean, dry leaves in food processor with garlic. Add nuts, cheese, Bragg Aminos, Sprinkle and olive oil while processor is running. Meanwhile, cook pasta. Place cooked pasta on dish and drizzle sauce over pasta. Now spray top with Bragg Aminos and shake Bragg Nutritional Yeast. Serves 4-6.

RAVIOLI WITH WALNUTS

36 vegetarian ravioli or
1 lb whole-grain pasta
½ cup soy cheese, grate
Bragg Liquid Aminos to taste
½ cup soy milk
1 cup shelled walnuts
2 Tbsp Bragg Organic Olive Oil
Bragg Sprinkle to taste

Chop nuts, add soy cheese, soy or rice milk, and olive oil to make a sauce. Add Sprinkle and Bragg Aminos to taste. Cook ravioli or pasta. Drain and coat with the sauce. Serves 4-6.

The desire for salty foods is an acquired taste. Your tastebuds can be retrained to appreciate the true flavors of foods & herbs. – Neal Barnard, M.D., President, Physicians Committee for Responsible Medicine (www.pcrm.org)

PASTA WITH SOY CHEESE AND WALNUTS

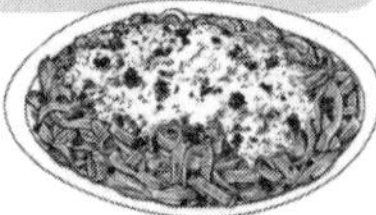

1 lb pasta of choice
3 cloves garlic, mince
1 cup walnuts, chop
3 Tbsp Bragg Olive Oil
¼ tsp Bragg Sprinkle
1 cup soy cheese, grate

Lightly sauté garlic in olive oil. Then add chopped walnuts to garlic and oil mixture. Stir 10 minutes. Remove from heat. Cook whole grain pasta. Toss drained pasta with grated soy cheese, walnut sauce and top with Bragg Aminos and Bragg Nutritional Yeast. Serves 4-6.

ITALIAN MACARONI AND BEANS

16 oz cooked Great Northern beans
½ cup red onions, chop
2 cloves garlic, mince
1½ cups cooked macaroni
4 Tbsps hard soy cheese, grated
1 tsp Bragg Liquid Aminos
¼ tsp Bragg Sprinkle
2 medium zucchinis, grate
½ cup tomato sauce
¾ cup distilled water

Preheat oven to 400°F. Combine all ingredients: zucchini, macaroni, beans, garlic and onion, except 2 tsps of grated soy cheese. Now pour macaroni, zucchini and bean mixture into lightly oiled casserole dish. Bake for 20 minutes. Last 10 minutes sprinkle top with grated soy cheese. Serves 4-6.

PASTA WITH GARLIC SAUCE

2 cups soy cheese
6 to 8 cloves garlic
2 tsps Bragg Liquid Aminos
8 oz cooked whole-grain thin spaghetti
4 Tbsps rice milk
¼ tsp Bragg Sprinkle
shake of Bragg Kelp
hard soy cheese, grate

Place all ingredients except cooked spaghetti in blender or food processor. Mix until completely smooth. Place in double boiler on medium heat. Bring to a simmer. Pour over cooked spaghetti, toss gently. Top with grated soy cheese. Serves 4-6.

BROCCOLI AND PINE NUT PASTA

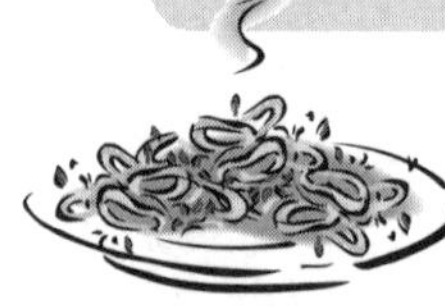

12 oz pasta
1 lb broccoli
pinch of cayenne
2 Tbsps pine nuts
½ tsp Bragg Liquid Aminos
3 cloves garlic, mince
1 Tbsp Bragg Organic Olive Oil
28 oz can crushed tomatoes
shake of Bragg Sprinkle (24 herbs & spices)

Cook pasta. Drain. Steam broccoli 10 minutes. Now sauté garlic, cayenne, pine nuts in olive oil in large wok for 1 minute, add tomatoes, cook medium heat 5-10 minutes. Stir in steamed broccoli. Serve over cooked pasta. Add Sprinkle, Bragg Aminos and Bragg Nutritional Yeast over top. Serves 6.

Sea vegetables (sea weed, kelp, etc.) are nutrient rich plants that can help rid the body of toxins and help us ward off cancer. Eating a mere ounce of seaweed a week can provide crucial minerals and healthy doses of vitamins C, E, B complex, plus beta-carotene and a reliable source of dietary iodine. – Delicious Living Magazine

PASTA WITH PEANUT SAUCE

12 oz pasta of choice
1 cup distilled water
3 green onions, mince
2 to 3 cloves garlic, mince
1 Tbsp Bragg Liquid Amino
1 tsp ginger, mince
1 Tbsp raw honey
shake of Bragg Sprinkle
⅔ cup creamy peanut butter
2 Tbsps Bragg Apple Cider Vinegar

Cook pasta. While pasta is cooking, whisk together remaining ingredients in saucepan. Heat slowly until sauce is smooth and slightly thickened. Add more water if sauce becomes too thick. When pasta is tender, drain and toss with sauce. Serves 6.

VEGGIE LASAGNE

12 oz whole-grain lasagne noodles
1 medium carrot, large grate
½ cup distilled/purified water
2 cups fresh mushrooms, slice
28 oz can of tomato sauce
½ tsp Bragg Sprinkle (24 herbs & spices)
½ cup fresh parsley, chop
½ tsp thyme and fennel seed
10 oz cooked spinach, chop
1 red onion, chop
3 garlic cloves, mince
15 oz can tomatoes, chop
shake of Bragg Kelp
pinch of cayenne
1 lb firm tofu, mash
1 Tbsp Bragg Liquid Aminos

Cook onion and carrot in distilled water in wok until tender. Add mushrooms and garlic; continue cooking until mushrooms are brown. Stir in tomatoes, tomato sauce, seasonings and simmer 10 minutes. Combine tofu, parsley, Bragg Aminos in a bowl. Preheat oven to 350°F. Spread 2 cups sauce in bottom 9x12" casserole dish. Now add layer uncooked noodles, then half tofu mixture and half of spinach. Spread half remaining sauce over this. Alternate layers with remaining noodles, tofu mixture, spinach and sauce. Cover casserole, bake 300°F for 1½ hours. Let stand 5 minutes before serving, then sprinkle on Bragg Nutritional Yeast. Serves 6.

STUFFED PASTA SHELLS

1 lb whole-grain pasta shells
1 lb soft tofu, drain, crumble
1 cup spinach, chop
2 cloves garlic, mince
½ cup soy cheese, (grated for topping)
½ cup fresh basil, chop
½ cup soy Parmesan cheese
⅓ tsp Bragg Sprinkle
⅓ tsp Bragg Sea Kelp
Egg Replacer equal to 2 eggs
2 Tbsps Bragg Organic Olive Oil

Cook pasta shells according to package. Meanwhile combine remaining ingredients in large bowl, mix thoroughly. Drain pasta shells, stuff each one with large spoonful of mixture, place in oiled 6x9" glass baking dish. Bake 350°F for 30 minutes. Top with grated soy cheese, return to oven 5 minutes. As serving sprinkle Bragg Nutritional Yeast on top. Serves 4-6.

Keep a rainbow in your heart and a smile on your face and live the Bragg Healthy Lifestyle and miracles will happen! – Beatrex Quntanna

ASPARAGUS - BEET GREENS — PASTA WITH ALMONDS

1 lb whole-grain spaghetti
2 cups beet greens
1 cup distilled water
2 tomatoes, chop
chili powder (to taste)
crushed red pepper flakes
1 Tbsp Bragg Nutritional Yeast
16 asparagus stalks, slice
1 tsp Bragg Organic Olive Oil
¼ cup slivered almonds
Bragg Sprinkle (to taste)
4 cloves garlic, slice

Cook spaghetti. Meanwhile, tear the beet greens into large pieces and cook in pot with 1 cup of distilled water for 2 minutes. Drain and save liquid. Lightly sauté garlic with olive oil in wok. Remove and set aside. Add almonds to wok and sauté. Reserve almonds. Steam asparagus for 5 minutes. Add beet greens, asparagus, tomatoes and ½ cup of reserved beet liquid to wok. Season with chili powder, Sprinkle and crushed red pepper flakes. Toss vegetables with cooked spaghetti. Sprinkle with reserved garlic, almonds and Bragg Nutritional Yeast. Serves 4-6.

SOBA — TOFU DINNER

5 garlic cloves, mince
1 tsp onion powder
½ lb soba noodles
freshly chopped parsley
½ cup Bragg Organic Olive Oil
¼ tsp Bragg Liquid Aminos
2 lbs firm tofu, cut bite-sized pieces
Bragg Sprinkle (to taste)

Lightly heat oil in heavy skillet. Add garlic, onion powder, tofu, Sprinkle, Bragg Aminos. Sauté about 5 minutes until garlic is golden, stir constantly. Prepare soba noodles according to package. Drain. Add noodles to garlic sauce, and cook 5 minutes. Sprinkle with parsley and Bragg Nutritional Yeast. Serve immediately. Serves 4-6.

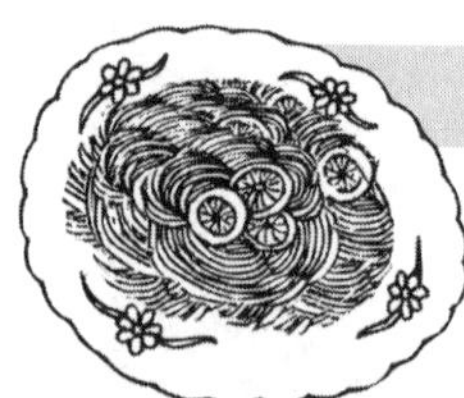

SPAGHETTI WITH CONFETTI

1 lb whole-grain spaghetti
½ cup mixed seeds (sesame, poppy, etc.)
1-2 cups soy cheese, grate
½ cup onion, mince
1 Tbsp garlic, mince
1 cup Bragg Olive Oil
Bragg Liquid Aminos
½ tsp Bragg Sprinkle (24 herbs & spice)

Cook spaghetti. Drain. Sauté onions and garlic in a small amount of olive oil. Add spaghetti to onion and garlic mixture. Sprinkle mixed seeds into wok, add remaining olive oil and Sprinkle and mix all ingredients together. Add grated soy cheese, lightly toss and serve immediately. Spray with Bragg Aminos to taste. *Variation:* Add minced vegetables, like carrots, turnips, scallions, eggplant, green pepper, etc. to onions and garlic. Serves 4-6.

Increasing intake of fruits and vegetables can help you prevent heart disease, cancer, and other chronic diseases. Surveys show those who increase their daily fruit and vegetable intake improve their health, vitality and well-being.
– UC Berkeley Wellness Letter • www.berkeleywellness.com

SPINACH PASTA WITH TOFU AND CORN

½ red onion, mince
1 lb spinach pasta
8 oz tofu, firm, cube
½ tsp chili powder
2 cups corn, fresh or frozen
1 qt vegetable stock (pg. 10)
1 tsp orange rind, grate
½ tsp Bragg Liquid Aminos
shake of Bragg Kelp
1 Tbsp Bragg Organic Olive Oil
1 bunch basil, cut for garnish
1 red bell pepper, thinly sliced
Bragg Sprinkle (24 herbs & spices), to taste

Cook pasta. Place onion, orange rind and vegetable stock in sauce pan. Bring to boil, simmer and reduce heat. Combine the tofu, chili powder, Sprinkle and Bragg Aminos. Heat skillet, add a little olive oil to prevent sticking and add tofu, peppers and corn, cook 5 minutes. Add vegetable sauce and bring to simmer. Add drained pasta to tofu mixture. Toss pasta mixture with sauce, continue to cook 1-2 minutes, until thickened. Garnish with basil and Bragg Nutritional Yeast. Serves 4-6.

TOMATO – LEEK LINGUINI

4 medium-sized leeks
28 oz can dice tomatoes
crumbled hard soy cheese
Bragg Liquid Aminos to taste
1 lb whole-grain linguini
1 tsp minced fresh thyme leaves
¼ cup Bragg Organic Olive Oil
Bragg Sprinkle (to taste)

Cook pasta. Cut leeks in half and slice into thin pieces. Heat olive oil in a large wok and sauté leeks over medium heat 5-10 minutes. Add tomatoes with juice, Sprinkle and simmer 10 minutes to thicken. Add Bragg Aminos to taste. Toss cooked linguini with tomato – leek sauce and soy cheese. Serves 4.

TOMATO SAUCE

3 cups cooked tomatoes, with juice
½ cup onions, finely chop, sauté
½ cup green pepper, chop
1 cup tomatoes, finely chop
1 Tbsp Bragg Organic Olive Oil
1 Tbsp raw honey
½ tsp Bragg Liquid Aminos
shake of Bragg Kelp
½ tsp Bragg Sprinkle
3 garlic cloves, crush

Place juice from 3 cups cooked tomatoes in sauce pan with sautéed onions and chopped pepper. Bring to a boil and let simmer, stirring occasionally, until volume is reduced by half. Add all remaining ingredients. Let simmer briefly or until mixture is thick and ready.

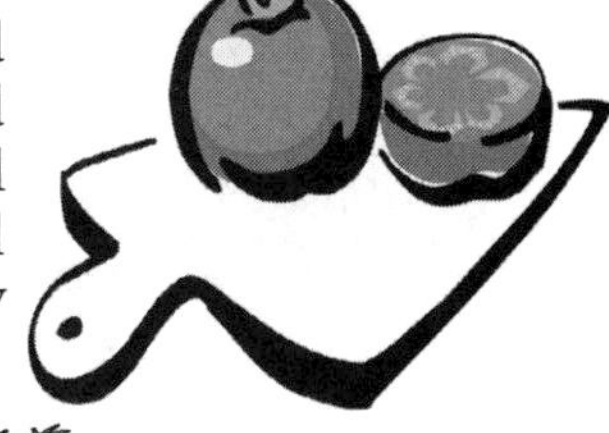

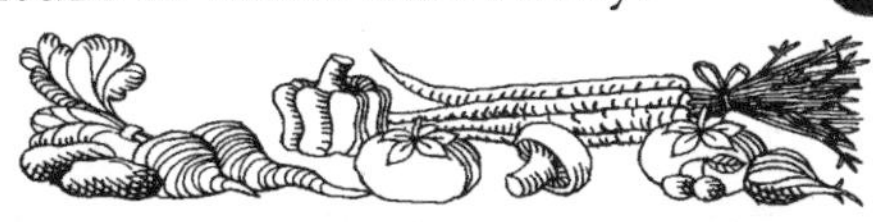

Tomatoes are rich in vitamins A and C and fiber and are cholesterol free. New medical research suggests that consumption of lycopene, the miracle that makes tomatoes red, may prevent cancer. Cooked tomatoes do have higher concentrations of lycopene than non-cooked tomatoes (see page 73).

PUMPKIN FILLED RAVIOLI

½ cup + 2 Tbsps tofu (extra firm), drain
1 cup pumpkin, canned or fresh cooked
Tomato-Basil Pasta (recipe below)
1 tsp Bragg Sprinkle (24 herbs & spices)
3 Tbsps prune purée*
1 Tbsp raw honey
¼ tsp nutmeg
1 Tbsp Bragg Olive Oil

Prepare one Tomato-Basil Pasta recipe (see below). Place tofu in food processor; add pumpkin and blend. Add remaining ingredients and process until smooth. Roll out 2 large sheets of Tomato-Basil Pasta. Place teaspoonfuls of filling at regular intervals on the first layer of dough. Cover with second layer of dough. Using thumbs gently press down spaces between mounds of filling. Dip rim of a 3-inch-diameter glass into flour. Use the glass to cut circles around each ravioli. Press the edges of each circle with fork to seal. Ravioli may be made a day before cooking. Drop into boiling water, to which 1 tablespoon olive oil has been added. Boil 10 minutes, stirring occasionally. Top with tomato sauce (recipe on page 111 and 163). Serves 6.

**To make Prune Pureé: combine 1/4 cup pitted prunes and 2 tablespoons warm water in food processor or blender. Pulse until prunes are finely chopped into purée texture. Take 3 tablespoons from this purée for above recipe.*

TOMATO – BASIL PASTA

½ cup tofu (extra firm), drain
1 Tbsp Bragg Organic Olive Oil
1 cup semolina flour
½ cup whole-grain flour
¼ tsp Bragg Liquid Aminos
1½ tsps dried basil
25 oz jar tomato sauce
6 Tbsps tomato paste
½ tsp garlic, finely mince
½ tsp Bragg Sprinkle

In food processor, mix tofu and tomato paste. Add flours, garlic, basil, Sprinkle and Bragg Aminos. Add olive oil and blend until dough sticks together. Turn dough onto board sprinkled with semolina flour. Knead until smooth, about 3 minutes. Place dough in plastic bag and set aside for 1 hour.

Divide the dough into 4 equal portions. If not using for hand made raviolis, place one portion on lightly floured board and return remaining portions to plastic bag for future pastas. Flatten dough into oval shape and roll dough into an oblong sheet, about 7x16". Dough should be thin, but not too translucent. Divide sheets crosswise and set aside to dry on wax paper in a warm place for about 30 minutes, or until it is dry and pliable, but not brittle.

For filled pasta, roll dough on floured board to about 8 inch thick. Sprinkle dough lightly with flour and roll up loosely. Use a sharp knife to cut type of pasta desired. Remember that pasta will swell about double when cooked, so make cuts about half the diameter desired. Allow the cut pasta to dry by tossing into a loose pile of flour laying flat on wax paper in the open air for at least an hour. This will prevent the pasta from sticking after it has been cut and keep it firm after cooking. To prepare pasta, cook in boiling water for 8-10 minutes. Serves 4-6.

PITA SANDWICHES

Pita bread is a substitute to serving sandwiches on sliced bread. It can be purchased at health stores or you can make it from scratch from the below recipe. We have included filling suggestions for delicious sandwiches for lunch and dinner treats that will delight children and people of all ages.

PITA BREAD

1 pkg active dry yeast
1 tsp raw honey
2 cups warm distilled water
1 tsp Bragg Sprinkle (24 herbs & spices)
4 cups organic whole-wheat flour

In a large bowl mix yeast, honey and flour together; then add water and Sprinkle and mix well. Cover and set aside in a warm place. Let rise until doubled. Punch down, divide into 12 balls. Put 2 cups flour on counter, roll balls out into circles about 8 inches thick. Place on un-greased cookie sheets to rise. Turn bread over gently with both hands while rising. Bake at 400°F for 5-10 minutes. Makes 12 delicious pitas.

Suggestions for Filling Pita Pockets:

- **Natural peanut or nut butters of choice & shredded carrots, apples alfalfa sprouts & tofunaise. (page 139) or Bragg Vinaigrette.**
- **Apple butter (made with honey & apples puréed), nut butter and sliced ripe banana.**
- **Hummus, sprouts & Bragg Sprinkle (24 herbs & spices).**
- **Nut butters, bananas & fruit slices or purées.**
- **Avocado, green pepper, onion, cucumber, sprouts & shred raw carrot & beet.**
- **Tahini (sesame paste, honey, wheat germ) and apple slices or sauce.**
- **Tomato, lettuce, red onion, soy cheese, sprouts, grated carrots topped with Bragg Organic Vinaigrette or Ginger Sesame Dressing.**
- **Quick Pita Pizza – spread pita with tomato sauce, add variety of chopped or grated vegetables. Place on cookie sheet, top with grated hard soy cheese, broil 5 minutes, until edges slightly crisp.**
- **Shred vegetables desired. Drizzle with Bragg Olive Oil, shake of Bragg Sprinkle, Kelp and dash of Bragg Aminos and Nutritional Yeast.**

HUMMUS FOR DIPS, PITAS & TOPPINGS

2 cups cooked garbanzo beans
¼ cup green onion, chop
1 Tbsp Bragg Organic Olive Oil
shake of Bragg Sprinkle
¼ tsp Bragg Liquid Aminos
2 cloves garlic, crush
¼ cup parsley, chop
½ cup tahini
paprika (garnish)
1 Tbsp lemon juice

Puree garbanzo beans, then add all ingredients. Sprinkle paprika for garnish. Delicious for dips, salads, and veggie toppings or serve with Pita chips: cut Pita in pie shaped pieces. Bake at 250°F for 15 minutes or until crisp. Serves 4.

VEGGIE ENTREÉS

BEAN STEW WITH HERB DUMPLINGS

FOR STEW:

3 Tbsps Bragg Organic Olive Oil
2-4 cloves garlic, mince
⅛ cup sweet basil, chop (garnish)
1 lb tomatoes, peel & chop
1 Tbsp Bragg Liquid Aminos
2 red onions, chop
3½ cups vegetable stock
2 celery stalks, chop
2 carrots, slice
Bragg Sprinkle
1 cup dried white kidney beans or black-eyed peas, soaked overnight in purified water

FOR HERB DUMPLINGS:

2 oz Bragg Olive Oil
1 tsp Bragg Sprinkle
1⅓ cups fresh whole-grain bread crumbs
6½ Tbsps self-rising whole-grain flour

Cook beans for 20 minutes. For stew, now heat olive oil in large pan over medium heat. Add onion and garlic, sauté 4 minutes. Stir in celery, carrots and cook 2 minutes longer. Add beans and remaining ingredients and bring to boil. Season with Sprinkle. Lower heat, cover and simmer 20 minutes. Meanwhile to prepare dumplings: mix dumpling ingredients with 5 Tbsp cold distilled water to make firm dough. Shape into 12 balls. Arrange on top of stew. Cover, continue simmering until dumplings are light and fluffy, about 20 minutes. Serve at once. Top with sweet basil and Bragg Nutritional Yeast. Serves 6.

BROWN RICE AND NUT PILAF

1¼ cups brown rice
2 cloves garlic, crush
2 Tbsps Bragg Olive Oil
1 tsp Bragg Sprinkle
½ cup unsalted raw nuts
fresh parsley, chop
1 onion, dice
1 large carrot, grate
2 cups veggie stock or distilled water
1 tsp mustard seeds (optional)
Bragg Liquid Aminos to taste

In a large shallow pan, gently sauté onion, garlic and carrot in olive oil for 3-5 minutes. Stir in rice and spices. Cook for a minute or two until grains are coated in oil. Pour in stock or water, add Bragg Aminos and Sprinkle. Bring to boil, cover, simmer gently 40 minutes. Remove from heat without lifting lid – this helps rice to firm up and cool properly. Set for 5 minutes. If rice is done there will be small steam holes in center. Stir in nuts. Season to taste. Sprinkle parsley and Bragg Nutritional Yeast on top. Recipe can be made ahead and reheated. Serves 4.

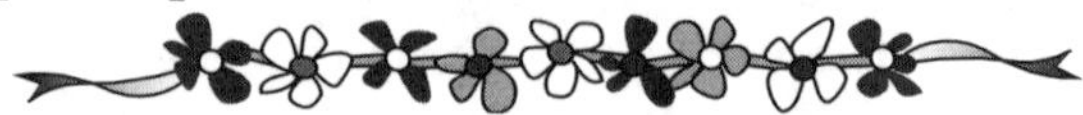

If you can't feed a hundred people . . . then feed just one. – Mother Teresa

---

Paul C. Bragg opened in New York City, the Macfadden's 7 famous "Penny Restaurants" during the big Depression Era. They fed millions of hungry people with healthy vegetarian meals for only a penny. Inspirational music & literature was given out to inspire and guide them.

CABBAGE AND SPROUTING BEANS

3 Tbsps sesame oil
2 cloves garlic, sliver
1 cabbage, slice
5 oz sprouting beans
3 green onions, slice
1 inch fresh ginger, grate
1 carrot, cut thin strips
½ cup unsalted cashews or almonds

SAUCE:

3 tsps Bragg Liquid Aminos
1 Tbsp sesame oil
shake of Bragg Sprinkle
⅔ cup cold distilled water
2 tsps raw honey
shake of Bragg Sea Kelp

Heat oil in large wok and sauté green onion, garlic, ginger and carrot for 2 minutes. Add sprouting beans and sauté for another 2 minutes, stir and toss together. Add cabbage and nuts. Stir-fry until cabbage leaves begin to wilt. Quickly mix sauce ingredients together and pour into wok; stir immediately, coating the vegetables with this delicious sauce and serve. Serves 2-4.

LENTIL AND NUT ROAST

1 cup lentils
1 large carrot, grate
1 large red onion, chop
1 Tbsp Bragg Olive Oil
2 celery stalks, mince
⅔ cup distilled water
½ cup each walnuts and hazelnuts
1 Tbsp Bragg Liquid Aminos
4 oz mushrooms, chop
½ tsp Bragg Sprinkle
Egg Replacer equal to 1 egg
2 Tbsps parsley and cilantro,

Soak lentils for 1 hour in cold water. Drain. Coarsely grind nuts in a food processor and set aside. Combine chopped carrots, celery, onion and mushrooms, pass through a food processor or blender until fine. Sauté vegetables lightly in olive oil for 5 minutes. Stir in Sprinkle and cook 1 minute. Mix soaked lentils with nuts, vegetables, Bragg Aminos, Egg Replacer, parsley, cilantro and water. Press mixture firmly into pan and smooth surface. Bake at 350°F for 30 minutes or until firm, covering top with lid or foil if it starts to burn. Allow mixture to stand for 15 minutes before removing from pan. This moist loaf will be soft when cut. Serve with Vegetarian Gravy (below). Serves 6.

VEGETARIAN GRAVY

1 large red onion, slice
3 turnips, slice
3 whole garlic cloves, crush
6 cups veggie stock or water
3 Tbsps Bragg Olive Oil
3 celery stalks, slice
½ tsp poultry seasoning
4 oz mushrooms, halve
⅓ tsp Bragg Sprinkle
1 tsp Bragg Liquid Aminos

Cook vegetables and garlic on moderately high heat with olive oil in a saucepan, stir occasionally until browned. Add stock or water, Bragg Aminos, Sprinkle; bring to boil. Cover, simmer 20 minutes. Purée (blend or mash) vegetables, adding a little of the stock and return to pan. Taste and season as needed. Freeze half of gravy in ice cube trays for future use and reheat remainder to serve with Lentil and Nut Roast (above). Serves 6-8.

HEALTHY STUFFINGS

WHOLE-GRAIN STUFFING

3 cups organic whole-grain, dried or toasted bread crumbs
1 tsp Bragg Liquid Aminos
1 cup red onion, chop
3 Tbsps Bragg Organic Olive Oil
1 cup celery, dice
⅓ tsp paprika
½ tsp poultry seasoning
½ tsp Bragg Sprinkle
a few celery leaves, mince

Sauté red onions, Bragg Aminos and seasonings in olive oil 2-3 minutes. Add celery and leaves and bread crumbs, mix. Put in baking pan, bake at 350°F until browned. Serves 6.

PECAN DELIGHT STUFFING

¼ cup Bragg Organic Olive Oil
1 red onion, mince
⅓ cup celery, mince
½ tsp poultry seasoning
½ tsp Bragg Sprinkle
⅓ tsp paprika
1 tsp Bragg Liquid Aminos
⅓ cup pecans, chop
⅓ tsp celery seeds
3 garlic cloves, mince
4 cups organic whole-grain dried bread crumbs

Sauté onion, celery, garlic and seasonings for 2-3 minutes in olive oil. Add bread crumbs and nuts. Mix thoroughly. Place in casserole. Bake at 350°F until thoroughly heated. Serves 6.

THANKSGIVING DRESSING

3 cups organic whole-grain, dried bread crumbs
Egg Replacer equal to 1 egg
4 tsps Bragg Organic Olive Oil
½ tsp Bragg Liquid Aminos
½ tsp Bragg Sprinkle
1 cup mushrooms, chop
1 cup celery, mince
1 tsp Bragg Liquid Aminos
½ tsp poultry seasoning
3 cloves garlic, mince
2 red onions, mince

Mix all ingredients together. If not moist enough, add a few tablespoons distilled water, or soy milk. Bake in casserole dish at 350°F until heated throughout and top is browned. Serves 6.

WILD RICE STUFFING

1 cup wild or organic brown rice
1½ qts boiling distilled water
Egg Replacer equal to 1 egg
½ tsp Bragg Liquid Aminos
2 Tbsps Bragg Olive Oil
⅓ cup mushrooms, slice
¼ tsp poultry seasoning
⅓ tsp Bragg Sprinkle

Rinse and cook organic rice in boiling water until done. Add Egg Replacer, the sliced mushrooms, olive oil, Bragg Aminos and seasonings to the rice. Blend thoroughly. Place in a casserole dish and heat at 350°F for 20 minutes. Serves 4-6.

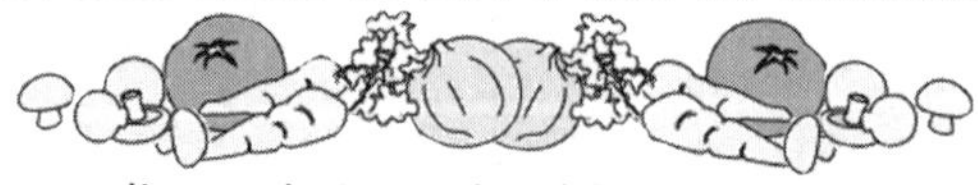

The closer you can live to being a healthy vegetarian, it's all the better.
– Gary Player, professional champion golfer

Chapter 10

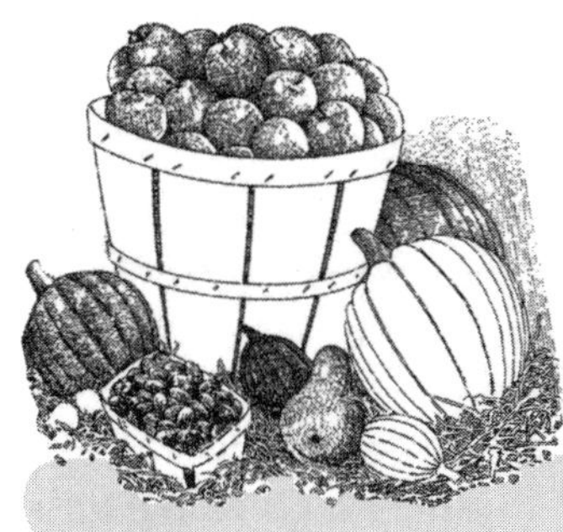

Vegetarian Entrées

BEAN PATTIES

1 cup whole-grain bread crumbs
2 cups cooked beans, mash
1 tsp Bragg Liquid Aminos
Egg Replacer equal to 1 egg
shake of Bragg Sprinkle
1 Tbsp parsley, chop

Mix all ingredients, form into patties. Bake at 350°F for 10 minutes. Any beans/legumes can be used in this recipe. Serves 4.

LENTIL LOAF

1½ cups cooked lentils
1½ cups whole-grain bread crumbs
1½ Tbsps parsley, chop
1½ cups soy milk
¾ tsp Bragg Liquid Aminos
shake of Bragg Sprinkle

Mix all ingredients well, place in oiled pan. Bake at 350°F for 20 minutes until firm. Beans or peas may be substituted for lentils. Also cooked organic whole-grain cereal (many varieties to choose from) instead of cooked lentils. Serves 5.

LENTILS WITH WILD RICE

1¼ cups lentils, purée
1½ cups cooked wild rice
2 Tbsps Bragg Organic Olive Oil
1 tsp Bragg Liquid Aminos
½ tsp poultry seasoning
1 red onion, mince
shake of Bragg Sprinkle
½ cup soy milk
Egg Replacer equal to 2 eggs
¼ cup chives

Combine lentils and wild rice; add olive oil, soy milk, Bragg Aminos and seasonings. Stir in Egg Replacer, add remaining ingredients. Place in oiled casserole. Bake at 350°F for 20 minutes, until lightly brown. Top with Bragg Nutritional Yeast. Serves 4.

VEGETABLE HASH

½ cup ripe olives, chop
½ cup red onions, chop
1 tsp Bragg Liquid Aminos
½ tsp Bragg Sprinkle
soy Parmesan cheese, grate
2 cups cooked soybeans
½ cup celery, chop
½ cup carrots, grate
½ cup beets, grate
tomato slices

Mix all ingredients together. Pour in a shallow, oiled pan. Cover with sliced tomatoes. Bake 400°F for 20-30 minutes until tender. Top with grated soy Parmesan cheese last five minutes. As serving add a shake of Bragg Nutritional Yeast. Serves 5.

When we eat vegetarian foods, we needn't worry about what kind of disease our food died from; this makes a joyful meal! – John Harvey Kellogg, M.D.

BEAN LOAF

- 1 cup dried lima beans, or any bean of your choice
- Egg Replacer equal to 1 egg
- 1½ cups whole-grain cracker crumbs
- 2 Tbsps Bragg Olive Oil
- 1 tsp Bragg Liquid Aminos
- 1 cup soy milk
- ½ tsp Bragg Sprinkle
- juice from 2 lemons, freshly squeezed

Wash and soak beans overnight. Cook until soft, drain, and rub through a coarse sieve. Add olive oil and lemon to make baste. Mix lima beans (or beans of choice) with other ingredients, place in oiled casserole and bake at 350°F for 30 minutes. Baste with lemon juice and olive oil. Serves 5.

SOYBEAN LOAF

- 3 cups cooked soybeans
- Egg Replacer equal to 3 eggs
- 3 Tbsps Bragg Organic Olive Oil
- 1 cup whole-grain cracker crumbs
- ½ cup celery, mince
- 1 cup soy milk
- ½ tsp poultry seasoning
- ½ cup red onion, mince
- 1 tsp Bragg Liquid Aminos
- shake of Bragg Sprinkle

Cook and mash soybeans. Mix all ingredients together. Place in oiled bread pan. Bake 30 minutes 350°F. Delicious served hot or cold. Top with Bragg Nutritional Yeast. Serves 6.

VEGETABLE AND SOYBEAN STEW

- 1 cup tofu, firm
- 2 cups fresh tomatoes
- 1 green pepper, chop
- shake of Bragg Sprinkle
- 3 cups cooked soybeans
- 2 red onions, chop
- 1 tsp Bragg Liquid Aminos
- 4 raw potatoes, chop

Cut tofu into small pieces and cook in a heavy skillet until slightly browned; remove from pan. Chop potatoes (with skins), onions and green pepper, put into skillet. Season with Bragg Aminos and Sprinkle (24 herbs & spices). Add soybeans and tomatoes. Cover. Cook for 30 minutes, or until done, adding water or liquid from soybeans as needed. Serves 5.

YELLOW CORN CROQUETTES

- 2 cups fresh or frozen corn kernels
- 2 Tbsps Bragg Organic Olive Oil
- 1 cup whole-grain bread crumbs
- 1 cup whole-grain cracker crumbs
- 1 tsp Bragg Liquid Aminos
- Egg Replacer equal to 1 egg
- 1 cup soy milk
- 1 Tbsp red onion, mince
- 2 Tbsps celery, mince
- shake of Bragg Sprinkle

Mix corn, onion, celery, soy milk, dried bread crumbs, Sprinkle and Bragg Aminos; shape into balls. Then add Egg Replacer over balls and roll in dry cracker crumbs. Sauté in olive oil or bake until golden brown. Serves 6-8.

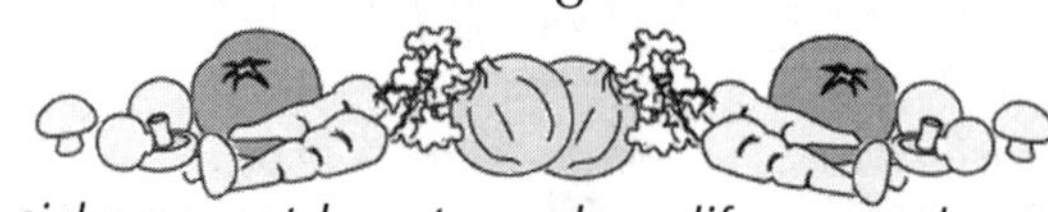

To avoid sickness, eat less; to prolong life, worry less. – Chu Hui Weng

POTATOES FLORENTINE

6 potatoes, slice
1 head cauliflower
3 Tbsps Bragg Olive Oil
3 Tbsps whole-grain flour
2 cups vegetable broth
1 Tbsp sesame seeds
2 cups soy cheese, grate
1 tsp Bragg Liquid Aminos
2 clove garlic, mince
½ tsp Bragg Sprinkle
1 lb spinach, chop
1 carrot, grate

Break cauliflower into florets and steam with potatoes for 10 to 15 minutes. Make a roux with olive oil and flour, add broth, then soy cheese and seasonings. In oiled casserole, layer ½ the potatoes and cauliflower, ½ spinach, ½ carrots and ½ sauce. Repeat layers. Sprinkle top with sesame seeds. Bake 350°F, 20 minutes. Garnish with Bragg Nutritional Yeast. Serves 4-6.

VEGETABLE POT PIE

1 cup vegetable broth
2 carrots, chop
2 cups potatoes, chop
1 cup turnips, chop
½ cup onion, chop
1 cup fresh or frozen peas
1 cup fresh or frozen corn
2 cloves garlic, mince
1 tsp basil
½ tsp Bragg Sprinkle
½ tsp Bragg Sea Kelp
1 tsp Bragg Liquid Aminos
2 Tbsps whole-grain flour
¼ cup distilled water
1 whole grain pie crust #2 (page 203)

Simmer carrots, potatoes, turnips, onions and seasonings in broth for 15 minutes. Combine flour and water in small bowl. Add to vegetables and cook over low heat, stirring until thickened. Remove from heat. Add peas and corn. Place half of whole-grain pie crust in bottom of pie plate, bake at 425°F for 15 minutes. Fill with vegetables and top with remaining crust. Fork vent holes and bake 15 more minutes at 375°F. Serves 6.

MOROCCAN STEW

3 Tbsps Bragg Organic Olive Oil
1 small red onion, chop
1 zucchini, slice
1 carrot, slice
1 celery stalk, slice
1 red pepper, chop
1 turnip, slice
roasted peanuts, chop
1 parsnip, slice
1 clove garlic, mince
2 cups tomatoes, chop
1½ cups cooked garbanzo beans
1 cup distilled water
1 Tbsp cumin
shake of Bragg Sprinkle
Bragg Liquid Aminos to taste

In medium pot, sauté onions in olive oil until golden. Combine all ingredients and seasonings with onions and simmer until vegetables are tender, about 30 minutes. Garnish with chopped roasted peanuts and Bragg Nutritional Yeast. Serves 6.

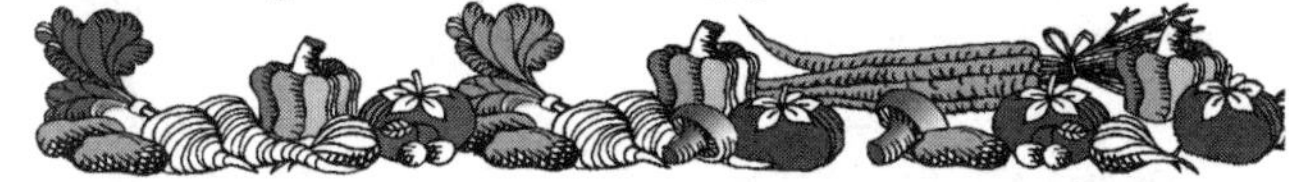

The cancer mortality rate was found to be 39% lower among vegetarians compared with meat-eaters. – Oxford Vegetarian Study

VEGETARIAN LOAF

1½ cups fresh cooked peas
3 Tbsps Bragg Organic Olive Oil
Egg Replacer equal to 3 eggs
2 cups tomato sauce (pg. 111 & 163)
¼ cup hot tomato sauce (topping)
1½ cups cooked beans
1½ cups cooked brown rice
pinch of celery seed
1 tsp Bragg Liquid Aminos
shake of Bragg Sprinkle
soy cheese, grated (for topping)

While hot, put cooked peas and beans through food processor. Add all other ingredients except ¼ cup hot tomato sauce, shape into loaf, adding more cooked brown rice if necessary. Bake at 350°F for 20 minutes. Top with grated soy cheese and hot tomato sauce. Garnish with Bragg Nutritional Yeast. Serves 8.

BAKED VEGETABLE LOAF

Egg Replacer equal to 1 egg
fresh ground peppercorn to taste
½ green pepper, chop
2 Tbsps Bragg Organic Olive Oil
1 cup fresh or frozen peas
1 tsp Bragg Liquid Aminos
1 cup whole-grain bread crumbs
1 cup soy milk
2 cups carrots, chop
½ red onion, chop
1 cup stewed prunes, chop
¼ cup unsulphured molasses
1 cup potatoes (with skin), chop
shake of Bragg Sprinkle

Steam carrots and potatoes for 15 minutes and mix with green pepper and onion. Add peas, prunes, ground pepper, Bragg Aminos, Bragg Sprinkle (24 herbs & spices), Egg Replacer, olive oil, soy milk, bread crumbs and molasses. Mix thoroughly, place in oiled pan, and bake at 400°F for one hour. Serves 6.

VEGETARIAN SAUSAGES

1 cup cooked lima beans
2 cups cooked soybeans
1 cup cooked navy beans
1 tsp Bragg Liquid Aminos
Egg Replacer equal to 1 egg
½ tsp Bragg Sprinkle
⅔ cup soy milk
⅛ tsp paprika
½ tsp poultry seasoning
1 cup cornmeal or whole-grain fine cracker crumbs
1 Tbsp Bragg Organic Olive Oil

Put all beans in food processor. Mix in seasonings. Shape seasoned beans into sausages. Beat Egg Replacer and soy milk. Now dip sausages in mixture, then cornmeal, and repeat. Place in pan with olive oil, and brown on all sides at 450°F. Serves 8.

Bragg Nutritional Yeast Flakes are Healthy and Tasty

Delicious added to many Vegetarian Recipes or garnish top when serving dish. Ideal for vegetarians, vegans and children, they have a delicious cheese-like flavor! Nutritionally, these yeast flakes contain high B-Complex Vitamins especially Vitamin B12. They also help boost your immune system! Delicious sprinkled over most foods, especially salads, vegetables, rice, pasta, dips, spreads and even popcorn. You can add flakes to vegetable juices, smoothies, cereals, soups and casseroles. Try Bragg Nutritional Yeast to garnish your vegetarian meals. For more info visit bragg.com

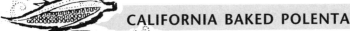

CALIFORNIA BAKED POLENTA

⅓ cup onion, chop
3¾ cups boiling distilled water
⅓ lb soy cheese, grate
2¼ cups cooked tomatoes, drain
4 oz fresh mushrooms, slice
1 small clove garlic, mince
¼ cup Bragg Organic Olive Oil
1½ cups yellow organic cornmeal
¾ cup cold distilled water
¾ tsp Bragg Liquid Aminos
¼ lb soy Parmesan cheese, grate
shake of Bragg Sprinkle

Wilt onion and garlic in hot olive oil; add Sprinkle and Bragg Aminos, sauté mushrooms lightly and add tomatoes. Simmer gently 30 minutes, stir occasionally and add more tomato juice if necessary. Prepare mush by combining cornmeal and cold water. Gradually add to boiling water and cook. Stir until thickened. Reduce heat and cook slowly for 10 more minutes. Spread a 2-inch layer of cornmeal in shallow baking dish; cover with 2 cups of sauce and add layer of thinly sliced or grated soy cheese. Repeat layers. Save some sauce for serving. Sprinkle top with grated Parmesan cheese. Bake at 300°F for 30 minutes. Garnish with Bragg Nutritional Yeast. Serves 4.

EGGPLANT – GARLIC BAKE

1 eggplant
4 cloves garlic, slice
Bragg Organic Olive Oil
1 cup distilled water
Bragg Liquid Aminos
shake of Bragg Sprinkle (24 herbs & spices)

Cut eggplant in half, stud with sliced garlic. Spray with Bragg Aminos and add Sprinkle. Place in casserole with water. Cover tightly, bake at 350°F for 30 minutes or until soft. *Variation:* last minutes add diced tomatoes and grated soy cheese. Serves 4.

ROASTED EGGPLANT ROLOTINI

1 eggplant, 1½" thick slices
3 Tbsps Bragg Organic Olive Oil
2 cloves garlic, mince
¼ lb cooked lasagna noodles
½ tsp marjoram
½ cup fresh basil, chop
1 tsp Bragg Liquid Aminos
½ lb crumbled firm tofu, drain
Tomato sauce (page 111 or 163)

Cut eggplant into 1½ inch thick slices. Place on oiled baking sheet. Combine minced garlic with olive oil and brush on slices. Bake at 350°F for 20 minutes or until tender. Cut lasagna noodles in half and place 1 eggplant slice on each piece. Noodles should be at 1-inch longer than eggplant. Mix tofu with herbs, Bragg Sprinkle and Bragg Aminos. Spread 1/6 of mixture on each eggplant slice. Top with tomato sauce, cook 30 minutes. Garnish with Bragg Nutritional Yeast. Serves 6.

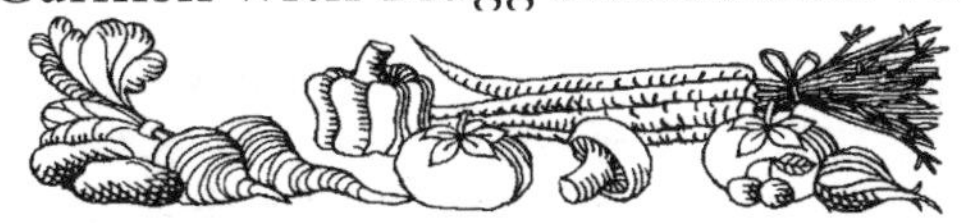

Use your will power and better judgement to select and eat only foods which are best for you, regardless of the ridicule of your friends . – Dr. Richard T. Field

MUSHROOM PROTEIN LOAF

3 Tbsps Bragg Olive Oil
Egg Replacer equal to 4 eggs
3 Tbsps whole-grain flour
1 Tbsp arrowroot
1 tsp Bragg Liquid Aminos
shake of Bragg Sprinkle
½ tsp dill seed
¼ cup celery, dice
2 lbs mushrooms, thinly slice
½ cup parsley, chop (garnish)

Add Egg Replacer to olive oil. Beat in flour and arrowroot. Add Bragg Aminos, celery, dill seed and mushrooms. Mix well, pour into an oiled pan. Bake one hour, at 350°F. Garnish with parsley and Bragg Nutritional Yeast Flakes. Serves 6-8.

VEGETARIAN CASSEROLE

3 cups distilled water
1 cup onions, chop
½ cup rice, brown or wild
2 cups gluten steaks, chop
1 tsp Bragg Liquid Aminos
2 cups carrots, grate
2 cups celery, mince
1 cup mushrooms, slice
2 Tbsps Bragg Organic Olive Oil
raw honey or molasses (optional)
shake of Bragg Sprinkle (24 herbs & spices)

Brown chopped gluten steaks or firm tofu in olive oil. Add onion, carrots, celery (or any vegetables desired) with uncooked rice, mushrooms, Bragg Aminos, Sprinkle and water. Sauté all together in skillet 5 minutes, then transfer to baking dish. Add honey or molasses to taste if desired. Bake at 350°F for 40 minutes. Gluten steaks available at health food stores, or use firm tofu. Garnish with Bragg Nutritional Yeast. Serves 6.

CHESTNUT CROQUETTES

2 cups chestnuts, ground
½ cup whole-grain cracker crumbs
1 cup celery, dice
3 slices pineapple, lightly broil
Egg Replacer equal to 1 egg
3 Tbsps Bragg Olive Oil
juice from 2 lemons
1 tsp Bragg Liquid Aminos
Optional: 1 tsp unsulphured molasses

Shell chestnuts, boil, then remove brown skins. Cool and put through food grinder. Add Egg Replacer, celery, cracker crumbs, 2 tablespoons olive oil and Bragg Aminos. (*Optional*: add 1 tsp unsulphured molasses.) Mix, shape as desired. Place in pan with olive oil. Bake at 400°F until brown. Baste with lemon juice, remaining olive oil. Last 10 minutes add pineapple slices. Garnish with Bragg Nutritional Yeast. Serves 6.

To reduce the risk of heart disease, boost your good blood cholesterol and reduce the bad. This can be done by following a low-fat diet and reducing your cholesterol intake. Exercise also boosts good cholesterol, as does being trim and fit, and of course, not smoking. Don't expect fast results overnight! It takes time for exercising and diet to bring about significant change in your cholesterol levels. Be faithful and diligent, it works! – UC Berkeley Wellness Letter

BOSTON MUSHROOM AND ONION PILAF

1½ cups rice, brown or wild
½ lb fresh mushrooms, slice
1 tsp Bragg Liquid Aminos
shake of Bragg Sprinkle
6 Tbsps Bragg Organic Olive Oil
2 large red onions, slice rings
1 tsp fresh ginger, grate
3 cups boiling distilled water

Wash, drain rice. Heat oil in heavy frying pan or wok. Add rice and cook over low heat until browned. Add mushrooms; brown lightly. Arrange onion rings over top. Pour boiling water and Bragg Aminos, Sprinkle and ginger over rice. Cover pan tightly. Reduce heat, steam, covered, for one hour or until liquid is completely absorbed. The rice should still be moist. Serves 6.

CINCINNATI MOCK TURKEY

1 cup each cooked soybeans & lentils
1 cup whole-grain bread crumbs
1 Tbsp Bragg Organic Olive Oil
¼ cup pecans, finely chop
1 cup whole-grain cracker crumbs
shake of Bragg Sprinkle
1 cup soy milk
¼ cup walnuts, finely chop
Egg Replacer equal to 1 egg
2 Tbsps onion, chop
2-3 Tbsps whole-grain flour
1 tsp Bragg Liquid Aminos

Optional: ½ tsp poultry herb seasoning

Place chopped onion and olive oil into small saucepan and heat for a few minutes, but do not brown or fry. Add soy milk. Warm mixture slowly and pour over cracker and bread crumbs. Sift whole-grain flour into pan and stir constantly over low heat until its color is light brown. Add chopped nuts, continue stirring until they are warm, but not browned. Beat Egg Replacer, add to mixture. Add nuts and browned flour. Process cooked soybeans and lentils through food processor. Add Bragg Aminos, Sprinkle and optional: poultry seasoning if desired. Mix all ingredients thoroughly. Pour mixture into oiled bread pan. Bake at 325°F for 30 minutes. Cool for 20 minutes. Then turn out into casserole dish. Serve with Gravy recipe below and homemade cranberry sauce. Serves 6.

CINCINNATI MOCK TURKEY GRAVY

1 Tbsp Bragg Olive Oil
1 Tbsp onion, finely chop
1¼ cups boiling distilled water
1 tsp poultry seasoning
1 tsp Bragg Liquid Aminos
2¼ Tbsps whole-grain flour

Mix ingredients to a smooth consistency and pour over baked mock turkey casserole. Place in oven 15 minutes. The recipe above makes a delicious vegetarian roast, served with this gravy recipe and cranberry sauce.

Healthy, healing dietary fibers are fresh vegetables, fresh fruits, salads, sprouts and whole grains. They help normalize blood pressure and the cholesterol levels. These healthy foods also promote healthy elimination.

Health and intellect are two blessings of life.
– Menander Monostikoi (342-292 BC) Greek comic playwriter

JAMBALAYA

3 cups cooked brown or wild rice
1½ medium onions, finely chop
16 oz firm tofu, cube
shake of Bragg Kelp
1½ Tbsps whole-grain flour
3 Tbsps Bragg Organic Olive Oil
1 green pepper, thinly slice
1 tsp Bragg Liquid Aminos
2 cups fresh/can tomatoes
1 tsp parsley, mince
½ tsp Bragg Sprinkle
1 clove garlic, mince

Heat olive oil in heavy pan. Add onion, brown. Blend in flour to make smooth paste. Cook until slightly brown. Add tofu, tomatoes, green pepper, parsley, garlic, Sprinkle and Bragg Aminos. Cook over low heat 30 minutes, stirring frequently. Add cooked rice. Simmer for about 7 minutes. Serves 8.

PROTEIN – MIXED NUT LOAF

½ cup walnuts, chop
½ cup blanched almonds, chop
Egg Replacer equal to 2 eggs
1½ cups whole-grain bread crumbs
shake of Bragg Kelp
½ cup pecans, chop
½ cup cashews, chop
½ tsp Bragg Sprinkle
2 cups tomato sauce
1 tsp Bragg Liquid Aminos
1½ cups crushed organic whole-grain cereal

Combine all ingredients, mix well, using only enough (about ¾ cup) tomato sauce to moisten. Place in oiled pan. Bake at 350°F for 30 minutes. Serve with remaining warmed tomato sauce, sprinkle of Bragg Nutritional Yeast. Delicious hot or cold. Serves 6.

NUT AND SOY CHEESE ROAST

1⅓ Tbsps Bragg Organic Olive Oil
1 cup whole-grain cracker crumbs
Egg Replacer equal to 2 eggs
1⅓ cups soy cheese, grate
juice from 1 lemon
2 red onions, finely chop
1 cup walnuts, chop
⅓ cup distilled water
1 tsp Bragg Liquid Aminos
Bragg Sprinkle (to taste)
2 tsps creamy organic, peanut butter or nut butter of choice

Brown onions lightly in olive oil. Add water and mix with cracker crumbs, reserving some for the topping. Add soy cheese, nuts, nut butter of choice, lemon juice, Sprinkle, Bragg Aminos and Egg Replacer. Mix well. Turn into an oiled casserole dish, top with crumbs and bake at 400°F for 30 minutes until brown. Garnish with Bragg Nutritional Yeast. Serves 4.

PECAN AND CELERY LOAF

1¼ cups pecans, chop
2 Tbsps Bragg Organic Olive Oil
¾ cup whole-grain bread crumbs
¾ cup whole-grain cracker crumbs
Egg Replacer equal to 2 eggs
2 tsps onion, chop
1 cup soy milk
1¼ cups celery, finely chop
½ tsp Bragg Liquid Aminos
shake of Bragg Sprinkle

Mix above ingredients. Bake in an oiled loaf pan for 30 minutes at 375°F. Garnish with Bragg Nutritional Yeast. Serves 6.

CREOLE PIZZA

2½ cups whole-grain cereal, cook
2 Tbsps Bragg Organic Olive Oil
4 Tbsps green pepper, chop
1 tsp Bragg Liquid Aminos
5 Tbsps red onion, mince
⅓ tsp chili powder
¾ cup soy cheese, grate
2½ cups canned tomatoes

Sauté green bell pepper and all but one teaspoon of the onion in olive oil. Add tomatoes and simmer until thickened. In a separate bowl, combine cereal, chili powder and remaining onion. Spread a thin layer of mixture in glass baking pan. Pour tomato sauce and Bragg Aminos on the cereal layer. Top with green pepper, sliced olives and soy cheese. Bake at 400°F for 20 minutes. Serves 6-8.

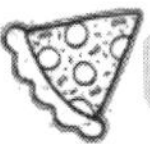

WHOLE-GRAIN VEGETARIAN PIZZA

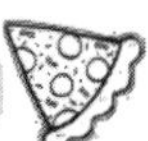

Use any bread dough for pizza crust. (see Breads, page 173) Mold dough into desired shape. Add mushrooms, tofu, sliced fresh veggies, onions, olives, pineapple, artichoke hearts, grated soy cheese, dash Bragg Aminos and Bragg Sprinkle. Bake at 400°F for 20 minutes. Garnish with Bragg Nutritional Yeast.

SPINACH AND NUT LOAF

2 Tbsps Bragg Organic Olive Oil
Egg Replacer equal to 2 eggs
1 cup whole-grain cracker crumbs
shake Bragg Sprinkle
1 lb spinach
1 red onion, finely chop
1 tsp Bragg Liquid Aminos
¾ cup walnuts, chop

Wash and steam spinach for 3 minutes. Chop and add to nuts. Mix in beaten Egg Replacer, onion and whole-grain cracker crumbs. Add Sprinkle, Bragg Aminos and olive oil. Turn into an oiled pan. Bake at 375°F for 20 minutes. Serves 4.

RATATOUILLE

1 large onion, chop
1 bell pepper, chop
1 eggplant, cut in 1″ slices
3 zucchini, cut in 1″ slices
3 medium tomatoes, chop
2 cloves garlic, mince
1 tsp Bragg Liquid Aminos
½ tsp Bragg Sprinkle
½ cup parsley, chop
3 Tbsps Bragg Organic Olive Oil

Mix all vegetables with olive oil, Bragg Aminos, garlic and Sprinkle. Spread in oiled baking pan and bake at 350°F for 30 minutes until cooked. Optional: serve over cooked millet, brown rice or other grains. Garnish with grated soy cheese, Bragg Nutritional Yeast Flakes and parsley. Serves 4-6.

Olive Oil is a perfect addition & has been proven to have anti-inflammatory properties which ease aches & pains of arthritis. – Great Life Magazine

TOMATO – SOY CHEESE – TOFU SAUCE

For Pasta, Corn Tortillas, Pitas and Veggies

½ lb soy cheese, grate
2 Tbsps Bragg Organic Olive Oil
Egg Replacer equal to 2 eggs
¾ cup warm tomato juice
½ cup whole-grain bread crumbs
½ cup soy cream
½ cup soft tofu, dice
shake of Bragg Sprinkle
soy parmesan cheese
Bragg Nutritional Yeast
Serve on: whole-grain toast, pasta, or warmed corn tortillas

Melt soy cheese with olive oil in double boiler; add toasted bread crumbs, soy cream and tomato juice, stirring constantly. Add Egg Replacer, tofu, and Sprinkle (24 herbs & spices). When mixture is thoroughly blended and melted, serve on organic whole-grain toast or pasta, warmed corn tortillas or pita bread, or over steamed fresh veggies. Garnish with soy Parmesan cheese and Bragg Nutritional Yeast Flakes. Serves 6.

SOY CHEESE SOUFFLÉ

2 Tbsps whole-grain or potato flour
4 Tbsps Bragg Organic Olive Oil
Egg Replacer equal to 4 eggs
⅛ tsp sweet basil
1 cup salt-free tomato juice
½ cup soy cheese, grate
½ tsp Bragg Liquid Aminos
shake of Bragg Sprinkle

Heat olive oil, add flour, stir over low heat for 3 minutes. Add warm tomato juice, Bragg Aminos, basil, Sprinkle and soy cheese. Stir until smooth and melted. Remove from stove and cool. Beat Egg Replacer and add to mixture. Turn into oiled casserole dish, bake at 325°F for 30 minutes. This will make the soufflé very firm. If softer texture is desired, decrease baking time and increase oven temperature. Serves 4.

SOY CHEESE CUSTARD

1 Tbsp Bragg Organic Olive Oil
½ tsp pure vanilla
1 cup soft whole-grain bread crumbs
Egg Replacer equal to 2 eggs
⅓ tsp almond extract
1 cup soy cheese, grate
½ cup soy milk
toast whole-grain bread

Heat olive oil, add soy cheese, soft bread crumbs, vanilla, almond extract and soy milk. Cook 5 minutes. Add beaten Egg Replacer and cook few minutes longer. Serve separate or on squares of toasted whole-grain bread or crackers. Serves 6.

SOYBEAN RICE LOAF

2 cups cooked soybeans, mash
1 cup brown rice, cook
Egg Replacer equal to 2 eggs
2 Tbsps tomato sauce
1 tsp Bragg Liquid Aminos
3 Tbsps red onion, mince
2 garlic cloves, mince
1 Tbsp lemon juice
⅓ tsp celery seed
shake of Bragg Sprinkle

Mix ingredients in the order given. Place in oiled loaf pan and bake in 350°F oven for 20 minutes. Garnish with Bragg Nutritional Yeast and soy Parmesan cheese. Serves 6-8.

MUSHROOM – BARLEY GOULASH OR SOUP

2 cups mushrooms, slice
2 cups carrots, dice
2 cups celery, dice
½ cup green pepper, dice
1 cup red onion, dice
⅓ cup Bragg Olive Oil
1 cup tomatoes, dice
2 Tbsps Bragg Liquid Aminos
3 cloves garlic, mince
1 cup unpearled whole barley
Bragg Sprinkle (24 herbs & spices)

Cover barley with distilled water. Add Sprinkle and Bragg Aminos and cover. Cook on low heat for 1 hour until almost done, stirring occasionally. Heat olive oil in a large wok and lightly sauté carrots, celery, green pepper, garlic and onion for 3 minutes. Add cooked barley, mushrooms and tomatoes. Cook for 10-15 minutes if you enjoy vegetables slightly undercooked. *Variations:* You can vary this recipe by adding other vegetables and grains desired and sprinkling grated soy cheese on top; or add more water to make a delicious, thick soup. Serves 4-6.

CHOP SUEY WITH TOFU

1 cup celery (slice diagonally)
1 cup red onions, chop
1 cup green pepper, chop
1 cup carrots (slice diagonally)
1 cup fresh or can mushrooms
1 small can water chestnuts, slice
1 cup firm tofu, cube
1 small can bamboo shoots
¼ cup Bragg Organic Olive Oil
2 Tbsps Bragg Liquid Aminos
2 cloves garlic, chop
1 cup Mung bean sprouts
½ tsp Chinese Five Spice*

Place olive oil, Bragg Aminos and Chinese Five Spice in skillet or wok over low heat until the oil is hot. Add all ingredients, except the tofu and mung bean sprouts. Use a wooden spoon to continuously sauté the vegetables (over medium heat to retain valuable vitamins, minerals, enzymes and nutrients). Once the mixture is thoroughly heated (about 10 minutes), gently place tofu in the skillet and mix with vegetables, being careful not to break up the little squares of tofu. After the tofu and vegetables are thoroughly warmed add a cup of fresh or canned mung bean sprouts. Serve with cooked brown rice. To enhance the protein content of this meal, add to each serving a heaping tablespoon of sliced almonds (pre-roast in oven). Serves 6.

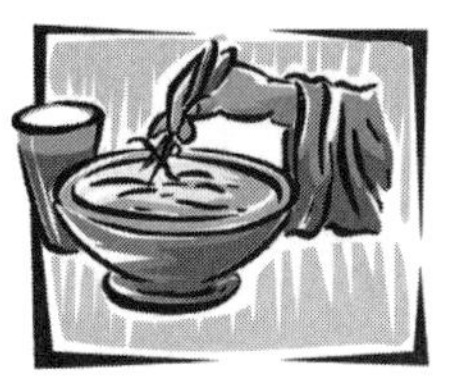

******Note: This popular Chinese Five Spice item is in the seasoning isle of most food markets. Choose a brand that contains no MSG or added salt!*

The Chinese believe it's important to incorporate principal of Yin and Yang into their meals, thus the heat of a dish should be counter-balanced by an equally cooling ingredient. When you try this Five-Spice Seasoning (cinnamon, cassia, anise, cloves and ginger) you will be surprised how delicious the flavors – sweet, warm, cool and spicy – blend. This versatile mixture is suited for rice, vegetables and any type of stir fry. – www.SpiceHouse.com

VEGETARIAN MUSHROOM CUTLETS

1 cup fresh mushrooms, slice
½ cup raw beets, finely grate
½ cup sunflower seeds, finely ground
2 Tbsps Bragg Liquid Aminos
Egg Replacer equal to 2 eggs
½ cup fresh carrots, grate
⅓ tsp Bragg Sprinkle
½ cup raw wheat germ
⅔ cup red onions, chop

Combine all ingredients and mix well. If mixture is too wet to form into patties, add more wheat germ. Place mixture in refrigerator for 30 minutes. Shape into patties. Sauté in lightly oiled skillet browning on both sides. Serves 4.

MILLET CASSEROLE

2 cups distilled water
1 cup hulled millet
½ cup celery, chop
½ Tbsp Bragg Liquid Aminos
2 cloves garlic, press
⅓ tsp Bragg Sprinkle
½ cup red onion, chop
1 cup mushrooms, chop
½ cup sunflower seeds, chop
1 cup zucchini, chop

Combine ingredients, mix well. Pour into casserole dish, bake 300°F, 1 hour until done. Garnish Bragg Nutritional Yeast. Serves 4.

MOLASSES – BAKED SOYBEANS

2 cups dried soybeans
½ bell pepper, chop
1 small red onion, chop
2 Tbsps Bragg Olive Oil
2 Tbsps blackstrap molasses
⅓ tsp Bragg Sprinkle
1 Tbsp raw honey
1 Tbsp Bragg Liquid Aminos
2 cups liquid from cooked soybeans or distilled water

Soak soybeans overnight. Cook on stove top or oven until tender (see page 84). Sauté onion and bell pepper in olive oil until tender. Combine ingredients in mixing bowl, transfer to covered casserole dish. Bake covered for 1 hour in preheated 350°F oven. Remove cover, bake 20 minutes or until done, stirring occasionally. Garnish with Bragg Nutritional Yeast. Serves 4-5.

KASHA, GREEN BEAN AND MUSHROOM CASSEROLE

Egg Replacer equal to 1 egg
½ cup brown buckwheat groats
1 Tbsp Bragg Liquid Aminos
1 large red onion, chop
2 cups fresh green beans, cook
1 cup grated soy cheese
½ cup celery, finely chop
½ cup green pepper, chop
2 cups sliced mushrooms
¼ cup Bragg Organic Olive Oil
1 clove garlic, chop
1 cup distilled water
½ tsp Bragg Sprinkle (24 herbs & spices)

Combine Egg Replacer, groats, and Bragg Aminos. Set aside. In medium fry pan, sauté onion, green pepper, garlic, celery and mushrooms in olive oil for 4 minutes. Stir in groats mixture, Sprinkle, green beans and water; bring to boil. Cook, partially covered, low heat 15 minutes. Place in serving dish, sprinkle grated soy cheese and Bragg Nutritional Yeast on top. Serves 6.

Each present day is a present to be treasured, spend it wisely! – Patricia Bragg

PEASANT'S PIE

2 tsps Bragg Organic Olive Oil
½ cup whole-grain bread crumbs
⅓ cup cashew nuts, chop
Egg Replacer equal to 1 egg
½ cup vegetable stock
or distilled water

1 red onion, chop
2 carrots, grate
shake of Bragg Sprinkle
½ tsp poultry seasoning
1 Tbsp soy or potato flour

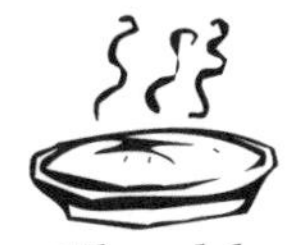

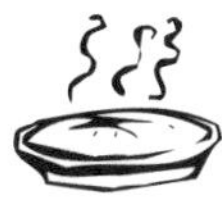

TOPPING:
1 lb mashed potatoes
Egg Replacer equal to 1 egg

Chop onions and sauté in olive oil until golden brown. Finely grate carrots. Crush dry bread crumbs, beat Egg Replacer and mix together with seasonings, nuts and flour. If mixture is dry, add vegetable stock or water until moist. Place in oiled baking dish and cover with mixture of mashed potatoes and beaten Egg Replacer. Bake for 30 minutes at 350°F. Serves 6.

CASHEW CASSEROLE

1 red onion, chop
2 tomatoes, chop
⅓ tsp poultry seasoning
½ cup soy cheese, grate
shake of Bragg Sprinkle

1 cup cashew nuts, chop
½ cup whole-grain bread crumbs
1 tsp Bragg Nutritional Yeast
Egg Replacer equal to 2 eggs
2 tsps Bragg Organic Olive Oil

Chop onion, sauté in olive oil 3 minutes. Skin tomatoes (see page 105) and chop. Mix chopped nuts, whole-grain dried bread crumbs, onions, tomatoes, seasonings, grated soy cheese, Bragg Nutritional Yeast and Egg Replacer. Place in an oiled baking dish. Bake at 400°F for 30 minutes. Serves 4.

BAKED BEANS

1 package dried navy beans
8 oz tomato purée
½ tsp mustard powder
1 tsp cinnamon powder
1 tsp Bragg Liquid Aminos

1 red onion, chop
¼ cup molasses
⅓ tsp clove powder
½ tsp Bragg Sprinkle
1 Tbsp fresh ginger, grate

Cover dried beans with 3 inches of distilled water and soak overnight. In the morning boil beans in the same water, adding more if necessary. Skim off foam as it comes to top. Boil until the skins break. Drain beans, reserve liquid and set aside. Pour beans in large glass casserole with onion and seasonings. Mix 3 cups of reserved liquid with rest of ingredients, add to beans, save remainder of water. Bake at 300°F until done, add more liquid as beans bake dry. Serves 6-8.

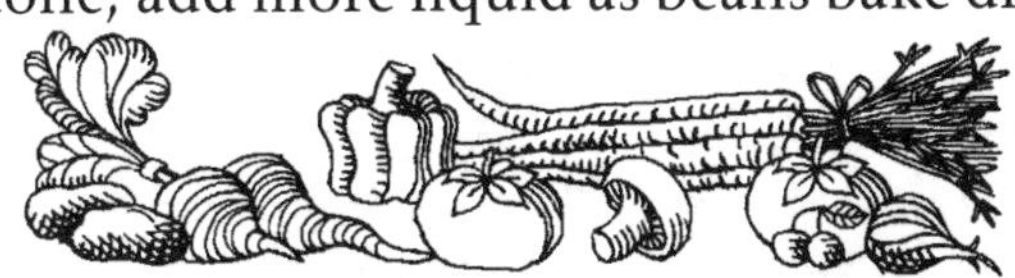

I used to say, "I sure hope things will change." Then, I learned that the only way things are going to change for me is when I change! – Jim Rohn

FISHLESS "TUNA" CASSEROLE

2 cups cooked brown rice
1 cup walnuts, chop
½ cup lemon juice
1 cup whole-grain toast, cube
1 Tbsp Bragg Liquid Aminos
3 Tbsps red onion, chop
3 Tbsps celery, finely chop
1 clove garlic, press
shake of Bragg Sprinkle
shake of Bragg Kelp

Thoroughly mix all ingredients except lemon juice together. Add soy milk or water if too dry. Bake at 350°F for 30 minutes. Add ½ cup lemon juice and allow to absorb. Serves 4-6.

BEAN - SQUASH CASSEROLE

½ lb dry white beans
2 lbs spinach or chard
3 Tbsps Bragg Olive Oil
3 crookneck squash, dice
2 Tbsps Bragg Liquid Aminos
¼ tsp Bragg Sprinkle
3 zucchinis, dice
2 cloves garlic, slice
½ cup soy Parmesan cheese, grate
soy yogurt or kefir (optional)

Cover beans with distilled water and soak overnight. Add more distilled water if needed and simmer until tender, about 1 hour. Add 1 tablespoon Bragg Aminos just before beans are done. Drain beans and sprinkle with 1 tablespoon of olive oil. Heat remaining olive oil in wok and add yellow crookneck, zucchini and garlic. Cook, stirring constantly to prevent scorching, until squash is tender. Transfer to an oiled casserole dish. Wash spinach thoroughly and shake off as much distilled water as possible. If using chard, tear coarsely. Spread spinach or chard over squash. Top with the beans and season with another tablespoon of Bragg Aminos and Sprinkle. Bake at 350°F for 30 minutes. When about half done, stir in soy Parmesan cheese. Serve hot or cold. Top with soy yogurt or kefir if desired when serving. Serves 6-8.

EGGPLANT CASSEROLE

2 medium round eggplants or
3-4 Japanese long eggplants
1 large red onion, mince
2 large garlic cloves, slice
1 large can tomato purée
4 oz soy cheese, slice thin
2 Tbsps Bragg Organic Olive Oil
½ tsp Bragg Sprinkle (24 herbs & spices)

Assemble in casserole dish in layers as follows:

½ Round eggplant (sliced 1-inch thick crosswise or long eggplant into 1" rounds), now add ½ Sprinkle, ½ garlic (sprinkle on top), ½ tomato purée, ½ minced onion, ½ soy cheese, ½ Bragg Olive Oil. Repeat with second layer. Bake at 350°F for 1 hour. Serves 4-6.

Think of yourself as a "battery" – you discharge energy and you must recharge yourself with proper food, exercise, rest and positive emotions.

Eggplants help block free radicals and are a source of folic acid & potassium.

PINTO CASSEROLE

2 cups dried pinto beans
3 cups distilled water
2 Tbsps tomatoes, chop
½ tsp poultry seasoning
2 tsps Bragg Liquid Aminos
2 cups green or sweet red bell pepper, chop
2 cloves garlic, mince
½ tsp Bragg Sprinkle
1 red large onion, chop

Soak beans overnight. Add distilled water. Bring to a boil, reduce heat, simmer covered, until the beans are tender, 1-2 hours. Add tomatoes, onion, green or red bell pepper, garlic, and seasonings. Place in oiled baking dish. Bake 325°F, 1 hour. Delicious garnished with Bragg Nutritional Yeast. Serves 6.

RICE PIZZA CRUST

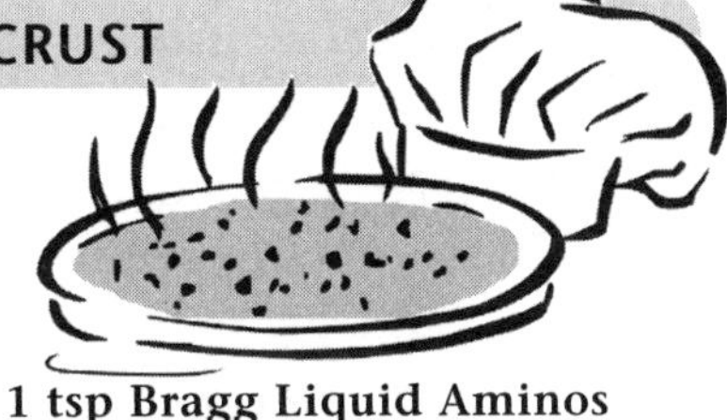

CRUST:
3 cups cooked brown rice
Egg Replacer equal to 2 eggs
1 cup soy cheese, grate

TOPPING:
16 oz fresh or can tomato sauce
⅓ tsp garlic powder
2 Tbsps soy Parmesan cheese, grate
1 tsp Bragg Liquid Aminos
½ tsp Bragg Sprinkle

To make crust, combine rice, Egg Replacer, and soy cheese. Press firmly into a 12-inch oiled pizza pan (or two 9-inch pie pans) by spreading evenly with a spatula. Bake at 450°F for 20 minutes. For topping, combine tomato sauce and seasonings. Spread evenly over rice crust. Top with soy Parmesan cheese. Bake 10 minutes longer. To serve, cut in wedges. If desired you may use these as additional toppings: finely sliced onion rings, mushrooms, red or green bell peppers, pineapple, and black olives. This entrée, with a big healthy salad, makes a delicious, nutritious meal. Serves 6.

SPAGHETTI PIE CASSEROLE

½ lb cooked and drained spaghetti
2 Tbsps Bragg Organic Olive Oil
½ cup hard soy cheese, grate
Egg Replacer equal to 2 eggs
1 lb firm tofu, drain and crumble
1 cup soy "mozzarella" cheese, shred
½ cup red onion, chop
2 tomatoes, chop
1 small can tomato paste
¼ tsp raw honey
2 cloves garlic, mince
½ tsp Bragg Liquid Aminos

Stir half the olive oil into cooked whole-grain spaghetti. Add grated soy cheese and Egg Replacer. Mix well. Press into an oiled casserole dish. Sauté onion in remaining oil for 3 minutes. Add remaining ingredients except soy mozzarella and cook 5 minutes. Pour over spaghetti and bake at 350°F about 20 minutes. Top with soy mozzarella and bake 10 minutes, until bubbly. Garnish with Bragg Nutritional Yeast. Serves 6.

Gardenburger Creator Thanks Bragg Books

Paul Wenner, the *Gardenburger* Creator, says his early years as a youth with asthma were so bad he would stand at the window praying to breathe through the night and stay alive. A miracle happened when as a teenager he read the Bragg *Miracle of Fasting, Bragg Healthy Lifestyle* and *Breathing* books and his years of asthma were cured in only one month. Paul Wenner became so inspired he wanted to be a health crusader like Paul C. Bragg and his daughter Patricia – and Paul Wenner has!!

Patricia with Paul Wenner

Now Gardenburgers are sold worldwide

GOURMET VEGGIE BALLS

VEGGIE BALLS:

1 cup walnuts
2 cloves garlic
1 red onion
1 Tbsp celery
1 carrot
2 Tbsps parsley
1 tsp Bragg Liquid Aminos
3 cups whole-grain bread crumbs
Egg Replacer equal to 2 eggs
3 Tbsps Bragg Organic Olive Oil

SAUCE:

1 can tomato paste
1 can tomato sauce
1 Tbsp Bragg Organic Apple Cider Vinegar
1 cup distilled water
2 Tbsps red onions, mince
2 Tbsps green pepper, mince
½ tsp Bragg Sprinkle
⅓ tsp Bragg Kelp
Serve over: cooked brown rice

Grind walnuts, garlic, onion, celery, carrot and parsley in blender. Add Bragg Aminos, dry bread crumbs and Egg Replacer. Shape into balls. Sauté balls in olive oil until browned on all sides. To make sauce, combine tomato sauce, tomato paste, vinegar, water, minced onions, green pepper, Sprinkle and Kelp. Put veggie balls in sauce, simmer on low heat for one hour. Serve over organic brown rice. Serves 6-8.

ECONOMY DELICIOUS "NO MEAT" HAMBURGERS

Egg Replacer equal to 2 eggs
½ cup walnuts, mince
1 cup raw oatmeal
½ cup distilled water
½ cup red onions, mince
1 tsp Bragg Liquid Aminos
½ tsp Bragg Sprinkle
2 cloves garlic, press
2 Tbsps Bragg Olive Oil
pinch poultry seasoning

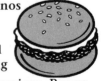

Combine Egg Replacer, walnuts, oatmeal, water, onion, Bragg Aminos, Sprinkle and garlic. Mix well and form into patties. Cook in Bragg Olive Oil for 15 minutes on both sides. Serves 4.

My years of asthma were cured in one month thanks to Paul Bragg and the Bragg Healthy Lifestyle. – Paul Wenner, Creator Gardenburger

SYRIAN THETCHOUKA

Egg Replacer equal to 6 eggs
3 red onions, chop
3 cloves garlic, mince
½ cup soy cheese, grate
3 tomatoes, chop
4 Tbsps Bragg Organic Olive Oil
1 carrot, coarse grate
3 green or red bell peppers, chop
1 Tbsp Bragg Liquid Aminos
shake Bragg Sprinkle (24 herbs & spices)

Sauté onions and peppers in the olive oil until golden brown. Add garlic, tomatoes, carrot and Bragg Aminos. Cover, cook slowly until all the vegetables are tender. Transfer the mixture to oiled glass casserole with a lid. Make 6 hollows in the mixture and carefully pour Egg Replacer into each one. Sprinkle with grated soy cheese and Bragg Sprinkle and bake at 350°F for 10 minutes or until set. Serves 4-6.

RICE – STUFFED CABBAGE

1 medium head cabbage
1 Tbsp Bragg Liquid Aminos
2 Tbsps Bragg Olive Oil
5 green onions, thinly slice
½ cup cooked brown rice
½ cup parsley, mince
2 cups distilled water
½ tsp cinnamon
½ cup walnuts, fine chop
½ tsp clove powder
6 carrots, long slice
2 tomatoes, dice

Place cabbage in deep pot of rapidly boiling water, cover and blanch for 5 minutes. Remove cabbage, drain well and carefully spread leaves to resemble opening flower petals. Cut large piece out of center. Heat olive oil in wok, add green onions, sauté until tender. Add rice and cook until it appears translucent. Add parsley, tomatoes, water, Bragg Aminos, cinnamon and clove powder. Cover tightly, cook 25 minutes. Most liquid should be absorbed, but rice will not be tender at this point. Chop center portion of cabbage, add to rice along with chopped walnuts. Carefully spoon stuffing into center of cabbage and between leaves. Shape into head again, tie securely with clean string. Place in steamer basket in deep pot. Slice carrots into 2-3 long pieces each, place around cabbage. Add 2 cups boiling water. Cover, steam on stove or bake at 325°F until tender. Cut into wedges, serve in bowls with liquid. Garnish with Bragg Vinaigrette Dressing and Bragg Nutritional Yeast. Serves 4.

CURRY RICE

3 cups brown rice (soak all day or overnight)
3 cloves garlic, press
shake of Bragg Sprinkle
½ tsp curry powder (or to taste)
1 Tbsp Bragg Organic Olive Oil
3¾ cups distilled water
1 tsp Bragg Liquid Aminos

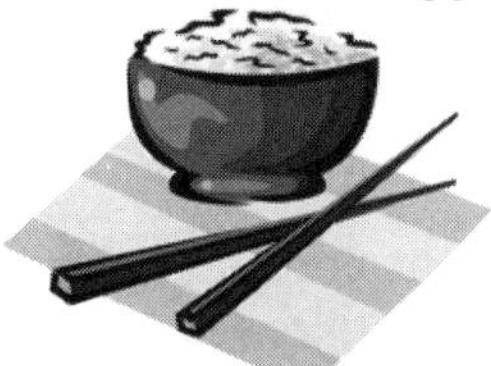

Bring above ingredients to a boil, then turn down heat, simmer 20-25 minutes. Serve with slice lemon, garnish with Bragg Nutritional Yeast and spray of Bragg Aminos. Serves 6-8.

LENTIL – SOY BALLS

½ lb cooked soybeans
½ lb cooked lentils
1 red onion, chop
1 cup cooked potatoes, mash
Tomato juice thickened with whole grain flour
3 Tbsps Bragg Olive Oil
2 Tbsps parsley, chop
½ tsp poultry seasonings
1 Tbsp Bragg Liquid Aminos
½ tsp Bragg Sprinkle
shake of Bragg Kelp

Add cooked soybeans to lentils and mashed potatoes. Sauté onion in half the olive oil and add soybean mixture. Now add all seasonings. Shape into size of golf balls, put on an oiled baking dish, top with remainder of olive oil, and bake at 350°F for 30 minutes until brown. Serve in a hot tureen bowl with a generous portion of thickened tomato juice. Serves 6-8.

LENTIL RISSOLES

2 cups cooked lentils
½ tsp Bragg Sprinkle
Egg Replacer equal to 1 egg
½ cup whole grain bread crumbs
2 red onions, chop
2 tsps Bragg Organic Olive Oil
4 oz soy cheese, grate
1 tsp Bragg Liquid Aminos
½ cup fresh toasted whole-grain bread crumbs

Sauté onions in olive oil until tender and golden. Mix all ingredients, (except toasted bread crumbs) and cool. Form cold mixture into small croquette, roll in toasted bread crumbs. Bake 425°F on pre-heated oiled baking tray 15 minutes. Turn over, cook another 15 minutes. Sprinkle on Bragg Nutritional Yeast. Serves 6.

BASIC KIDNEY BEANS

1 cup red kidney beans, pre-soaked
1 Tbsp Bragg Olive Oil
1 tsp Bragg Liquid Aminos
3 cloves garlic, chop
½ tsp Bragg Sprinkle
1 red onion, chop

Combine ingredients in large pot, cover with water. Cook 1 hour or until tender. Works well with any beans. Serves 4.

MUSHROOM BURGERS

1 cup cooked garbanzo beans, drain
½ cup red onion, finely chop
⅓ tsp Bragg Sprinkle
Egg Replacer equal to 1 egg
¾ cup wheat germ
1 tsp Bragg Liquid Aminos
1½ cups fresh mushrooms of choice, chop

Mash garbanzos in medium-size bowl with fork, add ¼ cup of wheat germ and all other ingredients. Mix thoroughly and form into burgers and roll in remaining wheat germ. Sauté in just enough olive oil to cover bottom of pan. Brown slowly on both sides over medium heat. Serves 4.

Kidney beans are good source of protein, folate, dietary fiber, iron magnesium, biotin, thiamine, copper, potassium & manganese.

NUT BURGERS

1 cup pecans, chop
½ cup pine nuts, chop
⅔ cup walnuts, chop
½ cup macadamia, chop
⅔ cup celery, finely chop
Egg Replacer equal to 2 eggs
1 cup cooked cornmeal
½ tsp poultry seasoning
½ tsp Bragg Sprinkle
2 tsps Bragg Liquid Aminos
Bragg Nutritional Yeast
2 Tbsps Bragg Organic Olive Oil

Mix all ingredients by hand, now shape into patties. Sauté in heated olive oil. When browned, remove, put on paper towel to absorb extra oil. Sprinkle with Bragg Nutritional Yeast. Delicious served hot or cold. Serves 6.

PASTA WITH GARBANZO SAUCE

1 lb pasta, any shape
1 Tbsp Bragg Olive Oil
1 red onion, dice
3 cloves garlic, mince
½ tsp Bragg Sprinkle
2 cups cooked garbanzo beans, mash
2 stalks celery, dice
1 tsp Bragg Liquid Aminos
pinch cayenne, to taste
1 cup tomato sauce (pg 111 or 163)

While pasta cooks, sauté in wok, onion, garlic and celery in olive oil until golden. Add cooked mashed garbanzo beans, tomato sauce, Sprinkle, Bragg Aminos and spices and simmer 10 minutes. Toss with cooked pasta, garnish with Bragg Nutritional Yeast and chopped parsley. Serves 4-6.

BAKED MILLET

4 cups vegetable broth
or distilled water
1 cup hulled millet
2 Tbsps Bragg Olive Oil
½ cup fresh mushrooms, chop
½ onion, chop
½ tsp Bragg Sprinkle
1 Tbsp Bragg Aminos

Heat olive oil in a large wok or saucepan. Add onion and mushrooms and cook until mushrooms are lightly browned. Add millet and cook over medium heat, stirring until well-coated with oil. Add Sprinkle, Bragg Aminos and the vegetable broth or water. Bring to a boil. Turn into an oiled 2-quart glass baking casserole. Cover tightly and bake at 300°F for 1 to 2 hours. (This makes a tasty main dish also using beans or peas instead of the millet.) Serves 4.

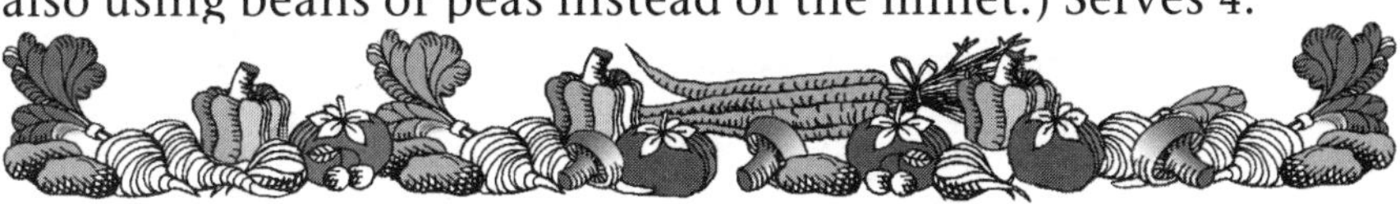

The use of antioxidant supplements and a diet high in antioxidant foods has been shown to reduce cancer and heart disease and increase life expectancy. Foods high in antioxidant vitamins include green vegetables, citrus fruits, nuts, whole grains, carrots, squash and cantaloupe. – U.S. News/Health Watch

---

The only way you get fat off is to eat less and exercise more. – Jack LaLanne

BUCKWHEAT GROATS OR KASHA

2 cups buckwheat groats (grains)
1 Tbsp Bragg Organic Olive Oil
⅓ cup parsley, chop
2 cups distilled water
½ tsps Bragg Liquid Aminos
Egg Replacer equal to 2 eggs
3 oz grated soy cheese
½ tsp Bragg Sprinkle

Bring water to boil in separate pot. Heat large frying pan with no oil. Mix buckwheat groats and Egg Replacer thoroughly. Put into heated pan and stir until toasted. Grains will separate when ready. Pour in actively boiling water, olive oil, Bragg Aminos, Sprinkle and stir. Cover and simmer on low heat 15 minutes, until water is absorbed. As a side dish, serves 4-6. For a main dish, cut 1 medium tomato into small pieces and mix in cooked groats. Top with grated soy cheese and parsley. Serves 2.

BUCKWHEAT OR KASHA CUTLETS

1 Tbsp Bragg Organic Olive Oil
1 red onion, chop
Egg Replacer equal to 1 egg
2 cups cooked kasha (buckwheat)
1 Tbsp Bragg Liquid Aminos
½ tsp poultry seasoning
1 Tbsp sunflower seeds, chop
½ tsp Bragg Sprinkle

Lightly sauté onion in olive oil. Add onion to kasha, Egg Replacer, Bragg Aminos, seasonings and sunflower seeds. Form into patties or drop by tablespoons onto heated skillet or wok, s`auté over low heat until both sides are nicely browned. Garnish with Bragg Nutritional Yeast. Serves 4.

PARSLEY PESTO WITH SOBA NOODLES

8 oz soba noodles
½ cup red onion, chop
3-4 cloves garlic
3 Tbsps fresh lemon juice
2 Tbsps Bragg Organic Olive Oil
⅓ tsp Bragg Sprinkle
2 bunches fresh parsley, stems removed

Cook soba noodles in boiling water until tender. Drain and rinse. Process onion and garlic in a food processor until finely chopped. Add parsley, lemon juice, olive oil and Sprinkle. Process until smooth. Add to noodles, toss to mix and serve. Serves 4.

QUICK BLACK BEAN CHILI

1 Tbsp Bragg Liquid Aminos
15 oz can diced tomatoes
½ tsp Bragg Sprinkle
1 Tbsp Bragg Olive Oil
⅓ tsp dried cumin
½ cup distilled water
4 oz can chilies, dice
2 red onions, chop
4 cloves garlic, crush
2 -15 oz cans cooked black beans, drain and rinse
¼ cup cilantro, chop

Heat water in large pan, add onions and garlic. Cook over medium heat until onions are soft. Add seasonings, Bragg Aminos and chilies. Cook 5 minutes over medium heat. Add tomatoes, black beans, and olive oil. Cover, simmer 10 minutes. Top with cilantro and Bragg Nutritional Yeast Flakes. Serves 4-6.

COOKING TIMES FOR BEANS

BEANS (1 cup uncooked)	COOKING TIME (hours)		YIELD (cups)
	Soaked	Unsoaked	
Adzuki	1 - 1 ½	2 - 3	2
Anasazi	2	2½ - 3	2
Black	1½ - 2	2 - 3	2
Black-eyed peas	½	1	2
Cannellini	1 - 1½	2	2
Chickpeas	2	3½ - 4	2½
Cranberry	2	2 - 3	2½
Great Northern	1½ - 2	2 - 3	2
Kidney	1½ - 2	2 - 3	2
Lentils	Not required	½ - ¾	2
Lima	¾ - 1	1½	2
Navy	1½ - 2	2½ - 3	2
Pinto	1½ - 2	2 - 3	2
Soybeans	2 - 3	3 - 4	2½
Split peas	Not required	¾	2

Legumes and Raw Nuts Improve Health

A recent report from the American Heart Association's Conference on Cardiovascular Disease Epidemiology and Prevention, has found that eating beans and other legumes at least four times a week lowered heart disease incidences by 19%, compared to those who ate legumes less than once a week. There are cardiovascular health benefits for those who increase non-meat protein sources in their diet. Eating a diet rich in raw, unsalted nuts and cooked beans improved their blood lipid levels in a clinical test given to 25 to 74 year-old participants.

Legumes are high-quality protein sources that are low in fat, high in dietary fiber and are cholesterol-free. In addition, legumes provide iron, folic acid, calcium, magnesium, potassium and B vitamins. Legumes include black-eyed peas, chickpeas, lentils, black, red, white, navy and kidney beans. Just a half a cup of cooked beans counts the same as an ounce of meat in the meat group of the Food Guide Pyramid as a source of protein. Legumes can be a delicious meat alternative in chili, pasta dishes, pitas, burritos, soups and even mixed in with salads.

The dietary fiber found in beans has been shown over time to decrease heart disease risks and helps lower cholesterol by binding bile while decreasing intestinal transit time. (see web: www.americanheart.org)

Vegetarian Protein % Chart

LEGUMES	%
Soybean Sprouts	54
Soybean Curd (tofu)	43
Soy flour	35
Soybeans	35
Broad Beans	32
Lentils	29
Split Peas	28
Kidney Beans	26
Navy Beans	26
Lima Beans	26
Garbanzo Beans	23

VEGETABLES	%
Spirulina *(Plant Algae)*	60
Spinach	49
New Zealand Spinach	47
Watercress	46
Kale	45
Broccoli	45
Brussels Sprouts	44
Turnip Greens	43
Collards	43
Cauliflower	40
Mustard Greens	39
Mushrooms	38
Chinese Cabbage	34
Parsley	34
Lettuce	34
Green Peas	30
Zucchini	28
Green Beans	26
Cucumbers	24
Dandelion Greens	24
Green Pepper	22
Artichokes	22
Cabbage	22
Celery	21
Eggplant	21
Tomatoes	18
Onions	16
Beets	15
Pumpkin	12
Potatoes	11
Yams	8
Sweet Potatoes	6

GRAINS	%
Wheat Germ	31
Rye	20
Wheat, hard red	17
Wild rice	16
Buckwheat	15
Oatmeal	15
Millet	12
Barley	11
Brown Rice	8

FRUITS	%
Lemons	16
Honeydew Melon	10
Cantaloupe	9
Strawberry	8
Orange	8
Blackberry	8
Cherry	8
Apricot	8
Grape	8
Watermelon	8
Tangerine	7
Papaya	6
Peach	6
Pear	5
Banana	5
Grapefruit	5
Pineapple	3
Apple	1

NUTS AND SEEDS	%
Pumpkin Seeds	21
Sunflower Seeds	17
Peanuts	16
Walnuts, black	13
Sesame Seeds	13
Almonds	12
Cashews	12
Macadamias	9

Data from Nutritive Value of American Foods in Common Units, USDA Agriculture Handbook No. 456. Reprinted with author's permission, from *Diet for a New America* John Robbins (Walpole, NH: Stillpoint Publishing)

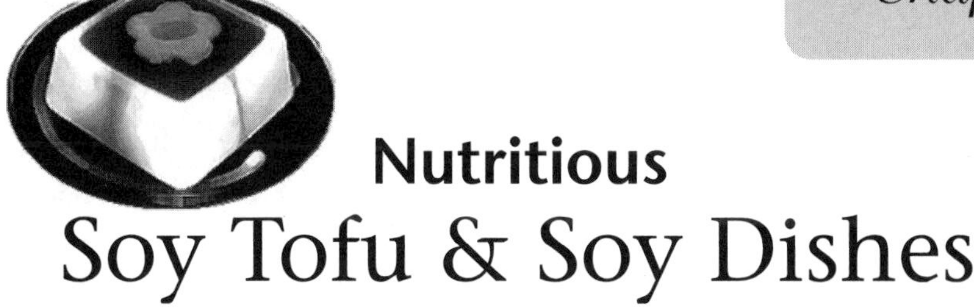

Chapter 11

Nutritious Soy Tofu & Soy Dishes

HOW TO PRESS & CARE FOR SOY TOFU

Put store-bought tofu in an airtight container, covered with new, purified water. Change the water daily. It will keep fresh for at least a week in the refrigerator. Soft tofu has a lot of water in it. The tofu becomes firm when it is pressed. To make firm tofu, pat with absorbent paper towel. Press tofu between baking sheets and paper towels. Put 5 lb weight on the top of baking sheet. Let stand 4 hours. The longer it is weighted, the drier it will become.

VEGGIE SOUP WITH TOFU CUBES

8 oz firm tofu, cube
1 cup mushrooms, slice
2 stalks celery, chop
½ tsp Bragg Sprinkle
1 cup zucchini, grate
1 cup carrots, grate
1½ tsps Bragg Liquid Aminos
2 cloves garlic, mince

Simmer vegetables in 3 cups distilled water for 20 minutes. Add tofu, garlic, seasonings and any other vegetables desired. Add enough water to cover. Simmer another 20 minutes. Serves 4-6.

TOFUNAISE

¼ cup distilled water
4 oz firm tofu, cut into pieces
shake of Bragg Sprinkle
1 Tbsp sesame oil
1 tsp Bragg Aminos, to taste
juice from lemon
1 tsp turmeric (optional for natural color)

Blend all ingredients in blender until smooth. Yields 2 cups.

CAJUN TOFU

2 tsps Bragg Olive Oil
½ cup red onion, dice
½ cup celery, dice
½ cup green pepper, dice
½ cup zucchini, dice
2 cloves garlic, mince
1 cup tomato sauce
½ tsp Bragg Sprinkle
1 tsp arrowroot powder
½ lb firm tofu, small cube
1 Tbsp Bragg Liquid Aminos
½ cup Bragg Apple Cider Vinegar

Sauté onion, celery, green pepper, zucchini and garlic in olive oil over medium-high heat for about 5 minutes. Add tomato sauce, Bragg Vinegar, Sprinkle and spices desired. Dissolve arrowroot and Bragg Aminos and add to vegetable mixture. Add tofu; cook 5 minutes, stir occasionally. Serves 4.

TOFU SCRAMBLE

2 tsps Bragg Organic Olive Oil
2 green onions (including tops), chop
½ tsp Bragg Sprinkle (24 herbs & spices)
½ tsp Bragg Liquid Aminos
¼ tsp turmeric
¼ tsp garlic powder
1 cup firm tofu, crumble
pinch cayenne pepper

In wok sauté onions in olive oil 3 minutes. Add all ingredients, cook 5 minutes. Sprinkle with Bragg Nutritional Yeast. Serves 4.

TOFU CHOW MEIN

¼ cup distilled water
pinch cayenne powder, to taste
2 cups bean sprouts
2 cups Chinese or sweet peas
1 tsp Bragg Liquid Aminos
1 cup firm tofu, cube
1 Tbsp Bragg Olive Oil
3 cups celery, thinly slice
½ tsp Bragg Sprinkle
½ cup water chestnuts, slice thin
1¼ Tbsps arrowroot, mix with water to make paste

In skillet combine: water, olive oil, Bragg Aminos, Sprinkle and cayenne. Add celery and tofu. Cover tightly, cook 10 minutes. Add bean sprouts, peas, chestnuts during last 5 minutes of cooking (add more distilled water if needed). Slowly add arrowroot paste. Stir until thickened. Pour over vegetables, serve with brown rice. Garnish with Bragg Nutritional Yeast. Serves 4.

TOFU CURRY – THAI STYLE

16 oz firm tofu, cube
2 Tbsps Bragg Liquid Aminos
2 Tbsps Bragg Organic Olive Oil

PASTE:

1 red onion
2 garlic cloves, chop
1 tsp lime rind, grate
1 tsp cumin
1 Tbsp Bragg Liquid Aminos
1 tsp raw honey
2 green chilies, seeded and chop
1 Tbsp grated fresh ginger
½ tsp Bragg Sprinkle
1 Tbsp fresh cilantro, chop
juice from 1 lime
1 oz coconut milk

GARNISH:

red chili or bell pepper, slice thin
fresh cilantro or parsley, chop

Toss tofu cubes in Bragg Aminos and let marinate while you prepare paste. Combine all paste ingredients into food processor, grind until smooth. Heat olive oil in wok until hot. Drain tofu cubes, stir-fry medium temperature until brown. Drain on paper towel. Wipe wok clean, now put in paste, stir. Return tofu to wok, mix in paste, reheating ingredients as you stir. Garnish with red chili or bell pepper, cilantro and Bragg Nutritional Yeast. This is delicious served with brown rice. Serves 4.

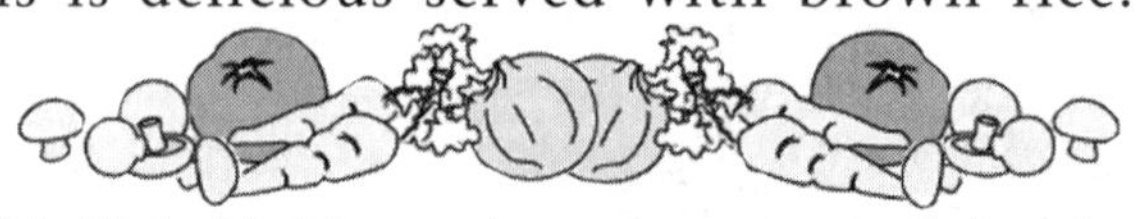

And God said, "Behold, I have given you every herb-bearing seed which is upon the face of the earth, and every tree in which is the fruit of a tree yielding seeds and nuts: to you it shall be as meat." – Genesis 1:29

TOFU CASSEROLE SUPREME

1 cup fresh tomatoes, chop
2 cloves garlic, chop
¼ cup Bragg Organic Olive Oil
1 cup zucchini or yellow squash
1-2 cups firm tofu cut 1" squares
1 cup red onion, chop
1 Tbsp Bragg Liquid Aminos
1 cup green pepper, chop
½ tsp Bragg Sprinkle
1 cup celery, slice

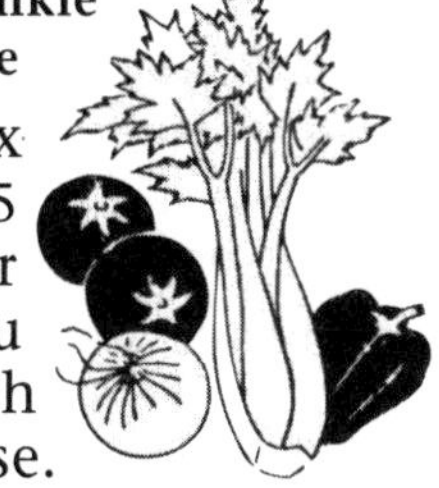

Combine all ingredients, except tofu and mix well. Place in casserole dish, bake 350°F for 45 minutes until almost done. Add tofu, gently stir with wooden spoon, careful not to break tofu squares. Bake 10 minutes longer. Garnish with Bragg Nutritional Yeast and grated soy cheese.

STIR-FRY ASPARAGUS AND TOFU

16 oz package firm tofu, cube
½ cup cucumbers, thin slice
1 tsp Bragg Liquid Aminos
2 cups asparagus, 1" cuts
½ tsp Bragg Sprinkle
⅓ tsp chili spice, to taste

Cut drained tofu into cubes. Add Bragg Aminos, Sprinkle (24 herbs & spices) and tofu to hot wok or skillet. Stir-fry for 5 minutes. Add asparagus and cucumbers. Sprinkle with chili spice as desired. Stir-fry 5 more minutes. Serve hot. Serves 2-4.

GARLIC TOFU SOUP

20 cloves garlic, peel
1 tsp Bragg Olive Oil
½ cup pea pods
1 Tbsp of Bragg Aminos
4 to 6 cups boiling distilled water
16 oz package tofu, cube
¼ cup parsley, chop
Bragg Sprinkle, to taste

Sauté garlic cloves in wok with olive oil. Add tofu cubes, water, parsley, pea pods and seasonings. Simmer 10 minutes. Spray with Bragg Aminos and garnish with Bragg Nutritional Yeast. Serves 4-6.

TOMATO, TOFU AND ONION SALAD

6 oz firm tofu, thin slices
½ cup red onion, thin slices
1 tsp Bragg Organic Olive Oil
shake of Bragg Sprinkle
1 medium tomato, thin slices
½ cup fresh basil
1 tsp Bragg Apple Cider Vinegar
shake of Bragg Kelp
Avocado slices (optional)

Arrange tofu, tomato, onion and basil on salad platter. Add avocado slices if desired. Combine Bragg Olive Oil, Bragg Vinegar and seasonings and drizzle evenly over salad, then sprinkle on Bragg Nutritional Yeast. Serves 3-4.

The beef industry has contributed to more American deaths than all the wars of this century, all natural disasters, and all automobile accidents combined. If beef is your idea of 'real food for real people,' you'd better live real close to a real good hospital. – Neal D. Barnard, M.D. President, Physicians Committee for Responsible Medicine, Washington, D.C.

TOFU KABOBS

MARINADE:
- ½ tsp Bragg Sprinkle
- 1 tsp Bragg Liquid Aminos
- ⅓ cup tomato juice
- 1 lb firm tofu, cut into cubes
- 1 cup distilled water
- ⅓ cup Bragg Apple Cider Vinegar
- pinch of cayenne pepper

VEGETABLES:
- red onion
- red and green bell pepper
- Japanese eggplant
- cherry tomatoes
- button mushrooms
- zucchini

Toast Sprinkle in large, dry wok over medium-low heat for 2-3 minutes. Add remaining marinade ingredients, (except tofu), stir to mix. Remove from heat. Cut firm tofu into 1-inch cubes and add to marinade. Allow tofu to marinate in pan for at least 1 hour, turning occasionally. Cut red onion in 1-inch chunks and peppers into large pieces. Clean and slice mushrooms, slice eggplant, zucchini and pineapple (optional) in 2-inch pieces. Stack variety of veggies, tomatoes and marinated tofu on skewers. Grill under broiler, over coals or campfire, turning regularly. Cook 10 minutes, or until vegetables are lightly browned. Serves 2-4.

TOFU TACOS

- 1 red onion, chop
- 1 bell pepper, dice
- ½ lb firm tofu, crumble
- 1 Tbsp Bragg Nutritional Yeast
- 1 Tbsp Bragg Liquid Aminos
- 6 corn tortillas
- 1 Tbsp Bragg Organic Olive Oil
- ½ cup tomato salsa
- shake of Bragg Sprinkle
- ½ tsp chili powder
- 2 garlic cloves, crush
- shake Bragg Kelp

Sauté half of onions, garlic and bell pepper in olive oil for 3 minutes, add tofu, chili powder, Bragg Yeast, Sprinkle, Kelp and Bragg Aminos. Cook 3 minutes. Add tomato salsa and simmer over low heat until mixture is nearly dry. Heat tortillas in an un-greased skillet or oven, turning from side to side until soft and pliable. Place small amount of tofu mixture in center, fold tortilla in half and remove from heat. Garnish with lettuce, raw onions, diced tomatoes, sliced avocado and top with salsa. Serves 2-3.

TOFU POTATO SALAD

- 5 steamed potatoes with skins, dice
- 2 cups firm tofu, crumble
- 2 stalks celery, dice
- 1 red onion, dice
- 1 Tbsp tofunaise (page 139)
- 1 tsp Bragg Liquid Aminos
- 1 Tbsp Bragg Apple Cider Vinegar
- 1 tsp raw honey (optional)
- 1 green pepper, dice

Combine ingredients. Refrigerate until ready to serve. Serves 8.

The secret of longevity is eating intelligently. – Gayelord Hauser

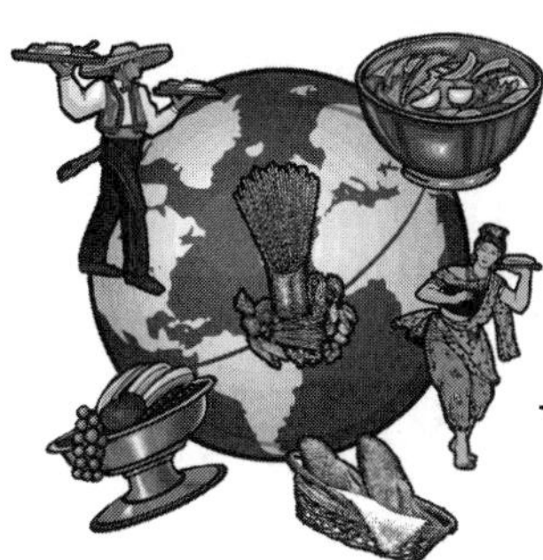

Chapter 12

International Vegetarian Cuisine

From the far corners of the world comes the heritage of good nutrition. Sometimes it is embodied in rare delicacies, but more often in the everyday foods of the common people. The peasants of many lands are often more skillful in their methods of preparing and flavoring nutritious food than are the famous chefs of the most exalted restaurants. Wild animals are more intelligent in their selection of foods than we, and earlier cultures followed in their footsteps. That is why the people closest to nature and natural living are instinctively more intelligent and intuitively adept with simple fresh natural foods grown locally and their preparation.

International foods as widely imagined, are not often heavy, rich and over-spiced. They are usually standard interpretations of fine foods, prepared delicately and hopefully many are prepared with intelligent, nutritional logic. Exciting the palate is not the least of their appeal and from the standpoint of health, not their entire value. Nutritionally speaking, foods and recipes stand firmly on their own healthy ingredients and health building principles, I've found in my 30 world trips.

We would be at a great loss if we ignored the marvelous combinations of vegetables of the Armenias, the ingenious uses of corn by the Mexicans, the full-bodied heartiness of the Russian interpretation, the symphonically-blended French foods, and the subtle, slightly "undercooked" offerings of the Chinese. In the world of good nutrition, we are not limited by differences of language, politics or boundaries. Our only required guide is the language of healthy common sense.

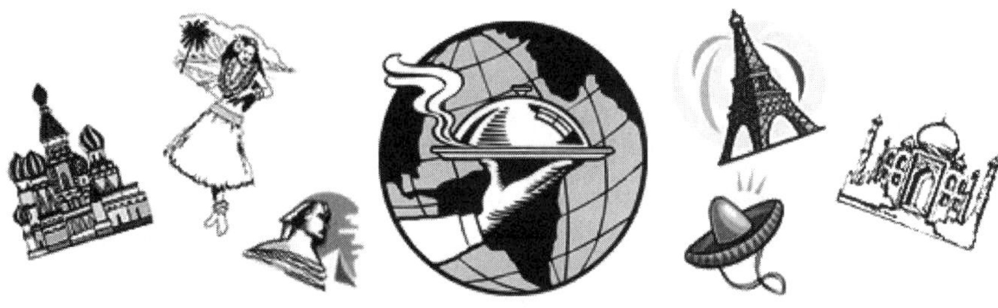

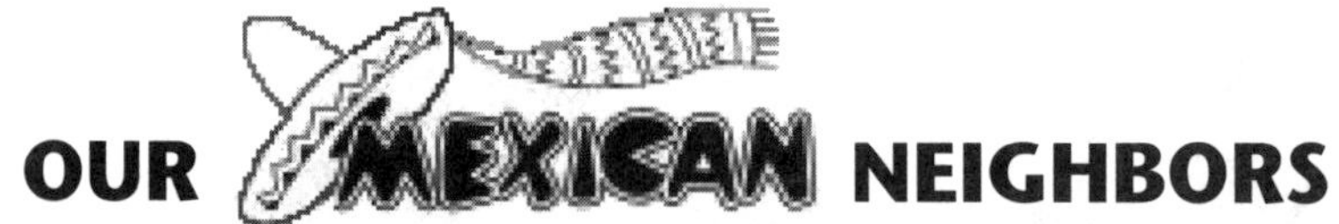

CORN TORTILLAS MADE WITH MASA HARINA

Corn tortillas are the foundation of classic Mexican dishes like enchiladas, quesadillas, tacos, fajitas, burritos and tostados.

Corn tortillas are made from a special flour called *masa harina*. The two most common brands are "Quaker" and "Maseca" that make excellent corn tortillas. Masa harina is corn flour that has been treated with calcium hydroxide which makes it more nutritious by releasing the niacin in the corn and makes it easier to digest. Masa harina can be found at Mexican markets or on-line at *www.mexgrocer.com*.

Fresh tortillas are quite easy to make. You will need a big cast-iron skillet or griddle and a tortilla press. You can find these at any kitchen-supply store. If you pay more than $20 for one you have paid too much. If you can't find a tortilla press, you can make the tortillas completely by hand, by forming a thin pancake with the dough between your hands. But unless you are somewhat experienced in this method, you will get more consistent results by using a tortilla press. It is possible to press your tortillas on a flat surface using a heavy, flat-bottomed dish.

Nothing beats the aroma of hot tortillas made from scratch. Home tortilla making is a delightful secret awaiting your discovery, give it a try and we believe that you will be hooked.

HOW TO MAKE CORN TORTILLAS

For 16-18 tortillas start with 2 cups of masa harina flour in a large bowl. Add 1 ½ to 2 cups of very warm purified water to the masa flour (according to directions on package, some brands may call for different water amounts). Mix in and let sit for 5 minutes. Begin working the masa with your hands. Press the dough as if you were kneading bread dough. If the dough seems too dry or too wet, add a little more water or masa to the dough.

Shape the masa dough into a ball about the size of a plum.

Take two pieces of wax paper and cut them to the shape of the tortilla press. Open the tortilla press and lay one piece of wax paper on the press. Place the masa ball in the center. Place another piece of wax paper over the masa ball. Gently close the press and press down, until the dough has spread to a diameter of 6 inches.

Heat a griddle or a large skillet on high. Working one at a time, carefully removing the wax paper on each side. Gently lay the tortilla down on the skillet. Cook the tortilla for about 30 seconds to a minute on each side. Remove and keep warm. Repeat.

HOW TO MAKE TAMALES FROM CORN MASA

Mix masa flour (available at Mexican markets) with oil and liquid. For liquid, use either distilled water or vegetable stock. Proportions must be experimented with because of the various types of corn, but the "floating test" will determine when you have the right consistency. If a small amount of corn masa dropped in water will float, it is satisfactory. However, here is a suggestion to use as the starting point of your experiment:

2 cups corn masa flour **1 cup corn oil or soy oil**
½ to ¾ cups vegetable stock or distilled water

The oil and liquid must be beaten into corn masa thoroughly and vigorously, but should be added only a little at a time until proper consistency is obtained. You need cornhusks to make the real Mexican tamale. You can buy them in the grocery store or in a Mexican grocery market in your city. Wash them thoroughly and use while they are still wet so they will be soft. Spread the cornhusks thick with masa, stuff with tamale stuffing, and fold or roll. Tie ends of cornhusk firmly to prevent leakage during cooking. Place in a pan suitable in size to the amount you are preparing and line the pan with cornhusks. Cook the tamales over steam for about one hour or until tender. When the masa breaks away from the cornhusks easily, the tamale is done.

USING CORN MASA FOR SWEET TAMALES

Some of the most delicious Mexican tamales are the "sweet" or fruit-filled ones. The corn masa for these tamales is prepared exactly as in the recipe above, except that the corn masa base should be compounded as follows:

2 cups corn masa **⅓ cup raw honey**
½ to ¾ cup fruit juice or distilled water

For filling, see Sweet Filling for Tamales (recipe below).

SWEET FILLING FOR TAMALES

Almost any cooked, sweetened fruit makes a delicious filling for sweet tamales. Pitted cherries, apricots, peaches, apples or pears (either dried or fresh), cooked and sweetened with raw sugar or honey, (diabetics use Stevia) make excellent fillings.

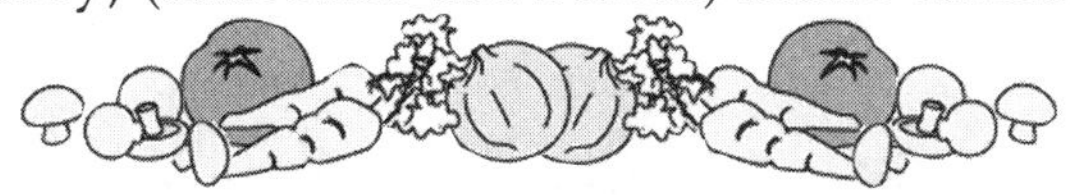

Corn tortillas can be made 2 hours in advance, wrapped and reheated. Bake at 350°F for 12 minutes. Put hot tortillas in covered Pyrex to keep warm.

HEALTHY TACOS

The taco is the Mexican version of the American sandwich, and to many is more delicious in every aspect. Healthy tacos are prepared by using a tortilla already baked on the griddle and filling it with some of the following combinations:

1. Sautéed and crumbled firm tofu, mixed with chopped olives, onions, tomatoes, and celery, moistened with a little green chili sauce, available mild, medium and hot.
2. Sautéed and crumbled firm tofu, mixed with fresh chopped onion, tomato, lettuce and green bell pepper, moistened with a little red chili sauce.
3. Sautéed and crumbled firm tofu, with chopped cucumbers, endive, tomatoes, onions and celery, moistened with a little chili or mushroom sauce.

Place fillings in the center of tortilla, fold and secure with two toothpicks, if necessary. Then place in 350°F oven for 5 minutes to brown. Or, cover with grated soy cheese and placed under the broiler long enough to melt cheese.

It would be worth your while to prepare the true native Mexican dishes given above, but you may not have the time or inclination for the various steps involved; however, you can still enjoy an excellent variety of enjoyable foods. Some of the more Americanized recipes are as follows:

RED CHILI SAUCE

3 cloves garlic
2 tsps Bragg Organic Olive Oil
¼ to ½ tsp oregano
4-6 red peppers (or of choice)
1 onion, finely mince
1 tsp Bragg Liquid Aminos
⅓ tsp Bragg Sprinkle
lemon juice for marinating

Marinate whole red peppers in fresh lemon juice and Bragg Liquid Aminos for 2 hours. Grind in food chopper using fine blade, then add remaining ingredients.

GREEN CHILI SAUCE

2 green chilies, small and hot
¼ green bell pepper
2 Tbsps boiling distilled water
6 small green tomatoes
½ of an onion
1 tsp Bragg Liquid Aminos
¼ tsp oregano powder (also a few fresh leaves, minced)
¼ tsp coriander powder (also a few fresh cilantro leaves, minced)

Blend all ingredients together. Add boiling water and mix.

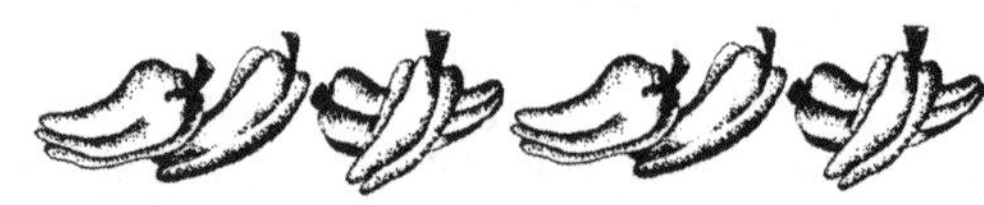

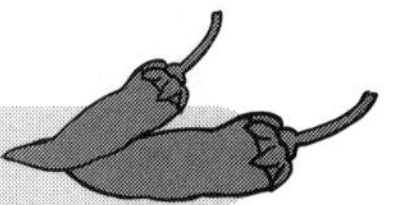

CHILI NON CARNE

- 2 cups dry kidney beans
- ½ red onion, mince
- 3 cloves garlic, mince
- 2½ Tbsps Bragg Olive Oil
- 3 cups tomatoes, dice
- distilled water (to cover beans)
- 1 tsp Bragg Liquid Aminos
- 2 Tbsps green pepper, chop
- ½ tsp chili powder or to taste
- 1 cup textured vegetable protein

Wash and soak kidney beans several hours or overnight. Drain water and rinse beans. Add fresh water, cook about 1 hour, or until tender. Sauté onion, green pepper in olive oil until tender. Add textured vegetable protein soaked in water and stir until separated and browned. Add tomatoes, Bragg Aminos, chili powder and garlic. Cook about 30 minutes on low heat. Add precooked kidney beans and cook an additional 10-15 minutes. Add more chili powder to taste. Serves 4-6.

TAMALE PIE

- 1½ cups organic cornmeal
- 2 red onions, chop
- 1 tsp Bragg Liquid Aminos
- 3 cups fresh tomatoes, chop
- 10 black olives, slice
- chili powder to season
- 6 cups distilled water
- 1 large green or chili pepper, chop
- 4 garlic cloves, mash
- 3½ Tbsps Bragg Organic Olive Oil
- 2½ cups firm tofu, crumble
- ½ tsp Bragg Sprinkle

Add organic cornmeal and Bragg Aminos to water in top of double boiler, cook 45 minutes. Chop onion and pepper, sauté in olive oil. Add tomatoes, tofu and chili powder; cook until thickened. Line an oiled baking dish with half of cornmeal mixture, pour in tofu and vegetable mixture, then cover with remaining cornmeal. Bake at 375°F for 30 minutes or until top is lightly browned. Serves 6.

AVOCADO MEXICAN SOUP

SOUP:

- 6 cups vegetable stock
- 2 red onions, minced
- 2 Tbsps parsley, mince

GARNISH:

- 2 green mild chilies, dice
- 2 medium avocados, mash
- ½ tsp Bragg Liquid Aminos

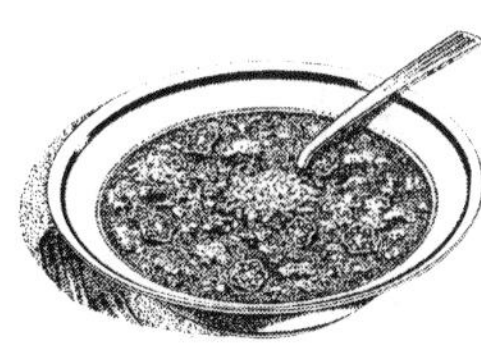

Cook onions in vegetable stock (see recipe page 10) until tender; add parsley. When serving, top soup with mashed chilies, avocados and Bragg Aminos. Delicious served with warm tortillas or pita bread. Serves 6.

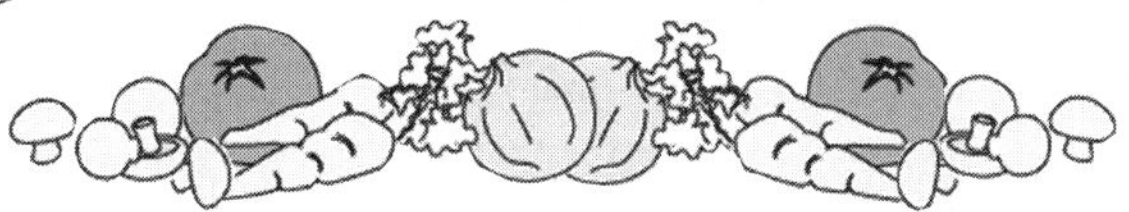

You can do almost anything with soup stock, it's like a strong foundation. When you have the right foundation, everything tastes good. – Martin Yan

---

The fruit of the avocado is the most tasteful & nourishing that grows out of the ground – it is the fruit of paradise! – See web: regenerativenutrition.com

PINTO BEANS

Soak 1 cup pinto beans overnight. Next morning, drain water and rinse beans. Add fresh water measuring 1-inch above the beans. Add following to beans:

2-3 cloves garlic, mince
2 red onions, chop
1 tsp chili powder
2 cups soy cheese, grate
½ tsp of Bragg Sprinkle
1 Tbsp Bragg Liquid Aminos
2 Tbsp Bragg Olive Oil
½ tsp Kelp

Bring beans to rolling boil, cook 1 hour or until beans are tender. Last 20 minutes add chili powder, Sprinkle, Kelp, Bragg Aminos, garlic and onions. Then mash the beans and add grated soy cheese. Stir well. Slowly sauté in olive oil. Serving suggestion: serve beans with enchiladas, tacos and a salad. This makes a perfect Mexican meal, ending with fresh papaya. Serves 6.

ENCHILADAS

First, prepare this simple enchilada sauce:

3 Tbsps mild chili powder
2 cups distilled water
8 oz can tomato sauce
3 Tbsps Bragg Organic Olive Oil
1 Tbsp organic yellow or white organic cornmeal

Brown cornmeal lightly in Bragg Olive Oil. Add the rest of the ingredients and cook for 10 minutes, stirring constantly to avoid lumps (this is enough sauce for 10-12 enchiladas).

1. When sauce is done, dip a corn tortilla in this sauce, remove it and place on a platter. Continue until all the corn tortillas have been dipped in the enchilada sauce.
2. Finely chop 1 cup red or green spring onions. Grate 2 cups soy cheese. Remove tortillas from plate (one at a time) and spread with onions, black olives and any finely grated veggies desired. Top with grated soy cheese. Roll all filled tortillas, place tightly in baking dish.
3. Pour any remainder of the enchilada sauce over the enchiladas in the baking dish and sprinkle with more grated soy cheese. Place the baking dish in 300°F oven for 15 minutes or until done and cheese has melted.

(In Mexican restaurants, enchiladas are served with a tossed green salad, rice and refried pinto beans).

I don't understand why asking people to eat a well-balanced vegetarian diet is considered drastic, while it is medically conservative to cut people open (cardiovascular/heart surgery) and put them on an expensive cholesterol-lowering drug (often with side effects) for the rest of their lives.

– Dean Ornish, M.D., Heart Disease Researcher who has proven Heart Disease is reversible on healthier low-fat vegetarian diet. *www.ornish.com*

FAJITAS

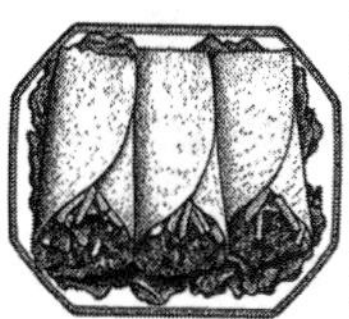

2 cups cooked pinto beans
1 red pepper, cut in strips
1 mild chili pepper, cut in strips
1 zucchini, thin slice
1 tomato, cut in thin wedges
Bragg Organic Olive Oil
1 onion, cut in strips
1 dozen corn tortillas
fresh cilantro, chop
spray of Bragg Aminos
tomato salsa
soy cheese, grated

Sauté vegetables in olive oil until cooked. Heat beans. Heat tortillas. Assemble by placing ⅓ cup beans in a tortilla and topping with cooked vegetables, salsa and cilantro. Serves 6.

FRIJOLES REFRITOS

2 lbs pinto or red kidney beans
6 Tbsps Bragg Organic Olive Oil
½ cups soy cheese, grate
3 cloves garlic, chop
1 onion, slice
distilled water
½ tsp of Bragg Sprinkle
2 tsps Bragg Liquid Aminos

Cover beans generously with water and soak overnight. Add Bragg Aminos, sliced onion, garlic and Sprinkle. Cook until beans are very tender, adding more water if needed, but beans should not be soupy. Drain beans of any excess liquid and save for soups or sauces. Heat 3 tablespoons of olive oil in a large skillet. Add beans and cook, stirring and mashing with back of spoon to make a paste. Gradually work in remaining oil. Sprinkle with soy cheese. This is a Bragg favorite, served with a big health salad first – then this bean dish. You can substitute any beans from soy beans to lima beans, they are all delicious!

MEXICAN BEAN STEW

1 cup dried pinto beans
1 cup dried garbanzo beans
1 red onion, dice
1 tsp ground cumin
14 oz can crushed tomatoes
black pepper, to taste
1 cup dried black beans
1 Tbsp Bragg Olive Oil
4 cloves garlic, mince
2 cups fresh corn kernels
½ tsp of Bragg Sprinkle
cayenne pepper, to taste

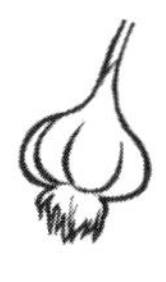

Rinse and sort pinto beans, black beans and garbanzo beans. Place in a large bowl and cover with water. Soak overnight. Drain beans and place in a large pot. Cover with distilled water. Bring to a boil and cook for 1 hour or until beans are tender. Add more water as needed to prevent drying out or scorching. Heat olive oil in a small saucepan over medium heat, sauté onion and garlic until onion is transparent. Stir in cumin. Add the onions, garlic and crushed tomatoes to the beans. Simmer for 20 minutes. Stir in fresh corn kernels and cook 15 minutes more. Add Sprinkle (24 herbs & spices), black pepper and cayenne to taste before serving. Serves 6.

Energy and persistence helps conquer all things. – Benjamin Franklin

FOOD FROM FRANCE

It is often said that the French can take leftovers and dress them up with superb sauces and herb flavorings until they are fit for a banquet. Whether that's true or not, the French do have a great gift with garlic, olive oil, and herb seasonings that has been handed down from generation to generation. Their salads are famed worldwide, probably because they favor variety. Salads are made with endive, escarole, watercress, romaine, etc. not just plain iceberg.

To top the list, they produce an innumerable amount of delicious soups, two of which are listed here because of their amazing delicious flavor and also nutritional value.

To the French, the art of eating, is one of the higher intellectual pursuits, a great deal more far-reaching than the general American concept of physical pleasure in food. It's no small wonder that France has produced the finest in the art of cooking with delicious flavor and food appreciation.

FRENCH ONION SOUP

4 cups consommé (pg. 54)
4 medium onions, thinly slice
3 Tbsps Bragg Olive Oil
2½ Tbsps dry soy cheese, grate
4 slices whole grain bread toast
½ tsp of Bragg Sprinkle

Sauté onions in olive oil and Bragg Sprinkle until golden and tender. Add to consommé stock. Simmer for a few minutes. Toast whole-grain bread until dry, then rub garlic over toast, and oil, and place at bottom of soup bowl; pour onion soup over it. Sprinkle with grated soy cheese before serving. Serves 4.

BRAGG RAW ORGANIC VEGETABLE HEALTH SALAD

2 stalks celery, chop
1 bell pepper & seeds, dice
½ cucumber, slice
2 carrots, grate
1 raw beet, grate
1 cup green cabbage, chop
½ cup red cabbage, chop
½ cup alfalfa or sunflower sprouts
2 spring onions & green tops, chop
1 turnip, grate
1 avocado (ripe)
3 tomatoes, medium size

For variety add organic raw zucchini, sugar peas, mushrooms, broccoli, cauliflower, (try black olives & capers). Chop, slice or grate vegetables fine to medium for variety. Mix vegetables & serve on bed of lettuce, spinach, watercress or chopped cabbage. Dice avocado and tomato, serve on side as a dressing. Serve choice of fresh squeezed lemon, orange or Bragg Ginger Dressing separately. Chill salad plates. Serves 3 to 5.

It's best to always eat salad first before hot dishes.

Seek out and choose whole foods, organic fruits, vegetables and organic whole grain cereals, breads, etc. rather than the commercial, canned, refined white flour and sugar products and other highly processed goods in the center aisles.

POTATOES NICOISE

1 lb small new potatoes, with skins, quartered
1 lb green beans
1 cup cherry tomatoes
¼ cup parsley, chopped
2 Tbsps capers
1 cup black olives, sliced

DRESSING:
4 Tbsps Bragg Organic Olive Oil
2 Tbsps Bragg Apple Cider Vinegar
2 Tbsps balsamic vinegar
1 tsp Dijon mustard
1 tsp Bragg Liquid Aminos
2 garlic cloves, minced

Steam potatoes and green beans until tender. To make dressing: mix olive oil, vinegars, mustard, Bragg Aminos, and garlic in bowl. Arrange lettuce leaves on platter. Top with cooked potatoes and half of dressing. Top with cooked green beans and remaining dressing. Arrange cherry tomatoes around outside of potatoes. Garnish platter with Bragg Nutritional Yeast, olives, capers and parsley. Serves 4.

FOOD FROM THE NEAR EAST

From Syria, Arabia, Armenia, Persia (Iran), Turkey and the Balkan countries come some of our greatest health foods. The thin, hard black breads and the honeys in generous abundance were the heritage of these people long before western civilization was dreamed of. Their specialties are the eggplant dishes, and delicious stuffings rolled in vine or grape leaves. Dates, figs and fruits of all kinds are as much a part of their national diet as are our potatoes. They use nuts and seeds of melons and sunflowers as we would confections, and most of their preserves are prepared with the natural sugars and honeys.

All these things are common to most Near Eastern countries. The differences among them are primarily in manners, customs and times of preparation and eating. They are beyond mastery in the use of whole-grains. Their desserts are usually simple: stewed fruits mixed with nuts, flavored with lemon juice and anise. Above all, their foods rank with the world's greatest dishes in delicious flavor.

ARMENIAN BULGUR GRAIN PILAF

2 cups Armenian Bulgur processed grain*
5½ Tbsps Bragg Organic Olive Oil
1 tsp Bragg Liquid Aminos
4 cups vegetable stock
1 large onion, mince
½ tsp Bragg Sprinkle

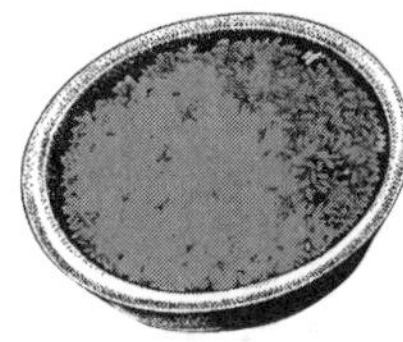

Place olive oil in very heavy skillet. Add grain and onion. Cook until slightly browned. Add Bragg Aminos, Sprinkle and stock. Now bake in 375°F oven 35 minutes. Then open oven, reach in and stir pilaf well. Close oven and continue baking for 15 more minutes. Serves 6.

* *This can be purchased at Greek or Armenian stores and is known as bulgur; it is precooked, sun-dried, whole-grain kernels.*

ARMENIAN RICE PILAF

Use the same recipe as Armenian Bulgur Grain Pilaf (page 151), using organic brown rice instead of the bulgur.

SYRIAN ROASTED STUFFED EGGPLANTS

2 eggplants, hollowed out
¼ cup pine nuts
1 stalk celery, mince
⅛ tsp pepper, freshly ground
½ tsp cinnamon powder
2 cups organic brown rice pilaf
1 carrot, mince
½ tsp Bragg Liquid Aminos
1 Tbsp Bragg Organic Olive Oil
½ tsp Bragg Sprinkle

Mince carrot and celery and mix with rice pilaf, pine nuts, Bragg Aminos, Sprinkle, pepper, cinnamon, olive oil and the chopped eggplant removed from the center. Moisten slightly with distilled water. Stuff eggplants with this mixture and brush with olive oil. Roast 375°F oven 45 minutes or until tender and brown. Garnish with Bragg Nutritional Yeast. Serves 4.

ARABIAN STUFFED EGGPLANT

3 eggplants, long 1½" slices
¾ lb firm tofu, crumble
4 Tbsps parsley, mince
½ cup Bragg Organic Olive Oil
2 cloves garlic, mince
¼ tsp Bragg Spinkle
2 tomatoes, chop
½ tsp cinnamon
Egg Replacer equal to 1 egg
½ tsp Bragg Liquid Aminos
1 small onion, mince
1 cup whole-grain bread crumbs

Cut eggplants into long, thick slices. Steam until almost tender. Do not allow to become mushy. The eggplants must hold their shape. For stuffing combine all other ingredients. Spread stuffing between every two slices of eggplant. Pierce with skewers to hold in place. Place in baking pan; pour oil over eggplant, bake until stuffing is cooked. Bake at 375°F 30 minutes. Garnish with Bragg Nutritional Yeast. Serves 6.

PERSIAN KEBAB

2 lbs firm tofu
½ tsp Bragg Liquid Aminos
½ tsp Bragg Sprinkle
2 Tbsps Bragg Organic Olive Oil
2 large onions
2 tomatoes
⅓ cup lemon juice
¾ tsp oregano

Cut tofu into 1-inch cubes. Slice onion in large wedges and place onion and tofu in a mixture of lemon juice, Bragg Aminos, olive oil and seasonings. Marinate 2 hours. Cut tomatoes in large wedges. On long skewers place one piece of tofu, then onion, tomato, etc. until skewer is half-filled. (*Options:* you can add mushrooms, pineapple, zucchini, etc.) Broil over moderate flame or campfire until done. Serves 6.

Vegetarians eat more fiber. Dietary fiber lowers risk of cancer and heart disease, helps control blood glucose levels, and reduces the risk for diabetes. Vegetarians on an average eat 50% to even over 100% more fiber than non-vegetarians.

STUFFED GRAPE LEAVES

FILLING:

2 Tbsps Bragg Organic Olive Oil
¼ cup raisins or pine nuts (optional)
2 cups cooked organic brown rice
¼ cup mint, mince
1 cup onion, chop
2 cloves garlic, mince

OTHER INGREDIENTS:

3 dozen young grape leaves, blanched and dried
2 cups vegetable broth (page 10) or distilled water
¼ cup Bragg Organic Olive Oil
½ cup fresh lemon juice

Sauté onion, garlic and brown rice in olive oil until golden. Add remaining filling ingredients. Line with grape leaves the bottom of a 3-quart pot. With remaining leaves, cut out tough stem and place bottom up, stem side facing you. Place 1 tablespoon of rice mixture in the middle and wrap sides over. Roll from bottom, and place snugly seam side down in pot. Mix broth or water, lemon juice and olive oil. Bring to a boil, then pour over top of rice stuffed grape leaves and weigh down with a plate. Cover and simmer 30 minutes. Serves 6-8.

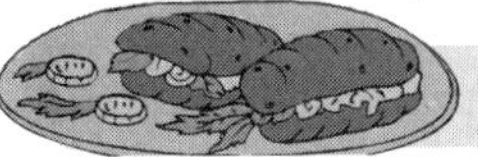

FALAFELS

1 cup garbanzo beans
½ cup onion
¼ cup parsley
2 cloves garlic, mince
1 tsp Bragg Liquid Aminos
1 tsp ground cumin
½ tsp ground coriander
¼ tsp Bragg Sprinkle
2 Tbsps whole-grain flour
1 Tbsp Bragg Olive Oil

Soak garbanzo beans overnight. Drain thoroughly. Combine in food processor with remaining ingredients, except olive oil. Shape mixture into small round patties and place on oiled cookie sheet. Bake at 350°F for 30 minutes. Serve 2 patties in a pita with shredded cabbage, carrots, chopped celery, and chopped tomatoes. Top with hummus (page 69). Serves 4.

TABOULI

2 cups wholegrain bulgur (pg. 151)
3 cups boiling distilled water
3 tomatoes, chop
½ cup green onions, slice
Bragg Liquid Aminos, to taste
¼ cup parsley, mince
¼ cup fresh mint, mince
¼ cup Bragg Organic Olive Oil
shake of Bragg Sprinkle
¼ cup lemon juice

Pour boiling water over bulgur, cover, and let stand for 30 minutes. Drain and chill. Add remaining ingredients and serve on a bed of fresh cabbage leaves or watercress. Serves 4-6.

Kind words can be short and easy to speak, but their echoes are truly endless. – Mother Theresa

---

Wherever there is a human being there is an opportunity for kindness. – Seneca

SERBIAN MUSHROOM VEGETABLE GOULASH

1 cup mushrooms, chop
1 cup red onions, chop
1 cup sweet green peppers, chop
2 Tbsps Bragg Organic Olive Oil
1 Tbsp Bragg Liquid Aminos
1 cup tomatoes, chop
2 cloves garlic (optional)
1 cup beets, grate
2 cups green or red cabbage (or mixed), coarsely slice

Mix all ingredients, place in oiled baking pan. Bake 30 minutes 350°F or until done. Garnish with Bragg Nutritional Yeast. Serves 3-4.

FOODS FROM THE FAR EAST

It is sometimes difficult to achieve the true Far Eastern flavoring because we do not always have the proper ingredients. It can be difficult to secure fresh ginger root, for instance, or the very young garlic bulbs such as the Chinese use that do not have the strong pungency of the more matured garlic bulb, or lotus leaves, small Chinese peas or bamboo shoots. Many of these ingredients are now becoming more available in the United States.

The Far East is the home of the soybean, the water chestnut, and the sesame seed, as well as some of the world's finest health foods. The people of East Asia, like their Western neighbors, have yielded too much to popular methods of fast food preparation. Too many of their foods are now prepared by deep-fat frying and other dietary practices that are unhealthy. However, if we look for the best in Far Eastern cookery, as we search for the best of our own, we will find a treasure trove to prepare of delicious, wholesome foods.

STUFFED PORTABELLA MUSHROOMS

4 large portabella mushrooms
½ tsp Bragg Liquid Aminos
2 tsps arrowroot or potato flour
½ lb firm tofu, crumble
2 tsps onion, mince
2 tsps lemon juice

Wash, cut off and mince the stems of mushrooms. Mix minced stems with tofu; add all other ingredients. Thoroughly wash mushroom caps. Stuff caps with mounds of tofu mixture. Place in regular steamer basket. Steam 10 minutes. Garnish each mound with small amount olive oil, sprinkle of soy parmesan cheese, place under broiler for few minutes. Serves 4-6.

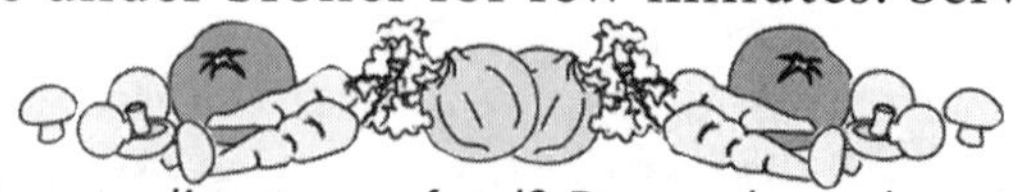

Do you know how to digest your food? Do you know how to fill your lungs with air? Do you know how to establish, regulate and direct the metabolism of your body . . . the assimilation of foods, so that it builds muscles, bones and flesh? No, you don't know how consciously, but your body has a miracle wisdom within you that does know how and does it! – Donald Curtis, Outstanding Leader in New Thought and Metaphysics for over 20 years.

MOO SHU

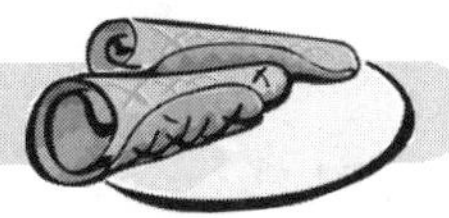

MANDARINE PANCAKES:

- 2 cups whole wheat flour
- 1½ cups soy milk
- Egg Replacer equal to 1 egg
- 1 Tbsp Bragg Olive Oil

Combine soy milk, olive oil, and Egg Replacer. Add soy milk mixture to flour, mix. Cover. Chill for 1 hour. Place a skillet coated with olive oil over medium heat until hot. Remove pan from heat and pour a ¼ cup batter into pan. Quickly tilt pan so batter covers bottom of pan. Cook about 1 minute. Turn pancake over; cook 30 seconds on the other side. Makes 12 pancakes.

FILLING:

- 1-oz bean thread noodles
- ½ cup shiitake mushrooms, slice (fresh or rehydrated from dried)
- ½ cup green onions, diagonally slice
- 1 cup bean sprouts
- 1 cup Chinese cabbage, thinly slice
- 2 cloves garlic, mince
- 1 tsp Bragg Liquid Aminos
- 1 Tbsp sesame oil
- 1 tsp fresh ginger, mince
- ½ cup firm tofu, shred
- Sweet & Sour Plum Sauce

Cover noodles and mushrooms with boiling water. Cover and let stand 30 minutes. Drain. Sauté with remaining vegetables and spices in oil until heated through and cabbage is limp.

Spread each pancake with 1 Tbsp of Sweet and Sour Plum Sauce (page 163) and ⅓ cup of filling. Roll up, folding in bottom end.

SWEET AND SOUR TOFU

- 1 lb firm tofu, drained and cubed
- 2 Tbsps Bragg Organic Olive Oil
- 1 carrot, diagonally slice
- 1 Tbsp Bragg Liquid Aminos
- 2 zucchini, slice thin
- 1½ cups pineapple chunks
- ¼ cup Bragg Apple Cider Vinegar
- 2 onions, slice
- 1 Tbsp arrowroot
- 1 red pepper, slice
- ¼ cup distilled water
- 1 cup pineapple juice
- 1 tsp ginger, mince
- 1 Tbsp raw honey

Brown tofu in olive oil. Add pineapple and vegetables and cook for 10 minutes. Make a paste with arrowroot, Bragg Aminos and distilled water. Add paste to vegetables, then add remaining ingredients and simmer until thickened. Serve with brown rice. Serves 4.

TOFU AND SPINACH WITH PEANUT SAUCE

- 1 lb firm tofu, drain and cube
- 1 Tbsp Bragg Liquid Aminos
- 1 clove garlic, mince
- 1 tsp fresh ginger, mince
- 2 Tbsps Bragg Organic Olive Oil
- 1 lb spinach, chop
- Peanut Sauce (recipe page 156)

Mix tofu with Bragg Aminos, garlic and ginger. Stir-fry in olive oil until brown. Remove from pan and keep warm. Add spinach to pan and heat just until limp. Arrange on a platter and top with tofu. Serve with Peanut Sauce (page 156). Serves 4-6.

PEANUT SAUCE

- 1 Tbsp Bragg Organic Olive Oil
- ½ cup onion, dice
- 1 Tbsp fresh ginger, mince
- ¼ tsp cayenne (optional)
- ¼ - ½ cup hot distilled water
- ½ cup organic peanut butter
- 1 tsp Bragg Liquid Aminos
- 1 Tbsp molasses
- juice of 1 lemon
- honey to taste

Sauté onion in olive oil 5 minutes. Add remaining ingredients and stir until blended. Add hot water to thin sauce. Makes 2 cups.

KUNG PAO TOFU

- 1 lb firm tofu, drain and cube
- Egg Replacer equal to 1 egg
- ½ tsp Bragg Liquid Aminos
- 2 tsps corn flour
- 2 tsps distilled water
- ½ tsp red pepper flakes
- 2 Tbsps Bragg Olive Oil
- 1 red pepper, slice
- 2 green onions, slice diagonally
- 2 Tbsps Sweet and Sour Plum Sauce (page 163)
- 1 Tbsp rice vinegar
- 1 tsp ginger, mince
- 1 cup cashews, chop

Mix together Egg Replacer, Bragg Aminos, corn flour and water. Add tofu and mix. Stir fry in 2 Tbsps olive oil until browned. Remove and add pepper flakes, red pepper, onion, ginger. Cook 2 minutes; add cashews, rice vinegar. Serve with Plum Sauce. Garnish with Bragg Nutritional Yeast. Serves 4-6.

CHINESE CABBAGE

- 1 lb green cabbage, shred
- 1 tsp Bragg Organic Olive Oil
- 2 green onions, slice diagonally
- ½ tsp Chinese 5 Spice (pg. 127)
- 1 Tbsp Bragg Liquid Aminos
- sesame oil to taste

Heat olive oil, add cabbage and green onions. Cook for 3-5 minutes, then add Chinese 5 Spice and Bragg Aminos and cook 3 more minutes. Stir in sesame oil to taste and serve.

RF

JAPANESE SALAD

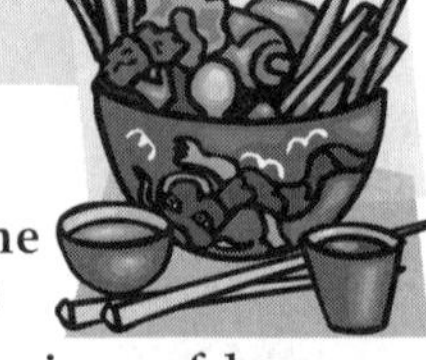

- 1 cup spinach leaves, tear
- ⅓ tsp fresh ginger, mince
- 2 Tbsps lemon juice
- 1 tsp Bragg Liquid Aminos
- 1 tomato
- 1 Tbsp raw honey
- 1 tsp toasted sesame seedc or to taste

Chop tomato, tear spinach leaves; prepare dressing of lemon juice, Bragg Aminos, honey, ginger root and toss with salad. Sprinkle with sesame seeds and Bragg Nutritional Yeast. Serves 4.

PHILIPPINE FRUIT COMPOTE & DRESSING

- 1 cup plums, dice
- 1 cup apricots, dice
- 3 Tbsps lime juice
- ⅛ tsp cinnamon

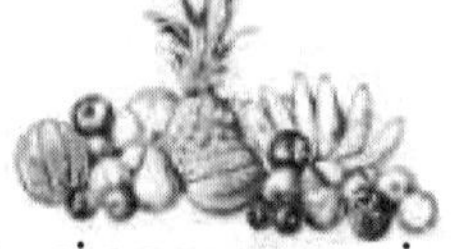

- 1 cup pears, dice
- 3 Tbsps raw honey
- 3 Tbsps pine nuts
- ¼ tsp ginger

Mix honey, lime juice, cinnamon, ginger and pine nuts. Thin with distilled water until runny. Use as dressing for the fruit compote, mixing thoroughly. Chill before serving. Serves 4.

FOOD FROM INDIA

A large portion of the people of India are vegetarians and are probably more adept at serving a wide variety of vegetarian foods than almost any other nation. They use coconut milk and ginger root abundantly and prepare many curry dishes. One of their basic foods, the lentil, is one of the healthiest legumes.

INDIAN EGGPLANT

2 cups eggplant, dice
1½ cups distilled water
¼ tsp Bragg Sprinkle
1 sprig lemon balm, mince
pinch cayenne pepper (optional)
½ tsp Bragg Liquid Aminos
¼ cup Bragg Organic Olive Oil
⅛ tsp sage
1 tsp parsley, mince
1 tsp mint, mince
4 Tbsps lemon juice
shake of Bragg Kelp

Place eggplant in water with sage, Sprinkle, parsley, mint and lemon balm and 2 tablespoons of lemon juice. Cook until eggplant is tender. Make sauce in bowl: olive oil with other 2 tablespoons lemon juice, Kelp, Bragg Aminos, and pinch of cayenne pepper (*optional*). Serve sauce over eggplant. Serves 6.

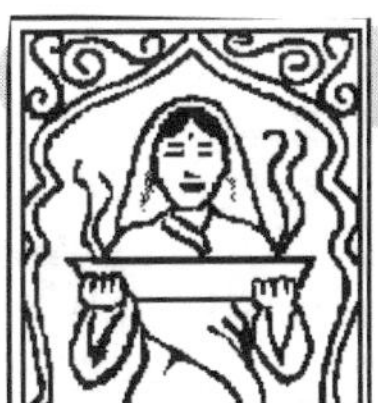

INDIAN CURRY POWDER

1 Tbsp turmeric powder
1 Tbsp coriander powder
½ tsp cardamom powder
⅓ tsp chili powder
½ Tbsp ginger powder
1 Tbsp cumin powder
½ tsp pepper
½ tsp fennel
½ tsp poppy seed

Try to buy all your ingredients ground to a fine powder. If you cannot, then mix all the ingredients thoroughly and grind them to a fine powder in a mortar yourself.

GOLDEN CURRY

1 Tbsp Bragg Olive Oil
1 onion, chop
3 stalks celery, chop
1 red pepper, chop
2 cloves garlic, mince
1 lb potatoes, cut in 1-inch cubes
1 cup cooked garbanzo beans
1 Tbsp curry powder (recipe above)
2 tomatoes, chop
2 cups vegetable broth
toasted coconut, cashews and raisins (as topping)

Sauté vegetables in olive oil for 5 minutes. Add remaining ingredients, cover and simmer for 30 minutes. Serve over Saffron Rice or grains of choice with Quick Chutney (recipe on page 158). Top with toasted coconut, toasted cashews and raisins (plump up with boiling water). Serves 6.

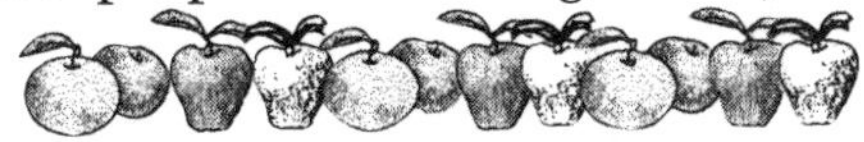

When speaking, ask: "Is it kind, is it truthful, is it necessary?" – Patricia Bragg

My pleasant, healthy thoughts bring me peace. – Paul C. Bragg

QUICK CHUTNEY

1 cup Peach Butter (page 191)
1 tsp Bragg Apple Cider Vinegar
½ tsp fresh ginger, mince
¼ tsp paprika powder
1 tsp Bragg Liquid Aminos
½ tsp garlic, mince
¼ tsp mustard powder

Mix Peach Butter with Bragg Aminos and Apple Cider Vinegar. Mix in minced garlic, ginger, mustard powder and paprika.

SAFFRON RICE

½ cup Bragg Organic Olive Oil
3½ cups of boiling distilled water
2 cups organic brown rice
pinch of saffron

Brown saffron in a dry skillet. Add to 1 cup boiling water. Sauté organic brown rice in olive oil until golden. Add remaining distilled water, bring to boil, cover and simmer 20-30 minutes until cooked. Best not to stir while cooking.

FOOD FROM HOLLAND

The Low Countries, the Netherlands and Belgium, have popularized the salad almost as much as has their neighbor, France. Years of trade with their colonies in the Far East has accustomed the culture to the use of spices for flavoring, and as a rule their food has hidden delicate fragrances and flavors. Like their Scandinavian neighbors, they are a little too fond of pickling, smoking and over-processing their foods, and perhaps also overcooking a great many of their foods. Their best health dishes are on the hearty side.

DUTCH VEGETABLE SOUP

1 cup tomatoes, chop
1 cup corn kernels
1 large turnip, dice
¼ cup soy or rice milk
½ tsp whole-grain flour
1 cup cabbage, chop
1 carrot, dice
1 onion, slice
½ tsp Bragg Liquid Aminos
1 cup dried lima beans (soak overnight)

Cook vegetables and lima beans in water until limas are soft. Season to taste with Bragg Aminos. Mix flour with milk, stir into soup. Serve hot. Garnish with Bragg Nutritional Yeast. Serves 4.

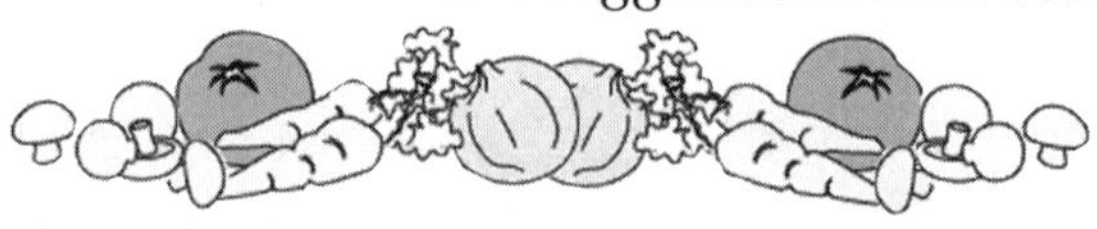

Studies prove free radicals are damaging substances that cause abnormal changes in cells that can lead to heart disease, cataracts and cancer and may be the cause of many of the effects attributed to premature ageing. Antioxidant compounds (like those found in fruits and vegetables) can trap and destroy these dangerous free radicals. Research shows that beta-carotene – a powerful antioxidant found in carrots, cantaloupe, squash and dark green vegetables – not only boosts the immune function, but is easily converted by the body to another important nutrient, vitamin A.

FOOD FROM RUSSIA

Russia affords more contrast in national foods than many other countries. Borscht, or beet soup with soy or rice sour cream; kasha, a sort of mush made with buckwheat; and the wonderful vegetable soups are delicious nutritional health delicacies! Yet these are the foods most often eaten by the peasants. Foods that are considered luxury foods in Russia, while good as a general rule, are often too rich and concentrated for the ordinary diet. But many of their national foods are delicious and we always enjoyed the Russian Tea Room in NYC.

BORSCHT

5 cups boiling distilled water
one bunch organic beet greens
¼ head green cabbage, shred
5 beets, cube
soy sour cream or soy yogurt
2 onions, slice
1 tsp Bragg Liquid Aminos
2 Tbsps lemon juice
½ Tbsp whole-grain flour
2 Tbsps Bragg Olive Oil
1 cup tomatoes, can or fresh, chop

Place beet greens, onions and Bragg Aminos in boiling water. Simmer until vegetables are tender. Strain. Put cut beets in separate pot with lemon juice and olive oil. Cook until tender. Add whole-grain flour to beets. Mix well; add to strained vegetable broth. Add tomatoes and cabbage and boil until cabbage is tender (3-5 minutes). Serve with one tablespoon of soy or rice sour cream or try soy yogurt on top of each Borscht. Serves 6.

FOOD FROM POLAND

Mushrooms with soy sour cream is a tasty vegetarian variation of this delicious dish from Poland.

MUSHROOMS WITH SOY SOUR CREAM

1 lb mushrooms, slice
1½ Tbsps soy milk
¼ cup onion, mince
paprika, sprinkle to taste
1 cup soy or rice sour cream
4 Tbsps Bragg Organic Olive Oil
⅓ tsp Bragg Liquid Aminos
1 Tbsp whole-grain flour

Sauté onion in olive oil. Add flour, blend and sauté until golden brown. Add soy milk. Simmer 5 minutes. Add mushrooms and Bragg Aminos. Add ½ cup soy sour cream and continue to simmer until mushrooms are tender. Add remaining soy sour cream and mix well. Sprinkle with paprika to taste. Best when served immediately. Serves 4.

To have love and joy one must share it. – Lord Byron

FOOD FROM SOUTH SEA ISLANDS

In the South Sea Islands, before the coming of the Europeans, Polynesians lived on an almost perfect health food diet. Nowadays, to a certain extent, that appetite has succumbed to depravity; but, the abundance of natural foods on the islands has made them almost an economic necessity in the diet. This is certainly fortunate for the Polynesians, who have only to draw from nature's generous supply to have their tables loaded with luxury.

TAHITIAN COCONUT CREAM

Drain milk from coconut. Grind the coconut meat. Combine coconut milk and ground coconut. Allow to stand for an hour. Mix thoroughly, re-grind or run through a juice extractor. Coconut cream is not only a delicious beverage, but can also be used as a topping on fruit desserts. Available Health Stores.

MALANA BANANA POI

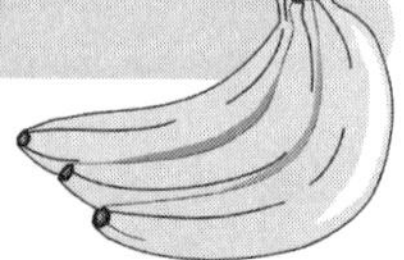

Mash banana; add grated coconut and raw honey to taste. Serve with cold coconut cream.

RAROTONGA COCONUT AND BANANA WHIP

Combine mashed banana and grated coconut, flavored with pure vanilla and raw honey (or Stevia) to taste. Whip with coconut cream, soy or rice cream to a frothy light consistency.

The word "vegetarian" is not derived from the word "vegetable," but from the Latin words, "homo vegetus," among the Romans meaning a strong, robust, thoroughly healthy man.

Study showed that patients with moderate-to-severe rheumatoid arthritis (RA), who switch to a low-fat, vegan diet can experience significant reduction in RA symptoms.
– Journal of Alternative & Complementary Medicine

A little more gentle sunshine might help you live longer! Sunlight spurs the body to produce vitamin D. Studies have found protective effects from higher vitamin D intake for some cancers and ailments as osteoporosis and diabetes. Modest sun exposure gives enormous vitamin D health benefits. – Reuters

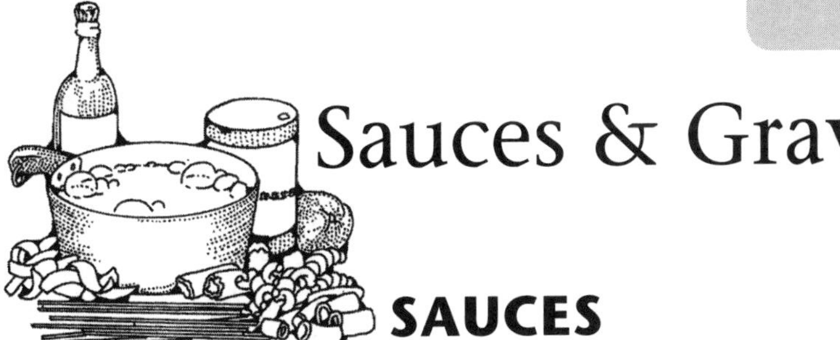

Chapter 13

Sauces & Gravies

SAUCES

HOLLANDAISE SAUCE

1½ cup firm silken tofu, crumbled
1 Tbsp Bragg Nutritional Yeast Flakes
1 Tbsp Bragg Liquid Aminos
¼ cup Bragg Organic Olive Oil
½ tsp Bragg Sprinkle
½ cup soy milk
2 Tbsps lemon juice
1 Tbsp Tahini
1 tsp turmeric

Place all the ingredients except for the olive oil in a blender and blend until very smooth and creamy. Slowly drizzle in the olive oil while continuing to blend. Transfer the blended sauce ingredients to a 1-quart sauce pan, and place it over medium-low heat. Slowly warm the sauce, stirring constantly until it is completely heated. Do not boil. Remove from heat. Serve at once. Serves 6.

BERNAISE SAUCE

To hollandaise sauce, add one tablespoon each of finely chopped fresh parsley and tarragon. If unable to obtain fresh tarragon, then add ½ teaspoon of dried tarragon.

CAPER SAUCE, HOLLANDAISE

To hollandaise sauce, add one to two tablespoons of capers.

CAPER SAUCE, MAÎTRE D'HÔTEL

4 Tbsps Bragg Organic Olive Oil
2 Tbsps capers
½ tsp Bragg Liquid Aminos
2 Tbsps lemon juice
1 tsp parsley, chop
shake of Bragg Sprinkle

Heat olive oil. Add lemon juice, capers, parsley and Bragg Aminos. Heat until sizzling. Serve with brown rice dishes.

CHEESE SAUCE

1½ Tbsps Bragg Olive Oil
¾ cup soy cheese, grate
⅓ tsp Bragg Liquid Aminos
1½ Tbsps whole-grain flour
¾ cup soy milk
shake of Bragg Sprinkle

Heat olive oil in double boiler. Stir in whole-grain flour. Add soy milk while stirring. Cook until smooth and thickened. Stir in soy cheese, Sprinkle and Bragg Aminos. Makes 1½ cups.

FRENCH MORNAY SAUCE

1 cup vegetable stock
¼ bay leaf
4 peppercorns
½ tsp Bragg Liquid Aminos
⅔ cup scalded soy milk
2 oz hard soy cheese, grate
1 slice onion
1 sprig parsley
⅛ tsp Bragg Sprinkle
½ cup carrot, grate
3 Tbsps Bragg Organic Olive Oil
5 tsps whole-grain pastry flour

Add onion, carrot, bay leaf, peppercorns, parsley, Bragg Aminos and Bragg Sprinkle (24 herbs & spices) to vegetable stock and cook slowly for 20 minutes. Then add olive oil to flour, blend in soy milk and strained stock gradually. Return to heat in double boiler for 15 minutes. Add soy cheese; whisk lightly through sauce. Put sauce on low heat for a few minutes to ensure melting of the soy cheese. Serves 4.

BERCY SAUCE

1½ cups vegetable stock
4½ Tbsps garlic infused oil
3 Tbsps whole-grain pastry flour
1½ Tbsps shallots, mince
1 Tbsp Bragg Organic Olive Oil
1 Tbsp lemon juice
¼ cup parsley, chop
¼ tsp Bragg Liquid Aminos

Gently sauté shallots in olive oil until thoroughly heated. Blend in flour until smooth. Add stock gradually and add the garlic infused oil, lemon juice, Bragg Aminos and parsley. Simmer over low heat for 5 minutes, stirring frequently. Serves 4-6.

ROBERT SAUCE

½ cup vegetable stock
3 shallots, mince
1 Tbsp lemon juice
1½ tsps black olives, chop
½ Tbsp Bragg Liquid Aminos
2 tsps Bragg Organic Olive Oil
1 tsp whole-grain flour
1½ tsps capers, chop
½ tsp mustard powder
shake of Bragg Sprinkle

Add minced shallots and flour to heated olive oil and cook about 5 minutes. Add other ingredients, continue cooking for about 12 minutes, stirring constantly. Prepare just before when needed. Do not reheat. Serves 4-6.

MUSHROOM HERB SAUCE

1 cup fresh mushrooms, chop
2 Tbsps Bragg Olive Oil
1 tsp Bragg Liquid Aminos
½ tsp Bragg Sprinkle
1 Tbsp soy flour
1 cup soy milk

Wash and chop mushrooms and stalks finely. Heat olive oil in a pan, add flour and stir well over gentle heat. Gradually add soy milk, stirring briskly, till a smooth sauce results. Add mushrooms, Sprinkle and Bragg Aminos; simmer for 10 minutes.

EGG REPLACER BUTTER SAUCE

Egg Replacer equal to 2 eggs
⅓ cup Bragg Organic Olive Oil
1½ tsps lemon juice
⅛ tsp paprika
1½ Tbsps soy cream

Add paprika to Egg Replacer; now gradually add the Bragg Olive Oil, soy cream and lemon juice. Makes ¾ cup sauce.

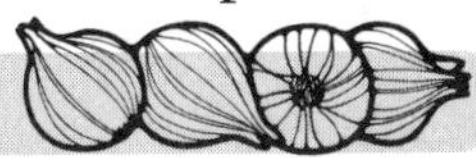

ONION SAUCE

3 Tbsps onion, finely chop
¼ cup Bragg Organic Olive Oil

Work onion into olive oil. Replace chives for the onion for a more delicate flavor; or, half of each can be used. Makes ½ cup.

TOMATO SAUCE

3 Tbsps Bragg Olive Oil
1½ cups cooked tomatoes
4 cloves garlic, chop
2 slices of onion, chop
½ cup tomato juice
¼ tsp of Bragg Sprinkle
½ tsp Bragg Liquid Aminos
3 Tbsps whole-grain flour

Combine all ingredients and simmer gently for 15 minutes. Blend this tasty sauce and serve hot. Makes 2 cups.

SWEET AND SOUR PLUM SAUCE

2 oz Asian pickled plums
2-3 large hot red chili peppers, seeded and mince
2 cups Bragg Apple Cider Vinegar
1¼ cups raw honey
1 red sweet pepper, seeded and mince
1¼ cups distilled water

Rub the plums through fingers to break up the flesh, but do not discard the pits. Put the honey and 1¼ cups of distilled water in a saucepan and bring to a boil over medium heat. When the syrup is boiling hard, add the chili peppers, the sweet pepper and the plums with their pits. Bring back to a boil and boil 2-3 minutes, then stir in Bragg Organic Apple Cider Vinegar. Let cool, then remove and discard the pits.

MUSHROOM SAUCE

2 medium onions, chop
2 cups mushrooms, slice
4 cup vegetable stock (page 10)
2 tsp unsulphured molasses
½ tsp thyme
2 cloves garlic, mince
3 Tbsps soy flour, toast
1 Tbsp Bragg Liquid Aminos
¼ tsp summer savory
shakes of Bragg Sprinkle

In a skillet, stir soy flour over medium heat until light brown. Set aside. Sauté onion and garlic 5 minutes using teaspoons of vegetable stock to prevent sticking. Add mushrooms, herbs and Sprinkle, cover, and simmer 5-10 minutes. Sprinkle flour over the mushroom mixture and blend. Stir in the rest of the vegetable stock, Bragg Aminos and molasses. Simmer until the sauce thickens. Delicious topping for vegetables, rice and bean dishes.

MEXICAN SAUCE

3 Tbsps onion, chop
⅓ lemon, thinly slice
1 Tbsp parsley, chop
1⅓ tsps raw honey
1⅓ tsps whole-grain flour
1 Tbsp Bragg Organic Olive Oil
1 tsp Bragg Liquid Aminos
2 cloves garlic (optional)
⅔ Tbsp celery leaves, chop
⅔ Tbsp lemon juice
⅔ cup tomato purée
⅓ tsp chili powder
¼ cup firm tofu, crumble
Egg Replacer equal to 2 eggs

Cook onion in olive oil until tender. Add whole-grain flour and allow to brown. Add the remaining ingredients except Egg Replacer. Simmer about 10 minutes. Add Egg Replacer, blend and serve over vegetables, rice or beans. Makes 2 cups.

TASSAJARA VEGETABLE SAUCE

1 cup white or brown sauce (see recipe below)
2 carrots, dice
thyme, sage, parsley to taste
2 stalks celery, dice
2 onions, dice

Make white or brown sauce following the recipe below. Sauté the diced vegetables and add them to the simmering sauce. Season with thyme, sage and minced parsley, to taste.

BROWN SAUCE

2 Tbsps Bragg Organic Olive Oil
1 cup heated liquid such as: distilled water or vegetable stock
2 Tbsps whole-grain flour
pepper to taste
⅓ tsp Bragg Sprinkle

Cook flour in Bragg Olive Oil several minutes, until well-browned. Meanwhile, boil water or vegetable stock. Pour boiling liquid into cooked flour; remove from heat. Stir mixture briskly with a whisk or fork. Use a spoon to scrape out the corners of the pan so that all the flour-oil mixture is incorporated into the water. Then put it back on the heat and let the sauce simmer for several minutes. Season lightly with pepper and Sprinkle.

WHITE SAUCE

2 Tbsps Bragg Organic Olive Oil
1 cup heated soy milk
2 Tbsps whole grain flour
white pepper, to taste

Cook flour slightly less time than for the brown sauce recipe. Follow directions for brown sauce (see recipe above).

TASSAJARA BROWN GRAVY

1 cup brown sauce (recipe above)
1 garlic clove, crush
pepper, to taste
shake of Bragg Sprinkle
1 onion, dice
Bragg Liquid Aminos, to taste
freshly grated ginger, to taste
1 Tbsp Bragg Organic Olive Oil

Sauté the onion in olive oil until golden brown and add it to the brown sauce. Season first with Bragg Aminos and then add the garlic, grated ginger, Sprinkle and pepper to taste.

DESSERT SAUCES

BUTTERSCOTCH SAUCE

2¼ cups raw honey
6 Tbsps Bragg Organic Olive Oil
½ cup distilled water
¾ cup nut meats, chop

Boil honey and water together to 235°F or until a small amount of the mixture forms a soft ball when dropped in cold water. Add olive oil and nut meats of choice. Makes about 3 cups.

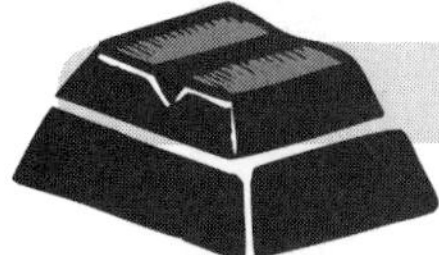

CHOCOLIKE SAUCE

4 oz carob bar
1⅓ cups raw honey
¾ cup cold distilled water

Combine water and carob and cook directly over medium heat for 4 minutes, stirring constantly. Add honey, then cook 4 minutes longer. Pour into an airtight jar and seal. Keep syrup and use as needed for desserts. Makes 1½ cups.

STRAWBERRY SAUCE

½ cup raw honey
1⅓ cups distilled water
1½ cups organic strawberries, crush

Boil honey and water together 12 minutes, add organic strawberries, and cook 1 minute, then cool. Makes 3 cups of sauce.

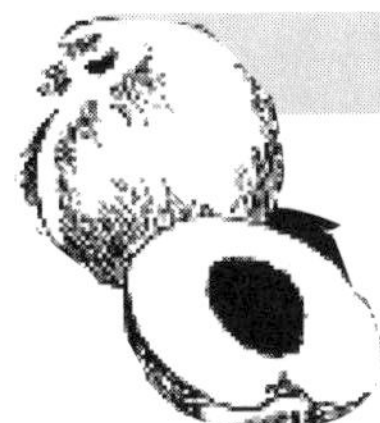

HONEY PEACH SAUCE

3 cups organic peaches, slice
¾ cup distilled water
½ cup raw honey

Cook the peaches in water until soft, then add the honey. Makes 4 cups of sauce.

ORANGE PUDDING SAUCE

1 cup raw honey
rinds of 2 organic oranges, grate
Egg Replacer equal to 2 eggs
1⅓ cups fresh orange juice
2 tsps lemon juice
4 Tbsps tapioca powder
1⅓ cups boiling distilled water
4 Tbsps Bragg Organic Olive Oil

Combine honey, tapioca and grated organic orange rinds; mix well. Add boiling water and cook in double boiler for 10 minutes, stirring occasionally. Remove from heat and pour some of the hot mixture over beaten Egg Replacer, blend well. Return to double boiler, add olive oil, cook for 2 minutes, stirring constantly. Add fruit juices and beat until well blended. Cool before serving. Makes 2⅔ cups.

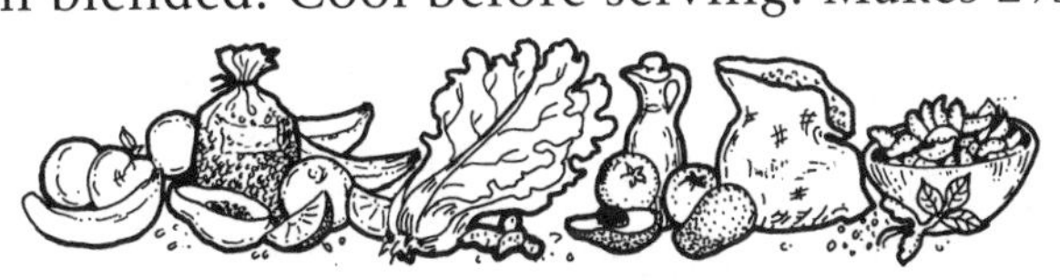

PINEAPPLE MINT SAUCE

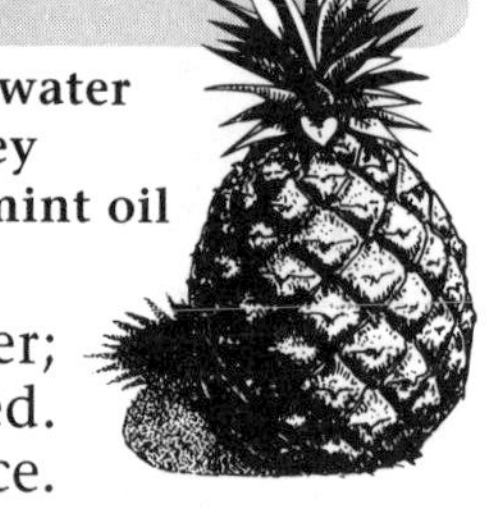

½ cup crushed unsweetened pineapple, drain
⅛ cup unsweetened pineapple juice
½ cup distilled water
⅓ cup raw honey
4 drops peppermint oil

Combine pineapple, juice, honey and water; simmer about 10 minutes or until thickened. Cool. Add peppermint oil. Makes 1¼ cups sauce.

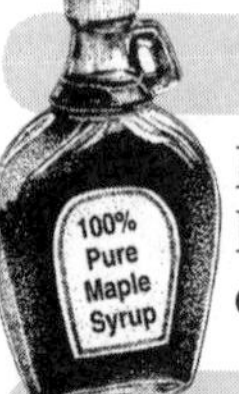

QUICK MAPLE SYRUP

Heat ½ cup of maple sugar. Add one teaspoon of Bragg Olive Oil. Serve hot in place of butterscotch or chocolate sauce for desserts, sundaes, pancakes, etc.

HOT CHOCOLATE FUDGE SAUCE

6 Tbsps carob powder
2 oz vegan chocolate, finely chopped
¾ cup rice soy milk
½ cup raw honey
6 oz soft tofu

In blender, combine tofu, soy milk, blend until creamy. Add carob powder, honey, blend until smooth. Pour mixture into medium saucepan, cook over medium heat, stirring continuously, until hot, but not boiling. Remove from heat, then add chopped chocolate, stir until chocolate melts. Serve hot for desserts, over soy or rice ice cream, waffles, etc. Makes 2 cups.

APPLE - CINNAMON SAUCE

¾ cup organic apple juice
⅛ tsp cinnamon powder
¼ cup distilled water
2 Tbsps kudzu root starch

Place all ingredients in saucepan, mix well, and bring to boil over medium heat, stirring constantly to avoid lumping. Just as boiling occurs, mixture turns into a clear, shiny sauce. Allow to cool. For use over a fresh fruit compote or fruit salad.

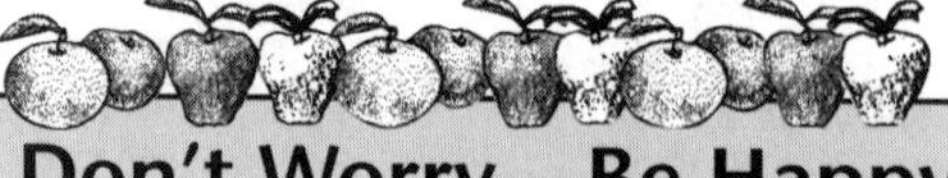

Don't Worry – Be Happy

Actions speak louder than words and can change your mood if you feel depressed. Take a walk outside – it often helps you sort out and solve your problems! Spend time with a young child - it simplifies life and puts everything in perspective. Find the comics section in the newspaper or something funny to read and laugh. If someone is upset, try to analyze the situation from that person's perspective. Make yourself physically smile and laugh, it opens the blood vessels in the back of your head and physically lifts your mood. Choose to be happy in spite of circumstances. No one "makes" you happy – it's an attitude that comes from within.

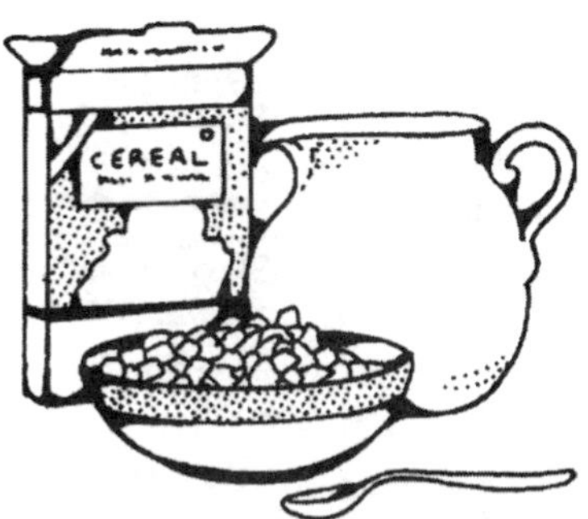

Chapter 14

Whole Grains, Cereals & Rice

One of nature's greatest gifts to mankind is the tiny, golden berry of grain. Whole wheat, rye, barley, oats – all nourishing nutlike grains – impart rich flavor to the menu and tremendous energy and healthy food nutrition value to the diet.

In modern civilization, one of the greatest crimes against food has been committed against the whole-grain! Since it contains elements that do not keep well in storage (for instance, the bran and the germ of the grains), the grain companies have established commercial practices of milling the bran and the germ right out of the grain and offering only a fraction of the original substance as an excuse for a rich, golden grain. They have robbed and refined the grains of much of their life, vitality, vitamins, and minerals, by removing part of their most precious substances! The tiny golden flake (the wheat germ), the rich, nutlike flavor of the bran, and the full-bodied flavor of the completely blended grain flavor, are lost forever in the refining processing!

Although organic, whole-grains have become more popular in recent years, they still do not take advantage of nature's rich variety of grain food. Wise, organic farmers never plant the same grain year after year. Doing so would deplete the soil. If you habitually eat only one whole-grain, such as whole wheat, you are not utilizing the food essentials in nature's grain variety. For this reason, I will give you a full range blend of grains to create an excellent basic cereal mixture (see page 168). You will note that most of the ingredients are thoroughly toasted.

COOKING TIMES FOR GRAINS

Grain (1 cup uncooked)	Liquid *(cups)*	Cooking Time	Yield *(cups)*
Amaranth	2½	20 - 25 minutes	3½
Barley (hulled)	3	1½ hours	3½ - 4
Barley (pearl)	3	50 minutes	3½
Bulgur	2	20 minutes	3
Couscous	2	5 minutes	3
Kamut	3	2 hours	2¾
Millet	2	25 minutes	3
Quinoa	2	15 minutes	3
Wheat Berries	3	2 hours	3

MY FAVORITE HEALTH BLENDED MEAL OR CEREAL

¾ cup cracked whole wheat
¼ cup cracked whole barley
½ cup cracked whole rye
½ cup raw wheat germ (vacuum-packed)
½ cup cracked whole oats
¼ cup raw rice bran
¼ cup raw oat bran

Grind wheat, barley, rye and oats in food processor or blender. Place in shallow pan, heat in oven at 150°F for 1½ hours or until almost done. Remove from oven, allow to cool to room temperature. Add last three ingredients (rice bran, oat bran and wheat germ) and blend thoroughly. This yields about 3 cups of delicious toasted multi grains that can be used in many ways.

METHODS OF BREAKFAST CEREAL PREPARATION

- Stir 1 cup blended meal into 2 cups boiling distilled water. Stir for 3 minutes. Cover, remove from heat. Allow to stand for 30 minutes.
- Soak ½ cup blended meal overnight in one cup cold distilled water. Cook in double boiler or heavy-bottomed pan 20-30 minutes.
- To one cup boiling distilled water, add ⅓ cup blended meal. Cook partially covered in double boiler for 20 minutes. Turn off heat, cover and let stand for several hours, preferably overnight. Reheat for 15 minutes.
- Soak ⅓ cup blended meal and raisins (optional) in 1 cup boiling distilled water, seal in large wide-mouth thermos overnight so it's ready in the morning. Allow 1-2 inches at top for expansion.

BREAKFAST CEREAL TOPPINGS

- Raw honey and nut milk (see page 41) or soy cream
- Sliced bananas, raw honey and non-dairy milk of choice, such as soy or rice milk
- Berries, raw honey and non-dairy milk of choice
- Slice fresh figs, raw honey and non-dairy milk of choice
- Chop dates, pecans and non-dairy milk of choice
- Dried, cooked or soaked unsulphured apricots, pears, peaches, prunes, figs with raw honey and non-dairy milk of choice
- Pecans, pine nuts or walnuts, chopped
- Flax oil or lecithin granules (for hot cereal)
- Any fresh fruit, natural sweetener and non-dairy milk
- Any fresh fruit, sweetener and fruit juice (try unsweetened apple, pineapple, grape or cranberry juice)
- Raw honey, 100% pure maple syrup, soy or nut milk (page 41)

While whole-grain products are an excellent source of magnesium - a vital element for maintaining healthy bone structure . . . studies have found that over 80% of magnesium is lost in the refining of the grains into white flour!

BAKING WITH CEREALS

NEW ORLEANS BREAD

7 cups blended 7-grain meal
2⅔ cups warm distilled water
½ cup brown rice syrup
½ cup Bragg Organic Olive Oil
1 pkg quick-rise yeast
shake Bragg Sprinkle (24 herbs & spices)

Mix yeast with the water according to directions on yeast packet. Add brown rice syrup or molasses and olive oil. Place in bowl. Add the meal and remaining water. Knead well on floured board for 10 minutes. Cover and keep in a warm place for several hours. Knead again. For variety in loaves, you may add 2 tablespoons grated hard soy cheese, a shake of Bragg Sprinkle or raisins. Place dough in well-oiled bread pans. Let rise until dough doubles in size (30-60 minutes). Bake at 350°F for 45 minutes until done. Makes 3 medium-sized loaves.

CALIFORNIA MUFFINS

2 cups blended 7-grain meal
2 tsps baking powder
1½ cups soy or rice milk
Egg Replacer equal to 1 egg
1 tsp brown rice syrup
2 ripe bananas (optional)
3 Tbsps Bragg Organic Olive Oil
1 Tbsp oat bran

Mix olive oil and rice syrup. Add beaten Egg Replacer, 7-grain meal, oat bran, baking powder, mashed banana and soy milk. Mix well and pour into muffin tin. Bake at 350°F until light brown. Makes 12 muffins. (*Variation:* Add 1 tsp pure vanilla extract, ¼ cup raisins or currants and 1 Tbsp chop nuts.)

SEVEN GRAIN MEAL WITH FRUIT

1 cup blended 7-grain cereal, cook
Egg Replacer equal to 1 egg
1 cup stewed fruit, fresh or dried
2 Tbsps raw honey
soy yogurt (as topping)

Combine 7-grain cereal with stewed fruit of choice. Stir in beaten Egg Replacer and honey. Bake in an oiled baking dish at 350°F for about 30 minutes until set in the center, as for custard. Serve hot or cold, top with soy yogurt. Serves 2.

HOT MILLET CEREAL

½ cup millet
2 cups distilled water
soy yogurt (as topping)
dates, raisins or figs
raw honey, to taste
maple syrup (optional)

Bring 2 cups water to boil in heavy pan with a tight lid. Stir in millet and continue stirring. Bring to a boil. Cover and cook over low heat 30 minutes. Add dates, raisins, or figs the last 10 minutes of cooking. Serve with soy yogurt and honey or 100% maple syrup. This makes a delicious meal. Serves 2.

You will never improve your life until you change to live a 100% Healthy Lifestyle!

BROWN RICE

One of our rich, nutritional cereal grains is organic whole brown rice – rice that has not been polished or processed to remove the golden bran. It is food that is easily digested because the starch grains are very small, and the delicacy of their shell walls makes it easy for the body to readily assimilate this healthy grain.

Delicious wild rice is more expensive than brown rice; but, it is a very palatable food, and one that has been relished by Native Americans. Wild rice is not truly a rice, but the seed of a tall grass that grows along the streams of the Mid-West, especially in the Mississippi Valley. It is expensive because it's difficult to harvest. Harvesters paddle slowly through the rice beds shaking the seeds into the bottoms of their boats or canoes. The grain does not ripen all at once and must be harvested in order to catch the seeds as they ripen at several different intervals.

WILD RICE CASSEROLE

1½ cups wild rice
3 cups boiling distilled water
Egg Replacer equal to 2 eggs
¼ cup Bragg Organic Olive Oil
1 cup parsley, chop
1 red onion, mince
1 cup soy cheese grated
1 tsp Bragg Liquid Aminos
1 small can of mushrooms with juice

Soak wild rice for 2 -3 hours. Cook in water for 30 minutes. Drain. Beat in Egg Replacer with olive oil, adding oil slowly. Add chopped parsley, onion and soy cheese. Add Bragg Aminos and small can of mushrooms with juice. Mix well and top with grated soy cheese. Bake 30-40 minutes at 350°F. Serves 4-6.

BROWN RICE BURGERS

1 red onion, mince
4 Tbsps whole-grain flour
Bragg Olive Oil
1 tsp Bragg Liquid Aminos
¼ cup soy milk
1 cup whole-grain cracker crumbs
shake of Bragg Sprinkle
2 cups cooked wild and/or brown rice

Add ½ cup of the whole-grain cracker crumbs, Bragg Aminos, soy milk, whole-grain flour, onion and Sprinkle to the cold cooked rice. Mix lightly. Shape into round balls and roll in remaining cracker crumbs. Brush lightly with olive oil. Place in oiled baking pan and bake at 350°F until golden brown. This may also be prepared with cooked whole-grain cereal, kasha or bulgur instead of brown or wild rice. Serves 4-6.

HEALTHY FIBER HABIT: *Have 3 tsp raw oat bran a day in juices, soups, herbal teas, pep drinks, cereals, muffins, etc., and have fiber in healthy salads, fresh fruits, vegetables, legumes and 100% whole-grains! Fiber helps reduce blood cholesterol and the formation of varicose veins. Fiber helps keep you regular and reduces hemorrhoids. It's also a natural body-weight normalizer.*

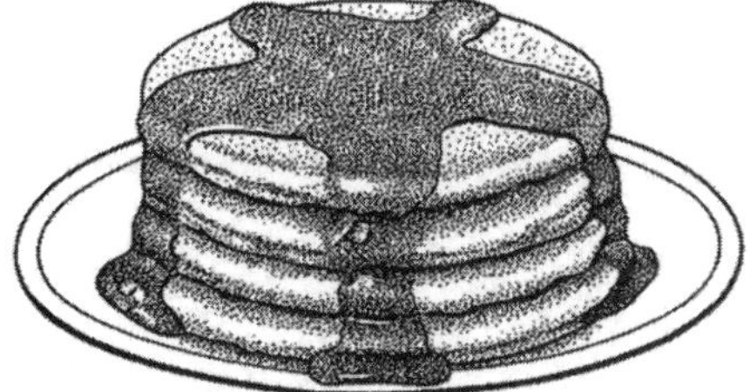

Chapter 15

Pancakes & Waffles

SUGGESTIONS FOR SOME INGREDIENTS:

- **Baking Powders** – that are without aluminum.
- **Vegetable oils** – olive oil or soy oils are best.
- **Sweeteners** – raw honey, molasses, 100% maple syrup, barley malt, Stevia herb powder or liquid, agave nectar, brown rice syrups, and fruit juice concentrates are the best. Use sparingly.
- **Eggs** – Egg Replacer by *Ener-G Foods, Inc.* It is a culinary egg substitute containing no eggs or animal products (see page 3). For 1 egg add: 1½ tsp *Ener-G Egg Replacer* plus 2 Tbsps warm water.

TOFU FRENCH TOAST

1 lb soft tofu
1 tsp vanilla extract
2 cups distilled water
10 slices of whole-grain bread
2 cups soy or rice milk
1 tsp cinnamon powder
Bragg Organic Olive Oil

Mix tofu, soy or rice milk, vanilla extract, cinnamon powder and water in a blender until you get the consistency of beaten eggs. Dip slices of bread into mixture. Cook in heated, oiled iron skillet until golden brown. Top with fresh fruit of choice and 100% maple syrup. Makes 10 delicious slices.

WHOLE/MULTI-GRAIN PANCAKES

¾ cup soy or multi-grain flour
1½ cups whole-grain flour
Egg Replacer equal to 2 eggs
3 Tbsps Bragg Organic Olive Oil
¾ cup wheat germ, raw
½ tsp baking powder
3 Tbsps molasses
3 cups soy or rice milk

Sift, measure flours. Re-sift with other dry ingredients. Add olive oil, molasses (*optional: 2 mashed bananas*), soy or rice milk to Egg Replacer. Stir into dry ingredients. Beat until smooth; don't over mix. Bake on hot oiled griddle. Serves 4-6.

WHOLE-GRAIN WAFFLES

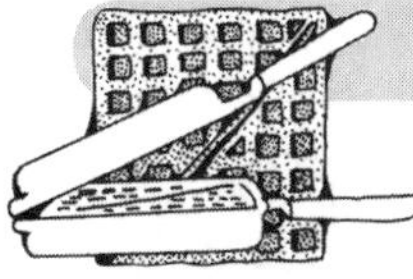

Egg Replacer equal to 2 eggs
½ tsp baking powder
3 Tbsps Bragg Organic Olive Oil
1 cup soy milk
1 cup whole-grain pastry flour

Beat Egg Replacer to a thick foam. Add soy milk. Fold in sifted flour and baking powder. Beat well; add olive oil and beat again. Bake in hot oiled waffle iron until golden. Makes 4 waffles.

BUCKWHEAT WAFFLES

1½ cups whole-grain pastry flour
1 cup soy milk or soy yogurt
Egg Replacer equal to 2 eggs
4 Tbsps Bragg Organic Olive Oil
¼ cup buckwheat flour
¼ cup raw wheat germ
½ tsp brown rice syrup
1 tsp baking powder

Sift whole-grain and buckwheat flour, wheat germ and baking powder together in large mixing bowl. Beat Egg Replacer; add rice syrup and mix with dry ingredients. Add soy milk (or soy yogurt) gradually and beat vigorously until batter is thin. Add olive oil last. Bake on a hot oiled waffle iron until golden brown, 3-5 minutes for crisp waffles. Serves 2-4.

BLENDED MEAL WAFFLES OR PANCAKES

1 cup whole-grain sifted flour
2 tsps baking powder
Egg Replacer equal to 2 eggs
3 Tbsps Bragg Organic Olive Oil
1 cup blended grain meal (pg. 168)
1 tsp brown rice syrup
1¼ cups soy milk
2 ripe bananas (optional)

Sift flour before measuring. Mix with blended meal, baking powder, olive oil and brown rice syrup. Beat Egg Replacer well. Add soy milk. Combine with flour mixture; beat until smooth. For variety, add mashed ripe bananas (our favorite). Bake in hot waffle iron or cook as pancakes. Makes 6 portions.

FRESH FRUIT OR NUTTY WAFFLES & PANCAKES

Add mashed bananas to whole-grain batter (our favorite), strawberries, blueberries or other fresh fruits alone or mixed, or add nut or seed meats of your choice (pecans, walnuts, almonds, cashews or sunflower, sesame or pumpkin seeds). Try experimenting to discover your favorite topping combinations. 100% pure organic maple syrup is our favorite topping.

Enjoy the natural healthy taste of your food without added refined sweeteners. By slowly removing sugar from your diet, you will find yourself enjoying the natural sweetness of foods like fresh fruit, fruit pies, apple sauce and fresh fruit juices. Over a period of time, by using natural sweeteners and fruit juice concentrates instead of refined sugar, your taste buds will enjoy natural flavors more.

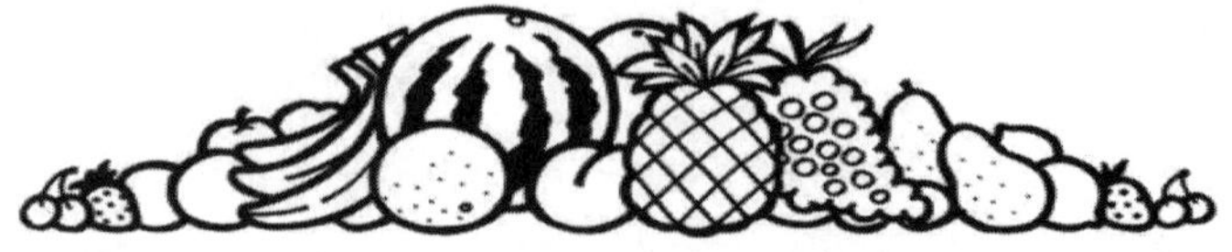

Living under conditions of modern life, it's important to bear in mind that the refinement, and over-processing of food products either entirely eliminates or partly destroys the vital elements in the original material.
– United States Department of Agriculture

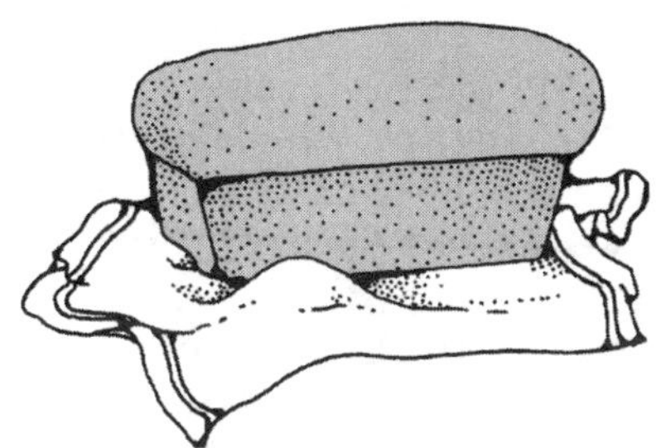

Chapter 16

Breads, Rolls & Muffins

HEALTHY STAFF OF LIFE: ORGANIC WHOLE-GRAIN FOODS

Whole-grains are one of nature's richest gifts, for their delightful taste and high nutritional value. Locked within the cells of golden grains are nature's vitamins and minerals.

At one time, the home and garden was the health factory for food production. People grew grains, and with primitive gristmills, ground it into flour and cereals. There was no milling or refining of any kind. People infused their bloodstream with everything nature had sown into the grain! Eventually people moved to congested communities, the thriving village and, finally, the industrialized city. Many were no longer able to produce their own food. This is where man ceased to eat healthy foods and began eating processed, devitalized foods. Perishable foods that are filled with vitamins and minerals providing health-building nutrients are more difficult to keep in storage. This is when a great crime was committed against food. With the introduction of the rolling mill, most of the life-containing elements were removed from whole grains. The energy element, B vitamins, were partially extracted. The germ, a vitamin rich component, was removed. Then the flour is less perishable. As humans make intelligent use of modern nutritional knowledge and healthy lifestyle living, their life will be lengthened with more vibrant health and longevity.

The difference between refined white flour and whole-grain foods is immeasurable. In commercial varieties, 99% of the taste sensation has been lost. The nutty flavor is gone, and with it the nutrients, vitamin E, iron and phosphorus, which are so important to maintaining super health! When you prepare rolls, breads, cakes, pastries and all baked dishes with rich, organic, whole-grains, you discover an entirely different taste appeal. Try it and prove to yourself how much more enjoyment you will receive from eating these natural whole-grains and products with the priceless germ (vitamin E) left in them. They are more nutritious and more satisfying! The reason for this is that you are getting what the master chemist put into the whole grain for your health!

Whole-grain bread strengthens man's heart and promotes health . . . that is why whole-grains are called the staff of life.

When using any of the recipes in this cookbook, especially in the baking section, be sure to use 100% organic whole-grain flours. Organic whole-grain pastry flours are best for cake, pie and cookie recipes. There are wonderful varieties of whole and multi-grain flours that are perfect for baked goods, pastries, pizzas, waffles, pancakes, etc. Some of our favorite flours are: multi-grain, rye, pumpernickel, spelt, quinoa, millet, soy, corn, oat and potato. Whole-grain bread flours are available in health food stores, and may be used for breads, rolls, biscuits, muffins, etc.

STORING WHOLE-GRAIN FLOURS

Whole-grain flours should be stored in an air-tight container and kept in the refrigerator or freezer. They absorb moisture and odors from other foods. Because they are "live" foods, they are perishable. They will not keep for long periods, as do refined, lifeless flours. It's best to grind your own flour as needed or buy from health food stores.

MEASUREMENTS

It is important to measure accurately. Baking with whole-grain flours and natural sweeteners is a process entirely different from using commercial, highly processed grains. With natural sweeteners you can adjust measurements to meet your "sweet desires"! For accurate measurements, all measurements are best level. Use a set of standard measuring cups and spoons.

Egg Replacer by *Ener-G Foods, Inc.* is a culinary egg substitute containing no eggs or animal products (see page 3). For 1 egg add: 1½ tsp Ener-G Egg Replacer plus 2 Tbsps warm water.

YEAST BREADS AND ROLLS

100% WHOLE-GRAIN OR MULTI-GRAIN BREAD

2 cups soy milk
2 Tbsps Bragg Olive Oil
7 cups whole-grain, multi-grain or pastry flour
4 Tbsps raw honey
2 Tbsps oat bran
1 pkg quick-rise yeast

Heat soy milk, add olive oil, yeast and honey or sweetener of choice. Cool. Beat in enough flour and oat bran to make a stiff dough. Knead for 10 minutes. Place in an oiled mixing bowl, cover and set in warm place. Let rise until double in size. Punch down and let rise again. Remove from bowl and shape into loaves. (*For variety it's fun to experiment and make different loaves. Try some grated soy cheese, zucchini, carrots, chopped nuts, seeds, raisins, a variety of whole-grain flours or herbs and spices.*) Place in oiled bread pans. Cover with a moist towel and let rise until double in size. Bake in preheated 375°F oven for 1 hour; cool on rack. Makes 3 loaves.

WHOLE-GRAIN & WHEAT-GERM BREAD

1 package quick-rise yeast
2 Tbsps Bragg Olive Oil
1 cup raw wheat germ,
⅓ cup raisins (optional)
4 Tbsps raw honey
1 Tbsp oat bran
6 cups 100% whole-grain flour
2 cups lukewarm soy milk

Sift and measure whole-grain flour. Combine yeast, soy milk, honey and olive oil. Beat in whole-grain flour, wheat germ and oat bran (gradually). Knead thoroughly, keeping dough soft. Cover, set in warm place, let rise 1-2 hours. When double in size, (*optional*: add raisins and ½ tsp cinnamon powder) form into loaves and place in oiled pans. Cover and let rise again for 1 hour. Bake in preheated 375°F oven for 1 hour. Makes 2-3 loaves.

WHOLE-GRAIN BREADSTICKS

Using the recipe above, make some ½-inch round ropes, cut into 6-9 inch lengths. Place on oiled cookie sheet and brush with Bragg Olive Oil. For variety, sprinkle sesame, poppy or chia seeds or crushed herbs. Bake 12-15 minutes at 300°F.

DUTCH RYE BREAD

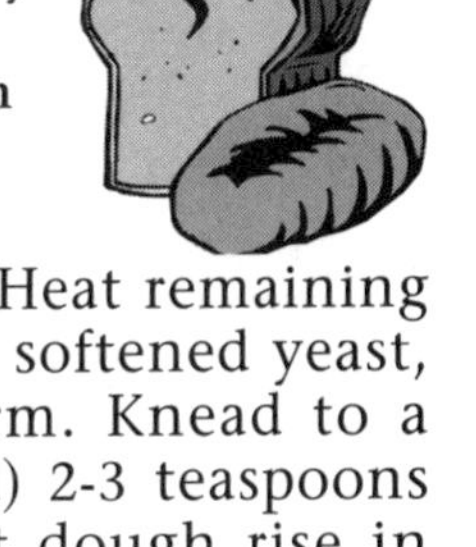

1 pkg quick-rise yeast
2 Tbsps Bragg Organic Olive Oil
1½ cups whole-grain bread or pastry flour
2-3 tsps caraway seeds (optional)
2 Tbsps raw honey
4 cups rye flour
1 cup wheat germ
3 cups lukewarm soy milk

Soften yeast in one cup lukewarm soy milk. Heat remaining soy milk to lukewarm. Add olive oil, honey, softened yeast, whole-grain and rye flours, and wheat germ. Knead to a stiff dough. While kneading, add (if desired) 2-3 teaspoons caraway seeds. Cover with moist cloth. Let dough rise in a warm place until double in size. Shape into loaves and place in oiled bread pans. Let rise again and bake at 375°F for 20 minutes; reduce heat to 350°F and continue baking for 40 more minutes. Makes two large or 4 small loaves.

BARLEY BREAD

2 cups whole-barley flour
2 Tbsps Bragg Organic Olive Oil
1 cup whole-grain bread or pastry flour
1 pkg quick-rise yeast
1 cup warm soy milk
1 Tbsp raw honey

Make a sponge by dissolving yeast in warm soy milk. To make a soft dough: stir in olive oil, honey and flours. Cover and set in warm place to rise for 1 hour. Punch down and knead for 10 minutes; let rise again. Divide into 2 loaves and place in oiled bread pans. Cover, let rise until light, and bake 35-40 minutes at 350°F. This bread bakes faster than others. Makes 2 loaves.

BROWN RICE BREAD

½ cup uncooked brown rice
1 Tbsp raw honey
1 pkg quick-rise yeast
6 cups whole-grain bread or pastry flour
1½ cups distilled water
1 Tbsp Bragg Organic Olive Oil
1 cup soy milk, lukewarm
1 cup whole-grain flour for kneading

Steam rice in a double boiler in water until soft and dry. Add honey and olive oil; heat to lukewarm. Dissolve the yeast in lukewarm soy milk and add to the rice. Stir in 2 cups of whole-grain flour. Cover and let stand until light. Add the remainder of flour; knead lightly. Let dough rise until it doubles in size. Knead. Shape into loaves. Place in oiled pans; cover. When the loaves have risen to loaf size, bake for about 50 minutes at 350°F. Makes 3 medium-sized loaves.

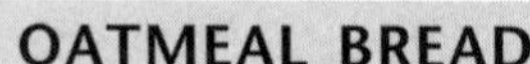

OATMEAL BREAD

2 cups rolled oats
2 pkgs quick-rise yeast
½ cup molasses
1½ cups boiling distilled water
½ cup lukewarm distilled water
1 Tbsp Bragg Organic Olive Oil
5 cups whole-grain bread or pastry flour

Cover oats with boiling water, let stand 30 minutes. Soften yeast in lukewarm water. Add softened yeast to oats, molasses, olive oil and whole-grain flour. Mix well. Turn out on floured board and knead until smooth. Place in oiled bowl. Oil surface of dough. Allow to rise until double in size (about 2 hours). Knead lightly, shape into two loaves and place in oiled pans. Drizzle olive oil on surface of loaves and allow to double in size (for 30 minutes). Bake at 400°F for 15 minutes, then reduce heat to 350°F and continue baking for 45 more minutes until done. Makes 2 loaves.

YEASTY CORN BREAD

1 pkg quick-rise yeast
1 Tbsp raw honey
4½ cups whole-grain bread or pastry flour
2 cups soy milk, lukewarm
1 Tbsp Bragg Olive Oil
2 cups yellow cornmeal
1 cup whole-grain flour for kneading

Soak yeast in ¼ cup of lukewarm water until dissolved. Heat soy milk and cool it to lukewarm. Add honey, dissolved yeast and olive oil. Make a sponge by adding 2 cups of the organic whole-grain flour, mix well, cover and let rise in a warm place until it doubles in size. Add organic cornmeal and remaining flour to make a stiff dough. Knead and let rise again. Shape into loaves. Cover, let rise in oiled pans until double in size. Bake 45 minutes at 350°F. Delicious with meals. Makes 2 loaves.

Whole-grain breads and cereals should be a good part of our daily diet according to USDA Food Pyramid.

BASIC DOUGH: THREE-IN-ONE BREAD RECIPE

3 cups lukewarm soy milk
1½ cups lukewarm distilled water
½ cup Bragg Organic Olive Oil
13½ cups whole-grain pastry flour
6 pkgs quick-rise yeast
⅜ cup raw honey
Egg Replacer equal to 3 eggs

Soften yeast in lukewarm water and soy milk. Blend in honey, olive oil and Egg Replacer. Gradually add sifted flour. Mix until dough is well-blended and soft. Split into thirds. Dough can be used for **lemon tea drops** (recipe below). Chill remaining dough for **cinnamon loaf** and **dinner rolls** (recipes below).

LEMON TEA DROPS

Use ⅓ unchilled basic dough (above recipe) to make 36 small tea muffins. Fill oiled 2-inch muffin pan halfway full. Mix 1 cup honey, 2 tsps lemon juice and 2 Tbsps grated lemon rind. Sprinkle about 1 tablespoon over each muffin. Cover with damp cloth and let rise at 80-85°F about 45 minutes. Bake at 375°F for 20 minutes.

CINNAMON LOAF

Use ⅓ chilled basic dough (above recipe). Roll dough into an 8x11 inch rectangle. Mix 2 cups brown sugar and one tablespoon cinnamon. Sprinkle dough and roll as a jelly roll, starting with 8-inch edge. Seal edges and place in oiled 9x4x3 inch pan. Cover with damp cloth, let rise in warm place (80-85°F) about 2 hours. Bake at 375°F for 1 hour.

DINNER ROLLS

Use ⅓ chilled basic dough (above recipe) to make 27 dinner rolls. Mold into crescents or any shape desired. Cover, let rise in warm place (80-85°F) about 2 hours. Bake at 425°F for 20 minutes.

PRUNE RING

Prune ring is a variation that may be used with the basic dough recipe (recipe above). Roll chilled dough to 12x16 inch rectangle. Spread with one cup cooked, chop prunes sweetened with raw honey if desired, and roll dough long as if for a jelly roll. Place in deep oiled 9-inch ring mold, joining ends to form a complete circle. Slash top of ring with deep, crosswise slices every 2 inches. Let rise about an hour or until doubled in size. Bake at 400°F for 25 minutes or until done.

Store your bread anywhere but the fridge. Well-wrapped in the freezer or green plastic bag at room temperature works well. – www.foodnetwork.com

WHOLE-GRAIN ROLLS

2 pkgs quick-rise yeast
¼ cup unsulphured molasses
¼ cup Bragg Organic Olive Oil
Egg Replacer equal to 1 egg
2 cups soy milk
¼ cup raw honey
1 cup wheat germ
1 cup whole-grain flour
5½ cups organic whole-grain pastry flour

Crumble yeast into mixing bowl. Add lukewarm soy milk. Stir in molasses and honey, let stand until thoroughly dissolved and bubbly. Add Egg Replacer, wheat germ and whole grain flour. Beat until elastic. Add pastry flour and olive oil to form soft dough. Turn out on floured board, let stand 10 minutes, then knead 7 minutes. Place in oiled bowl, oil surface of dough, cover with damp cloth, let rise until double in size (2 hours). Knead lightly and shape as desired. Place in oiled pans, brush with olive oil. Let rise again until double in size. Bake 425°F for 15 minutes. (If less needed cut amounts). Makes 48 rolls.

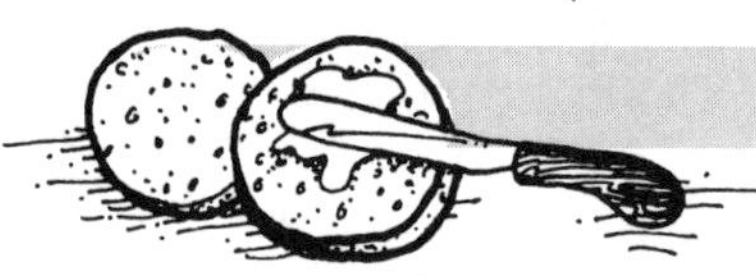

FLUFF ROLLS

1 cup soy milk, lukewarm
1 pkg quick-rise yeast
⅛ cup lukewarm distilled water
1 Tbsp raw honey
3 Tbsps Bragg Organic Olive Oil
3 cups whole-grain flour

Make a sponge of lukewarm soy milk, olive oil, honey and 1½ cups of the flour. When sponge is cool, add yeast dissolved in warm water. Add remaining flour. Stir until dough is stiff, but can still be stirred with a spoon. Cover with damp cloth; set to rise in a warm place. When double in size, stir down and let rise again. Put in oiled muffin tins. Cover and when double in size, bake at 375°F for about 25 minutes. Makes about 20 rolls.

SPEEDY PAN ROLLS

1 cup lukewarm soy milk
1 Tbsp raw honey
4 cups whole-grain pastry flour
⅓ cup Bragg Olive Oil
2 pkgs instant yeast
Egg Replacer equal to 1 egg

Mix soy milk, olive oil and honey. Add yeast and mix well. Add Egg Replacer. Gradually add sifted whole-grain flour and mix until dough is well-blended and soft. Roll out on floured board, cut dough into 1x4 inch rectangles. Brush cut sides with olive oil. Place in oiled 12 x 8 inch pan, cover with a damp cloth and let rise in a warm place (80-85°F) about 30 minutes. Bake at 425°F for 20 minutes. Makes 24 rolls.

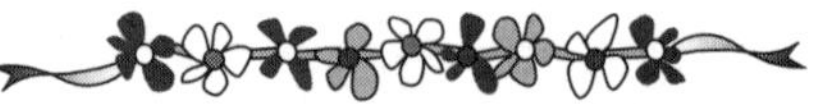

There is much false economy: those who are too poor to have seasonable fruits and vegetables will yet have pie and pickles all year. They cannot afford apples, yet can afford tea and coffee daily. – Health Calendar 1910

SOY LEMON BUNS

¾ cup lukewarm soy milk
6 Tbsps raw honey
½ tsp mace
Egg Replacer equal to 2 eggs
½ lb soft tofu, crumble
¼ cup Bragg Organic Olive Oil
2 tsps organic lemon rind, grate
1 pkg quick-rise yeast
3¼ cups whole-grain pastry flour
½ cup organic raisins

Mix soy milk, olive oil, 4 tablespoons honey, organic lemon rind and mace. Add crumbled yeast. Stir until dissolved. Add half of the Egg Replacer and enough flour to make a soft dough. Turn onto floured board, knead until smooth—about 5 minutes. Place in an oiled bowl; cover and let rise in a warm place (80-85°F) until light, or about 1 hour. Punch down; turn onto floured board and shape into balls 2-3 inches in diameter. Place 2 inches apart in shallow oiled pans. Cover with damp cloth; let rise. Meanwhile, combine tofu, raisins, remaining 2 tablespoons honey and beaten Egg Replacer. When balls are double in size (about 30 minutes), make a large dent with the back of a spoon in center of each roll, fill with raisin and tofu mixture. Bake 425°F for 15 minutes. Makes 12 buns.

HOT-CROSS BUNS

1 cup soy milk
1 cup raw honey
2 pkgs quick-rise yeast
1 cup wheat germ
1 tsp cinnamon powder
⅓ cup Bragg Organic Olive Oil
4 cups whole-grain pastry flour
¼ cup lukewarm distilled water
Egg Replacer equal to 2 eggs
1 cup raisins or currants

Mix soy milk, olive oil and honey and heat to lukewarm. Soften yeast in lukewarm water; stir and add to milk mixture. Add cinnamon, Egg Replacer and half of flour. Beat well. Work in enough of the remaining whole-grain flour and wheat germ to make a soft dough. Turn out onto a lightly floured board and knead 10 minutes or until smooth. Place dough in a warm, oiled bowl; brush surface with oil; cover with a damp cloth. Let rise in a warm place (80-85°F) about 2 hours until doubled in size. Turn onto floured board. Lightly knead in the raisins. Shape into balls about 1½ inches in diameter. Place in oiled pan close together for soft buns, farther apart if individual round buns are desired. Slice top in form of a cross. Brush with Egg Replacer; cover and let rise 45 minutes or until doubled in size. Bake at 375°F for 30 minutes. Makes 24 buns.

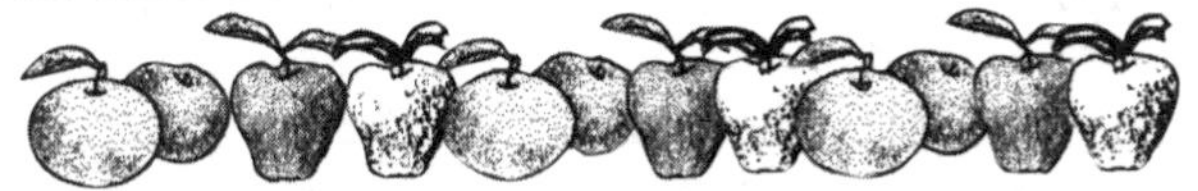

Organic whole-grains are rich in complex carbohydrates, protein, vitamins, minerals, polyunsaturated fatty acids and healthy fiber.

You are what you eat, drink, breathe, think, say and do. – Patricia Bragg

DATE AND NUT BREAD

- 2 cups dates, coarsely chop
- ½ cup unsulphured molasses
- 4 cups whole-grain pastry flour
- 1 cup whole-grain bread flour
- 2¼ cups pineapple juice or organic apple juice
- 1 cup nuts, coarsely chop
- 1 cup currants or raisins
- 3 Tbsps Bragg Olive Oil
- 2 pkgs quick-rise yeast
- 1 cup wheat germ

Soften yeast in 2 cups lukewarm organic apple or pineapple juice. Add remaining pineapple or apple juice, olive oil, then molasses. Beat in flours and wheat germ to make a stiff dough. Brush surface very lightly with olive oil; cover with a damp cloth and let rise in a warm place (80-85°F) for about 2 hours, or until doubled in size. Turn out on lightly-floured board. Dredge dried fruit with flour, mix with nuts and raisins, and knead into dough. Knead for about 10 minutes, or until smooth and satiny. Divide dough into two equal portions. Cover and let stand 10 minutes. Shape into loaves. Place in oiled loaf pans (about 9½ x 5½ inches). Brush tops with olive oil, cover, and let rise about 1 hour, or until double in size. Bake at 375°F for 45-55 minutes. Makes 2 loaves.

JINGLE BREAD

- 2 pkgs quick-rise yeast
- ⅓ cup raw honey
- ¼ cup Bragg Organic Olive Oil
- 4 cups whole-grain pastry flour
- 1⅔ cups lukewarm soy milk
- 1 cup wheat germ
- Egg Replacer equal to 2 eggs

Soften yeast cakes in ¼ cup of soy milk. Add sweetener, olive oil and remaining milk. Mix; add beaten Egg Replacer. Beat in wheat germ and whole-grain flour for soft dough. Place dough in an oiled, covered bowl. Let rise in warm place for 1½-2 hours. Jingle filling recipe follows. Serves 8.

JINGLE FILLING

- ½ cup raw honey
- ½ cup nuts, chop
- 1 tsp cinnamon powder
- ½ cup dates, chop
- ½ cup raisins
- ¼ cup orange or lemon rind, grate
- 2 Tbsps fresh orange or lemon juice

Mix all above ingredients well. Roll out Jingle Bread dough into about an 18-inch square; spread with Jingle fruit filling. Roll up as a jelly roll. Cut into 1-inch slices and arrange disks in well-oiled round pan. Cover and let rise in warm place about 30 minutes. Bake 350°F for 1 hour. Remove from pan at once, cover top with syrup or sauce desired. Makes 2 cups.

Statistics show that degenerative illnesses are increasing at alarming rates and attacking people at increasingly early ages. It is time to recognize that diet is largely responsible for this increase, and that sugar, coffee, salt, refined and chemical-loaded foods, and lack of exercise are the major culprits!

QUICK BREAKFAST RING

1 cup soy milk
½ cup raw honey
¼ cup Bragg Olive Oil
¼ cup warm distilled water
2 pkgs instant yeast
Egg Replacer equal to 1 egg
½ cup raisins, softened
3¾ cups whole-grain pastry flour

TOPPING:
mix ¼ cup raw honey, ¼ tsp cinnamon and ¼ cup chopped nuts

Mix soy milk, honey, olive oil, and water. Heat to lukewarm. Stir in yeast – softened in water, Egg Replacer, 1 cup flour. Beat well with spoon. Add remaining flour and raisins, beat 3 minutes. Line a bottom-oiled angel-cake pan with waxed paper. Fill with batter. Mix topping and sprinkle over batter. Cover with damp cloth; let rise in warm place (80-85°F) until doubled in size, about 1 hour. Bake at 375°F for 40 minutes. Makes one ring.

PUMPERNICKEL BREAD

MIX THOROUGHLY:
2½ cups warm distilled water
2 pkgs quick-rise yeast
1 Tbsp caraway seeds
2 cup blackstrap molasses
2 Tbsps Bragg Olive Oil
1 Tbsp raw honey
1 Tbsp dill seeds

THEN ADD:
1 cup branflakes
1 cup wheat germ
1-2 Tbsps Bragg Yeast
½ cup soy flour
2 cups whole-grain flour
2½ cups rye flour

Mix together, kneading about 5 minutes. Cover and set in a warm place and let rise 1-2 hours. When double in size, form into loaves and place in oiled pans. Cover and let rise again for 1 hour. Bake 375°F for 45 minutes. Makes 2-3 loaves.

PUMPKIN BROWN BREAD

2 cups soy milk
1 cup distilled water
¼ cup 100% maple syrup
½ cup raw honey
1 cake fresh yeast
2¼ cups cornmeal
2 cups cooked pumpkin
1 Tbsp Bragg Organic Olive Oil
3 cups whole-grain pastry flour
dates, nuts and raisins (optional)

Mix soy milk, maple syrup, water, olive oil, honey and pumpkin together. Dissolve yeast in ¼ cup lukewarm water, add to mixture. Beat in half the flour and cornmeal. Add rest of flour, cornmeal, beat again. (*Optional*: add chopped dates, nuts or raisins if desired). Cover with damp cloth; set in warm place to rise until it has doubled in size. Stir down. Put into oiled bread pans. Cover; let rise. Bake at 375°F for 1 hour. Place some water in a pan in the oven with the bread. This gives bread a glossy appearance. Makes 2-3 delicious loaves.

Home-baked breads have long history for a reason. Healthy bread baking is a happy family time with delicious aromas and nutritious meal time treats.

ALFALFA SPROUT BREAD

2 small potatoes with skins
1 qt distilled water
½ cup plus 2 Tbsps raw honey
1 Tbsp Bragg Liquid Aminos
1 tsp Bragg Sea Kelp
2 pkgs quick-rise yeast
¼ cup Bragg Organic Olive Oil
4 cups young alfalfa sprouts
8-10 cups whole-grain or soy flour or a combination of these

It is important to use young sprouts; older sprouts have a high water content and will make the bread soggy. Wash potatoes, cut into small pieces and cook in 1 cup water until done. Liquefy in blender with 2 cups cold water. Put through strainer to remove skin particles. Measure and add enough warm water to make a total of 3½ cups liquid. Add ½ cup honey, Bragg Aminos, Sea Kelp and olive oil. Dissolve yeast and 2 tablespoons honey in ½ cup warm water. Let stand 10 minutes and add to potato liquid. Stir in 5 cups of whole grain or soy flour. Add sprouts, and additional flour to make a stiff dough. Knead well until smooth and elastic. Cover with damp hand towel. Let rise in warm place until double. Punch down, form into loaves. Place in oiled pans, bake 350°F oven 1-1½ hours until done. Makes 2 loaves.

BANANA CORNBREAD

1 pkg quick-rise yeast
Egg Replacer equal to 2 eggs
¾ cup whole-grain flour
3 Tbsps Bragg Organic Olive Oil
2 Tbsps raw honey
1 cup organic cornmeal
¼ cup soy flour
2 medium bananas

Dissolve yeast in ½ cup warm water and add honey. Set aside. In a mixing bowl, combine cornmeal and flours. In another bowl, mash bananas and add olive oil and Egg Replacer. Stir well. Add banana mixture to yeast. Combine dry and liquid ingredients, stirring well. Pour into an oiled 8-inch square pan. Let dough rise in a warm place 30 minutes. Bake 350°F for 30 minutes. Delicious with meals.

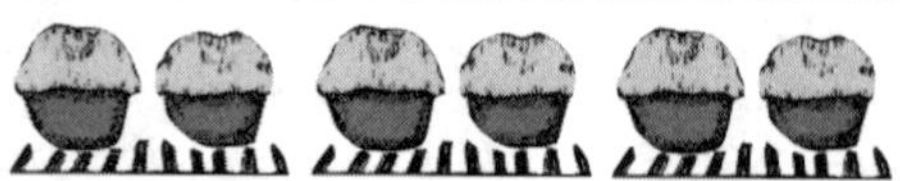

You don't get old from living a particular number of years; you get old because you have deserted your ideals. Years can wrinkle your skin, renouncing your ideals wrinkles your soul. Worry, doubt, fear & despair are the enemies which slowly bring us down to the ground and turn us to dust before we die. – Douglas MacArthur

---

Whole grains have been shown to lower cholesterol & supply vitamins & antioxidants that may help the heart. In fact, a recent study showed that people who eat two servings a day of whole grains are about one-fifth less likely to have heart disease than those who pass on whole grains. – www.CBSNews.com

---

Alfalfa sprouts are a very good source of Dietary Fiber, Vitamin C, Vitamin K, Thiamin, Riboflavin, Folate, Pantothenic Acid, Iron, Magnesium, Phosphorus, Zinc, Copper and Manganese. – www.nutritiondata.self.com/facts/vegetables

MUFFINS & QUICK BREADS

DELICIOUS WHOLE-GRAIN MUFFINS

1⅓ cups rolled oats
⅓ cup raw honey
Egg Replacer equal to 1 egg
½ cup nuts, chop
1 cup soy milk
½ cup whole-grain pastry flour
2 tsps baking powder
½ cup raisins or currents
½ cup dates, chop
3 Tbsps Bragg Organic Olive Oil

Sift together flour and baking powder; add rolled oats, dried fruit and nuts. Add honey, soy milk and Egg Replacer stirring lightly. Fold in olive oil. Fill oiled muffin pans ⅔ full. Bake at 425°F for 15-25 minutes, depending on the size of the muffins. Delicious with breakfast or main meals. Makes 18 muffins.

DATE BRAN MUFFINS

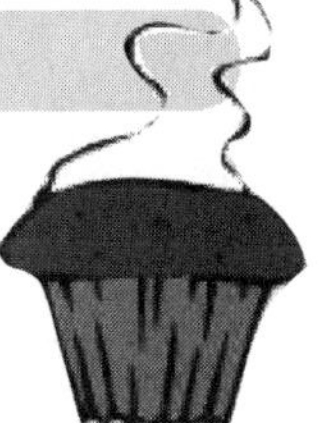

1 cup 100% oat bran
Egg Replacer equal to 1 egg
6 dates, halve
¼ cup Bragg Organic Olive Oil
¾ cup whole-grain pastry flour
1 cup soy or rice milk
¼ cup molasses
2 tsps baking powder
½ cup dates, chop

Mix bran and soy milk; let stand five minutes. Beat Egg Replacer; add molasses to bran mixture. Sift dry ingredients and add to mixture. Quickly stir in Bragg Olive Oil. Add chopped dates. Fill oiled muffin pans ⅔ full. Place half a date on top of each muffin. Bake at 375°F for 30 minutes. Makes 12.

APPLE CORN MUFFINS

⅓ cup yellow cornmeal
3 tsps baking powder
⅓ cup soy milk
3 Tbsps Bragg Organic Olive Oil
Egg Replacer equal to 1 egg
¼ cup raw honey
¼ cup raw apple, grate or finely slice
¾ cup whole-grain pastry flour

Sift whole-grain flour, cornmeal and baking powder together. Mix Egg Replacer, soy milk and raw honey and add to dry ingredients, stirring only enough to completely moisten. Stir in olive oil. Fold in apple. Fill well-oiled muffin tins ⅔ full and bake at 375°F for 25 minutes. Makes 12 medium-sized muffins.

RYE MUFFINS

2 cups rye pastry flour
4 tsps baking powder
2 Tbsps Bragg Olive Oil
4 Tbsps raw honey*
1 cup distilled water*
For variation: fruit or fruit juice

Sift dry ingredients together. Add in olive oil and honey. Stir in water until large lumps are blended, but do not beat. Place in oiled muffin pans. Bake 35 minutes at 400°F. Makes 12.

**Variation: Using half the honey, stir in 4 tablespoons of fruit, such as berries or pineapple, or use organic fruit juice instead of water.*

RYE BISCUITS

2 cups rye pastry flour
6 Tbsps Bragg Organic Olive Oil
3 tsps baking powder
6 to 8 Tbsps distilled water

Sift and blend dry ingredients. Add in olive oil and water. Put on rye-floured board and roll to about 2-inch thickness. Cut with biscuit cutter. Place on an oiled baking pan and bake at 400°F for about 15 minutes. Watch biscuits during the last 3 minutes to see that they do not over-brown. Makes 12 biscuits.

BUCKWHEAT CORN MUFFINS

1 cup buckwheat flour
½ cup cornmeal
2½ tsps baking powder
1 tsp Bragg Liquid Aminos
1 Tbsp raw honey
Egg Replacer equal to 4 eggs
1¼ cups soy or rice milk
¼ cup Bragg Olive Oil

Preheat oven to 400°F. Mix buckwheat flour, cornmeal and baking powder. Combine Egg Replacer, soy or rice milk, Bragg Aminos, honey, olive oil. Stir into dry ingredients until moistened. Fill muffin tins ⅔ full and bake 15-20 minutes. Makes 12.

BANANA RAISIN MUFFINS

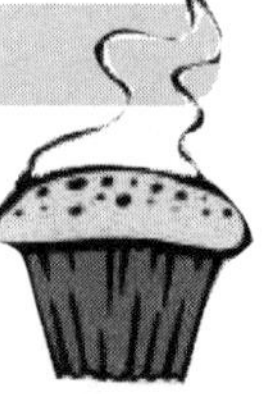

1½ cups whole-grain flour
½ cup organic raw honey
¼ cup soy milk
1 tsp vanilla extract
¼-½ cup chop nuts (optional)
1 tsp baking soda
¼ cup Bragg Olive Oil
1 cup bananas, mash
½ cup organic raisins

Stir baking soda and flour into a bowl. Add honey, olive oil, soy milk, mashed bananas and vanilla extract. Mix until flour is just moistened. Fold in raisins and nuts if desired. Fill oiled muffin tins ¾ full with batter. Bake 375°F for 15 minutes or until golden brown. Remove from pan immediately. Makes 12.

WHOLE-GRAIN POPOVERS

Egg Replacer equal to 3 eggs
1 cup whole-grain flour
3 Tbsps Bragg Organic Olive Oil
1½ cups soy or rice milk
¼ tsp sea salt

Preheat oven to 475°F. Combine Egg Replacer, soy or rice milk, flour and sea salt in a mixing bowl and beat vigorously about 2 minutes. Add olive oil. Oil muffin tin and place in oven for 2 minutes. Remove muffin tin and fill each cup ¾ full and bake 15 minutes. Turn temperature down to 350°F and bake 25 minutes longer until golden brown. Makes 12 popovers.

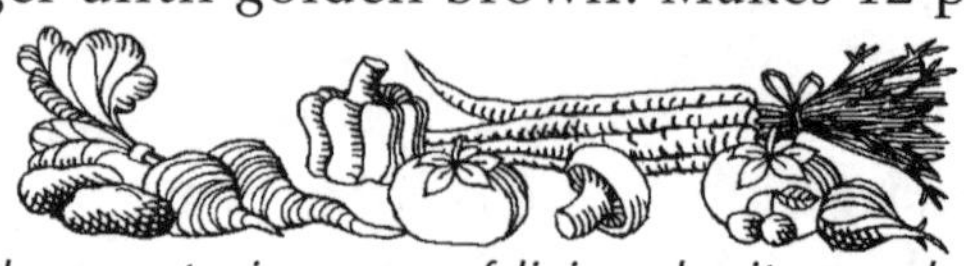

It is my view the vegetarian way of living, by its purely physical effect on the human temperament, would beneficially influence all mankind.

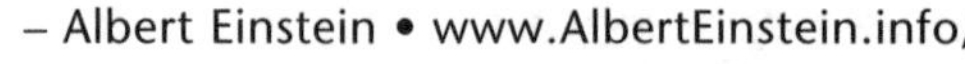

– Albert Einstein • www.AlbertEinstein.info/

BROWN BREAD – QUICK AND EASY

2 cups whole-grain flour
1 cup whole-grain pastry flour
½ cup blackstrap molasses
2 cups soy yogurt
½ cup raisins
2 tsps baking soda

Preheat the oven to 325°F. In a large mixing bowl, stir dry ingredients together. Add yogurt, molasses and raisins. Stir the batter until completely mixed. The batter will be very stiff and sticky. Spoon the batter into an oiled pan. Bake at 325°F for 1 hour. Delicious topped with rice dream ice cream.

PUMPKIN BREAD

1½ cups organic, whole-grain flour
1½ cups mashed or puréed pumpkin
½ cup Bragg Organic Olive Oil
1 tsp spiceberry or allspice
Egg Replacer equal to 2 eggs
½ cup raw honey
½ cup dried cranberries
1 tsp baking powder
½ cup pecans or walnuts, chop

Preheat oven to 350°F. Combine flour, pumpkin, honey, olive oil, Egg Replacer, baking powder and allspice in a bowl. Stir just until combined. Stir in nuts and cranberries. Pour batter into an oiled 6x9 inch bread pan. Bake 1 hour or until done in center. Remove loaf from pan and let cool on a baking rack. Serves 8.

WHOLE-GRAIN WALNUT BREAD

2 cups whole-grain pastry flour
2 tsps baking powder
Egg Replacer equal to 1 egg
1 cup walnuts, coarsely chop
1 cup wheat germ
1 cup raw honey
1 cup soy milk

Sift whole-grain flour, wheat germ and baking powder into mixing bowl. Add Egg Replacer mixed with soy milk and honey. Beat well. Stir in chopped walnuts. Pour into well-oiled loaf pan and let stand 20 minutes. Bake at 350°F about 65-70 minutes. Turn out on rack to cool. Makes one loaf.

GINGERBREAD

⅓ cup raw honey
Egg Replacer equal to 1 egg
2½ cups whole-grain flour, sift
1½ tsps baking soda
1 tsp ginger, grate or powder
⅓ tsp cloves, powder
½ cup Bragg Organic Olive Oil
1 cup molasses
½ cup raisins
1 tsp cinnamon
1 cup soy milk

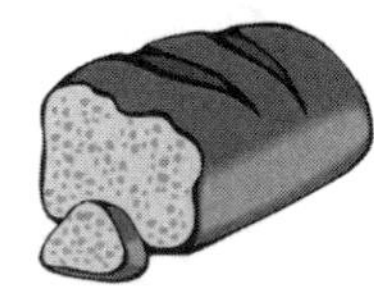

Sift dry ingredients together. In a separate bowl combine olive oil and honey. Add Egg Replacer and molasses. Add soy milk, beat until smooth. Add to dry ingredients. Add raisins. Batter will be soft. Bake in oiled shallow pan for 35 minutes at 325°F. Delicious topped with sauce (page 165). Makes 15 servings.

When you realize each cell is a small factory, needing constant recharging through the food you eat, you'll begin to think about what you eat. – Dr. J.D. Nolan

HONEY NUT BREAD

2 Tbsps Bragg Organic Olive Oil
Egg Replacer equal to 1 egg
2½ cups whole-grain pastry flour
½ tsp baking soda
¾ cup fresh orange juice
1 cup raw honey
2 tsps baking powder
rind of organic orange, grate
¾ cup walnuts, chop
½ cup raisins or currants

Combine olive oil and honey and mix well. Add Egg Replacer and orange rind; beat until creamy. Mix and sift whole-grain flour, baking powder, baking soda, currants and walnuts. Add flour mixture and orange juice alternately to first mixture, mix well between each addition. Bake in oiled, ovenproof glass loaf pan at 350°F for 1 hour. Loaf tastes better the second day. Makes 1 loaf.

CORN BREAD

1 cup whole-grain flour
¼ Tbsp raw honey
Egg Replacer equal to 1 egg
3 Tbsps Bragg Organic Olive Oil
4 tsps baking powder
1 cup organic cornmeal
1 cup soy milk

Sift whole-grain flour and baking powder together. Add organic cornmeal. To Egg Replacer add soy milk, honey and olive oil. Beat in whole-grain flour mixture just until blended; do not over-mix. (*Variety*: try ½ tsp Bragg Sprinkle and ⅓ cup raisins or currants.) Bake in a shallow oiled pan at 350°F for 20 minutes or until golden brown. Serves 6-8.

GRAHAM PINEAPPLE LOAF

1 qt crushed pineapple
1 lb whole-grain graham crackers, crumbled
2 bananas
1 Tbsp lemon juice
¼ lb coconut or nuts, ground

Drain pineapple and mix with graham crackers. Use some of the pineapple juice to moisten if necessary. Form in loaf pan and let set. Remove from pan. Mash bananas with lemon juice. Frost the loaf with mashed banana. Sprinkle coconut or ground nuts on top. Any desired fruit (peaches, strawberries, kiwi, apricots, etc.) may be used instead of the pineapple. Serves 6.

GARLIC WHOLE GRAIN FRENCH BREAD

⅓ cup Bragg Organic Olive Oil
1 loaf whole-grain French bread
¼ cup soy Parmesan cheese, grate
1-2 cloves garlic, mash
¼ tsp Bragg Liquid Aminos
shake Bragg Sprinkle

Add garlic to olive oil and mash lightly with fork. Let mixture stand 30 minutes until garlic flavor permeates oil. Slash bread diagonally into thick slices, being careful not to cut the bottom crust. Spread garlic oil generously between slices and on top of loaf. Spray loaf with Bragg Aminos. Sprinkle soy cheese and Sprinkle. Bake 375°F for 10 minutes, then cut slices apart. Serve immediately. Serves 8.

Chapter 17

Jams, Preserves, Jellies & Marmalades

CALIFORNIA FIG JAM

5 cups fresh organic black mission figs, unpeeled, quarter
1 organic lemon, very thinly slice
2¼ cups raw honey

Boil fruit, lemon and 1 cup honey exactly 5 minutes. Add 1 cup honey and boil again for 5 minutes (time after boiling point is reached). Add rest of honey and boil again for 3-5 minutes. Bottle hot into sterilized jars and seal.

QUICK GRAPE JELLY

3 cups unsweetened grape juice
1½ cups distilled water
2 cups raw honey
1½ pkgs powdered pectin

Combine organic grape juice and water; stir in pectin. Heat to the boiling point and add honey. Bring to full rolling boil, and boil exactly 2 minutes. Remove from stove, skim and pour into sterilized glass jars and seal.

APRICOT BUTTER

6 lbs organic apricots
cinnamon sticks (if desired)
1 lb raw honey
whole cloves (if desired)
juice and rind of organic orange, grate

Pit organic apricots. Cut into small pieces. Add honey, orange juice and rind. Bring to boil and cook, stirring frequently until desired consistency (usually thick). Watch carefully to prevent burning. If spices are desired, tie cinnamon sticks and whole cloves (or add ¼ tsp in powdered form) in a cheesecloth bag, add to mixture while cooking. Remove before pouring into jars. Pour into hot, sterilized jars, fill to top and seal.

TOMATO PRESERVES

5-10 lbs tomatoes
2 organic lemons, thinly slice
1 cup raw honey
½ tsp Bragg Sprinkle (optional)

Dip tomatoes in boiling water for a few minutes. Plunge into cold water. Peel off skin and gently cut tomatoes into quarters, and add honey and sliced organic lemons. Simmer until thick (about 20-30 minutes), stirring frequently to prevent burning. Pour hot into sterilized pint or quart glass jars and seal.

BLUEBERRY OR RASPBERRY JELLY

6 cups berry juice, made from fresh blueberries or raspberries
3 Tbsps fresh lemon juice
1½ cups liquid pectin
2 cups raw honey

To prepare juice, wash berries and crush. Place in jelly bag; squeeze out juice. Mix berry juice, lemon juice and honey in large saucepan. Bring to a boil as quickly as possible and add pectin at once, stirring constantly. Bring to full rolling boil and boil hard for exactly 30 seconds. Remove from heat; skim and pour into hot, sterilized jars. Seal at once.

STRAWBERRY AND RHUBARB JELLY

3 cups strawberry and rhubarb juice, made from fresh fruit
1½ cups raw honey and 6 oz liquid pectin (¾ of 8 oz bottle)

To prepare fruit, cut about ¾ pound fully ripe, reddish rhubarb in one-inch pieces and put through food processor, using medium blade. Thoroughly crush about 1½ quarts fully-ripe, washed strawberries. Combine fruits, place in jelly cloth spread over a colander, and squeeze out juice. Measure honey and juice into large saucepan and mix. Bring to a boil over high heat, and immediately stir in the liquid pectin. Bring to a full rolling boil, and boil hard 30 seconds. Remove from heat, skim, and pour quickly into clean, freshly-sterilized jelly glasses to within ½-inch of top. Seal at once. Makes six 6-ounce jars.

WHOLE STRAWBERRY JAM

3 cups raw honey
3 Tbsps lemon juice
6 cups (3 lbs) prepared fruit
6 oz liquid pectin (¾ of 8 oz bottle)

To prepare fruit, use about 3 quarts small, fully ripe organic strawberries. Spread ¼ of berries at a time in single layer, on flat surface or in pan and with bottom of a tumbler, press gently to a ½-inch thickness. This crushes centers of berries without breaking skins. Put layer of pressed berries into large kettle and cover with layer of honey. Continue to alternate layers of pressed berries and honey until all have been used, pouring honey on top. Add lemon juice. Let stand for at least 5 hours. Mix well. Then bring to a full, rolling boil. Boil hard 60 seconds. Remove from heat and stir in liquid pectin. Ladle off into glasses hot, clear syrup for jelly. (To separate syrup from fruit, press a sieve into jam.) Stir and skim jam alternately for 5 minutes; cool slightly to prevent floating fruit. Pour into clean, freshly-sterilized jelly jars to within ½-inch of top. Remove from heat; skim and pour into hot, sterilized jars. Seal at once. Makes eight 6-ounce jars of jam.

One cup strawberries contains over 100 mg of vitamin C. Strawberries also adds calcium, magnesium, folate and potassium. – www.nutrition.about.com

STRAWBERRY RELISH

- 3 quarts organic strawberries
- ½ tsp allspice
- ¾ tsp cinnamon powder
- ½ tsp clove powder
- 1½ cups raw honey
- 3 Tbsps lemon juice
- 6 ounces liquid pectin (¾ of 8 oz bottle)

Wash and stem strawberries. Crush or put through food processor, using coarse blade. In a large kettle, combine crushed berries (should be 6 cups), spices (adjust amount to suit taste), honey and lemon juice; mix well. Bring to a full, rolling boil over high heat; boil 3 minutes, stirring constantly. Remove from heat; stir in liquid pectin. Then, stir and skim alternately for 5 minutes. Cool slightly, then pour into freshly-sterilized jelly glasses to within ½-inch of top. Seal. Makes about ten 6-ounce jars.

RHUBARB CONSERVE

- 10 lbs rhubarb
- 2 - 20 oz cans crushed pineapple
- 6 ounces liquid pectin
- 6 small whole oranges, dice
- 1 cup broken walnuts
- 2 cups raw honey

Wash rhubarb; cut into ½-inch pieces. In kettle, combine all remaining ingredients, except the liquid pectin. Bring to a boil, keep stirring constantly. Reduce heat; simmer uncovered over low heat for 1½ hours or until a consistent texture. Stir occasionally the first hour and more often during the last 30 minutes. Remove from heat; stir in liquid pectin. Pour immediately into clean, freshly sterilized pint reserve glass jars; seal. Makes about 8 pint jars.

GREEN TOMATO MARMALADE

- 8 lbs green tomatoes (about 12 medium tomatoes)
- 8 organic lemons
- 1½ cups raw honey
- 2 cups distilled water
- 2 tsps ginger powder

Slice green tomatoes in ½-inch crosswise slices; slice organic lemons paper-thin. Bring honey, water and ginger to a boil. Add tomato and lemon slices. Bring to a boil then simmer uncovered for 15 minutes. With a skimmer, carefully remove the fruit. Boil the liquid down until it measures 6 cups. Boil it slowly stirring frequently so as not to scorch it. Replace fruit in liquid and bring to boil. Immediately place in clean, hot preserve jars. Adjust covers as directed by manufacturer. Set on wire rack in covered, deep kettles with boiling water to cover top by one-inch. Process 30 minutes, counting time from moment active boiling resumes. Remove; immediately adjust seal according to manufacturer's directions. Serve this as spread or dip for crackers or bread. Makes about 4 pints.

Rhubarb is 95% water and is low in sodium. Rhubarb's crisp thin stalks are rich in vitamin C, dietary fiber and calcium. – www.rhubarbinfo.com

SLICED ORANGE MARMALADE

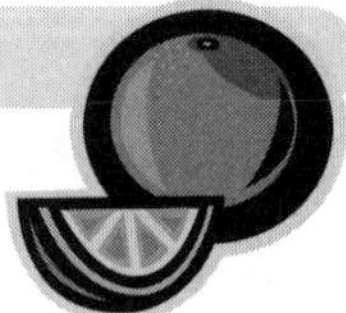

3 cups organic oranges, 1/8-inch thick slices
2 1/2 cups distilled water
2 cups raw honey
3/8 cup lemon juice
12 oz liquid pectin

Cut unpeeled organic orange slices in halves or quarters (or leave whole), as preferred. Remove seeds. Put in saucepan with water, 1 1/2 cups honey, and lemon juice. Cover; bring to a boil. Reduce heat and simmer 30 minutes. Measure fruit and liquid into large kettle, using additional water as necessary to make 5 1/4 cups. Add remaining honey. Mix well, bring to full, rolling boil over hot heat, stirring constantly. Boil hard for 1 minute. Remove from heat and stir in liquid pectin. Stir and skim alternately for 5 minutes. Pour into freshly-sterilized jelly glasses to within 1/2-inch of top. Seal. Makes ten 6-ounce jars.

CALIFORNIA TANGERINE MARMALADE

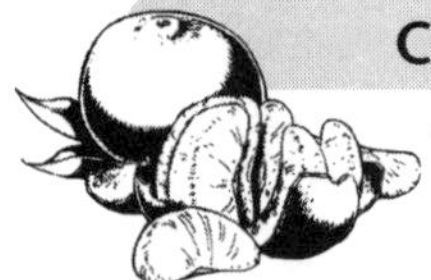

6 medium tangerines
1 1/2 cups organic lemons very thinly sliced
1 1/2 cups raw honey
3 Tbsps lemon juice
distilled water

Separate peeled tangerines into sections and cut into small pieces; there should be about 3 cups. Remove seeds. Cut lemon into very thin slices. Measure tangerine pieces and lemons into saucepan. Add four times as much water. Bring to boil; cook uncovered until tender, 30-35 minutes. Measure 3 cups of this mixture into a saucepan; add 1 1/2 cups honey. Boil vigorously, uncovered, stirring constantly for about 10 minutes or until syrup reaches jelly stage. To test for jelly stage, dip large spoon into boiling mixture, then lift spoon so syrup runs off side. When syrup no longer runs off spoon in a steady stream, but separates into two distinct lines of drops that cling together, stop cooking. Add lemon juice; boil about 1 minute or until syrup again reaches jelly stage. Pour hot quickly into sterilized jelly jars and seal.

CRANBERRY - ORANGE MARMALADE

4 whole medium organic oranges, quarter and remove seeds
4 cups fresh, washed cranberries
3 cups raw honey
4 1/2 cups distilled water

Place organic oranges and cranberries in food processor, catching juice in bowl (there should be about 6 cups ground fruit). Combine fruit, juice, water and honey in saucepan. Cook, uncovered, until thick (about 30 minutes) stirring frequently. Pour hot quickly into sterilized jelly jars and seal. Makes about ten 8-ounce glasses.

Oranges are a great source of vitamin C, calcium and folate. Oranges are also a great source of fiber and antioxidants. – nutrition.about.com

PEACH BUTTER

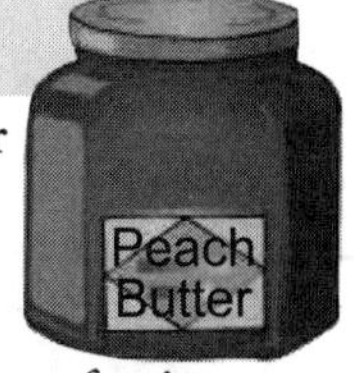

6 lbs organic peaches or apricots
3 cups distilled water
3 tsps cinnamon powder
juice and rind of one lemon
1½ tsps clove powder
¾ tsp allspice
⅔ cup raw honey

Wash, peel, pit and quarter peaches or apricots (or other fruits desired). Cook in water slowly until soft. Put fruit through a strainer. To each cup of fruit pulp, add honey, cinnamon, cloves, allspice, juice and grated lemon rind. Cook fruit butter slowly until it is thick and clear. Pour into sterilized jars and seal.

GRAPE CONSERVE

6 lbs organic Concord grapes
1 large orange
6 oz liquid pectin
1½ cups raisins or currants
1⅛ cups nut meats, chop
2 cups raw honey

Wash, drain and stem Concord grapes. Remove skins and reserve for later use. Place pulp in kettle, bring to boiling and cook slowly about 10 minutes. Press through strainer to remove seeds. Put orange through the food processor. Combine grape pulp and orange in large kettle, add honey, pectin and raisins. Cook rapidly until mixture thickens, add chopped grape skins and cook 15 minutes more, stirring constantly. Stir in chopped nut meats (of choice). Pour into hot, sterilized jars and seal.

PINEAPPLE - STRAWBERRY SPREAD

6 cups organic strawberries
6 cups pineapple, chop
3 cups raw honey

Pour half the honey over the pineapple and half over the strawberries; let stand for 4 hours. It can stand overnight without too much juice forming. Put all together in a large kettle, mix well and cook 25 minutes after rolling boil is reached. Pour in sterilized glass jars and seal.

DATE AND NUT SPREAD

⅓ cup walnuts, chop
¾ cup dates, chop
1¼ Tbsps orange juice
¾ cup pineapple juice

Mix all ingredients in saucepan and cook together until mixture thickens slightly (about 5 minutes). Serve on whole-grain toasted bread or crackers, or as dessert with berries. (*Optional:* Top with soy yogurt.) Makes 1½ cups.

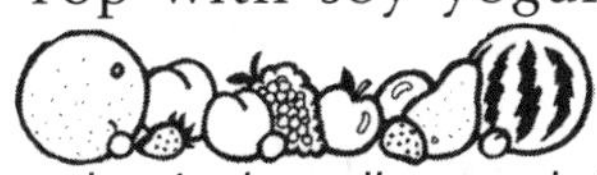

An important fact to remember is that all natural diets, including vegetarian diets without a hint of dairy products, contain amounts of calcium that meet your nutritional needs. Calcium deficiency caused by an insufficient amount of calcium in a diet that meets caloric needs is not known to occur in humans.
– John McDougall, M.D., author (drmcdougall.com) See calcium chart page 52.

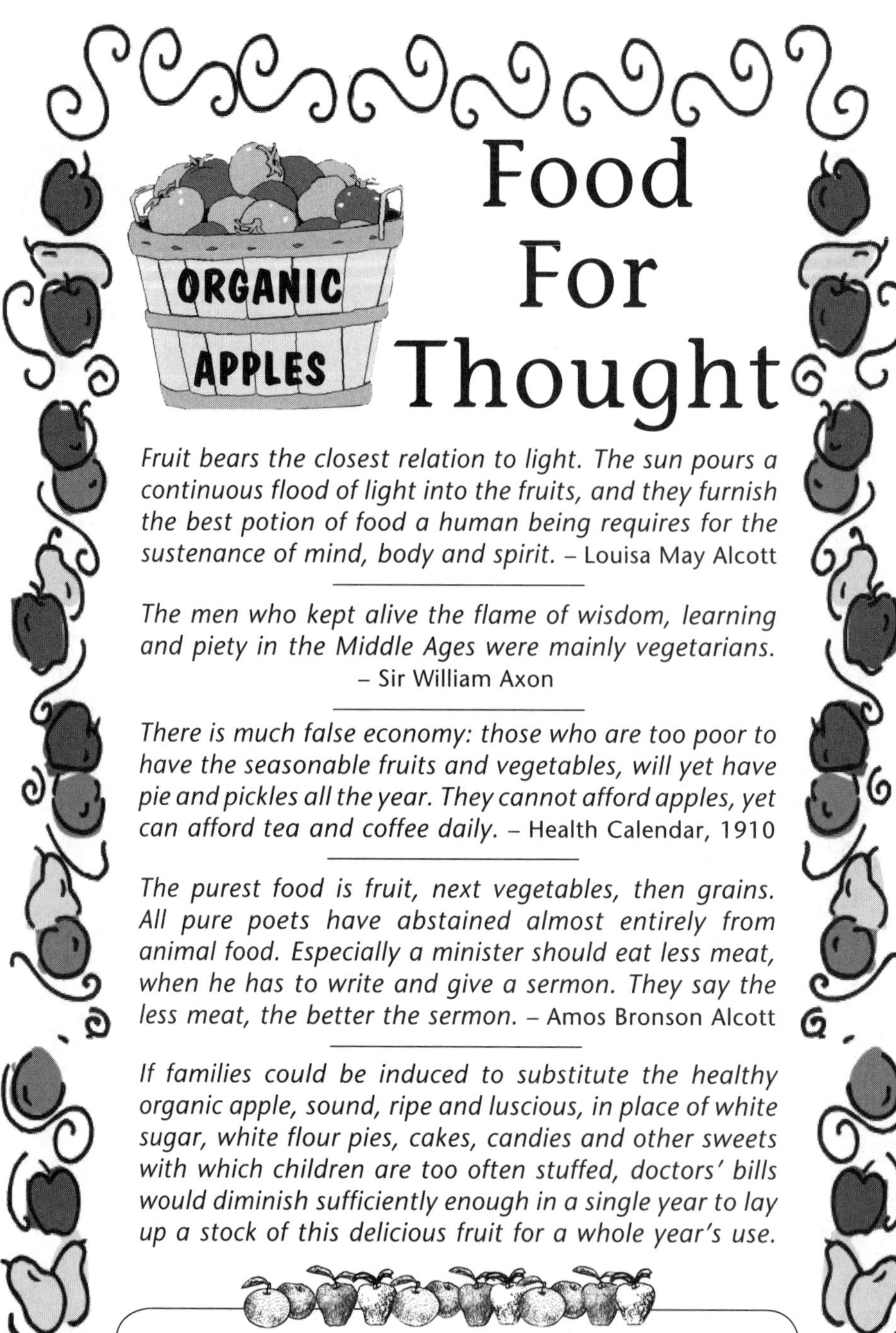

Food For Thought

Fruit bears the closest relation to light. The sun pours a continuous flood of light into the fruits, and they furnish the best potion of food a human being requires for the sustenance of mind, body and spirit. – Louisa May Alcott

---

The men who kept alive the flame of wisdom, learning and piety in the Middle Ages were mainly vegetarians. – Sir William Axon

---

There is much false economy: those who are too poor to have the seasonable fruits and vegetables, will yet have pie and pickles all the year. They cannot afford apples, yet can afford tea and coffee daily. – Health Calendar, 1910

The purest food is fruit, next vegetables, then grains. All pure poets have abstained almost entirely from animal food. Especially a minister should eat less meat, when he has to write and give a sermon. They say the less meat, the better the sermon. – Amos Bronson Alcott

---

If families could be induced to substitute the healthy organic apple, sound, ripe and luscious, in place of white sugar, white flour pies, cakes, candies and other sweets with which children are too often stuffed, doctors' bills would diminish sufficiently enough in a single year to lay up a stock of this delicious fruit for a whole year's use.

DO MORE TO MAKE LIFE SUCCESSFUL

Do more than preach, practice.
Do more than think, ponder.
Do more than sympathize, empathize.
Do more than scold, set an example.
Do more than criticize, praise.
Do more than dream, make it a reality!

– Rev. Paul Osumi, Honolulu, Hawaii

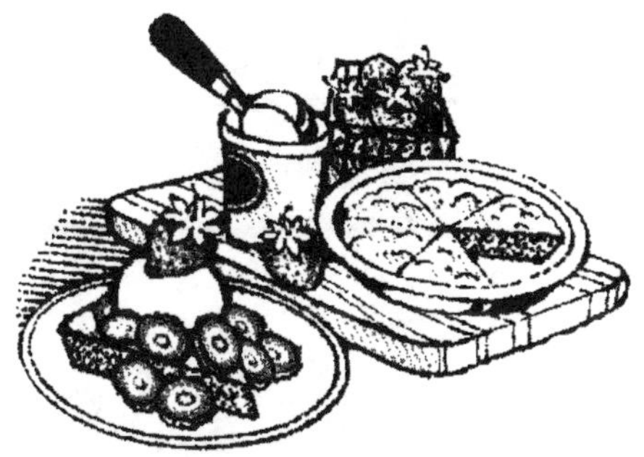

Chapter 18

Healthy Desserts

FRESH FRUITS FOR DESSERT

There is no finer dessert than organically grown fresh fruit. In Europe, fresh fruit is served with thin slices of natural cheeses. We suggest using the scrumptious , delicious non-dairy soy cheeses. A fruit bowl on the family table is graceful, beautiful and appetizing. Luscious pears, peaches, grapes, bananas, nectarines, plums, apricots, kiwis, persimmons, pineapple, pomegranates, cherries, oranges and apples cannot be surpassed as a delicious, wise finish to a gracious, healthy meal. (Watermelons and melons are best served alone as a fruit snack, and not mixed with other fruits or food.)

When your favorite fresh fruit is not in season, there are other fruits available year-round, like bananas, apples, oranges, etc. or organic frozen fruits. Also delicious sun-dried fruit desserts you will enjoy.

SUN-DRIED, UNSULPHURED FRUITS

The natural, unsulphured, sun-dried fruits are rich in iron and other minerals and vitamins. Health Food Stores carry a wide selection of these popular health enhancers.

All sun-dried fruits, before being used, should be scrub-washed and soaked in hot water for 3 minutes (to remove any mold that might have developed during the drying process). To prepare sun-dried fruit, just cook or soak overnight (until tender) in distilled water or unsweetened pineapple or fruit juice. Many dried fruits need no sweetening, cooking or soaking. If desired, add small amounts of raw honey, barley malt or brown rice syrup. If dried fruit is not to be cooked, but eaten raw, store unwashed in a tightly covered jar in the refrigerator, cellar or cold room.

Enjoy the natural, healthy taste of your food without added sweeteners. By gradually removing refined sugar from your diet you will enjoy the natural sweetness of foods such as fresh fruits, fruit pies, apple sauce & fresh fruit juices. Sugar can be replaced with unrefined, natural sweeteners, such as raw honey, maple syrup, agave nectar, barley malt, concentrated fruit juice and Stevia powder.

FRESH FRUIT COMPOTE

You can vary or add to any of these combinations and serve as a fruit compote. If desired, sweeten with raw honey, natural sweeteners, or unsweetened pineapple or fruit juices. Garnish with soy yogurt and/or grated coconut.

* Apricots and red cherries
* Black cherries and peaches
* Berries and pineapples
* Pears, plums and bananas
* Dates, peaches and nectarines
* Persimmons and pineapples
* Berries, bananas and peaches
* Melon balls from your favorite melons
* Peaches, nectarines, orange and grapefruit sections
* Halves of bananas, apples, plums and seeded grapes

PINEAPPLE DELIGHT

1 cup crushed pineapple, fresh or unsweetened if canned
1 cup soy or rice cream or non-dairy whipping cream

Fold crushed pineapple into the non-dairy whipped cream. If more sweetening is desired, add 1 tablespoon raw honey or barley malt sweetener. Chill. Serves 2.

FRUIT WHIP

1 cup soy cream or non-dairy whipping cream
1 Tbsp raw honey
1 tsp pure vanilla extract
2 cups mixed diced fresh fruit, such as bananas, strawberries, apples, pears, peaches, apricots, pineapples, and grapes
½ tsp arrowroot powder

Whip cream. Add arrowroot powder. Fold in vanilla extract, and the honey and mixed fruit. Chill and serve. Serves 2-4.

GRAPEFRUIT, FRESH OR BROILED

Cut grapefruit in half. Remove fruit from skin, taking out in one whole section by cutting carefully around perimeter and bottom. Carefully section fruit. Serve fresh or put under broiler for a few seconds until heated. Delicious as is, or top with diced fresh fruit and soy yogurt.

Fruits are generally high in fiber, water and vitamin C. Fruits also contain phytochemicals which research indicates are required for proper long-term cellular health and disease prevention. Healthy consumption of fruit is associated with reduced risks of cancer, cardiovascular disease, and stroke.

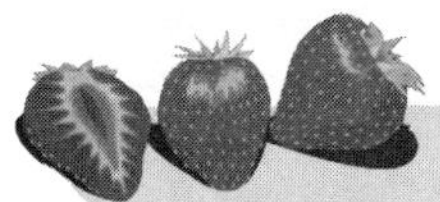

FRESH STRAWBERRY SPONGE

¼ cup hot distilled water
½ cup strawberries, juice and pulp
½ Tbsp arrowroot powder
¼ cup soy cream or non-dairy whip cream for garnish
Egg Replacer equal to 1 egg
¼ cup raw honey
½ Tbsp fresh lemon juice
berries for garnish

Crush organic strawberries; add honey, allow to stand 30 minutes. Dissolve arrowroot in water, add to strawberries and lemon juice. Cool. When it starts to thicken, fold in whipped soy cream and Egg Replacer. Put in sherbet glasses. Chill. Garnish with berries, delicious non-dairy cream or non-dairy yogurt (rice, soy or nut creams) if desired. Serves 3.

DATE AND NUT CRUMBLE

Egg Replacer equal to 2 eggs
2 Tbsps whole-grain flour
¼ tsp pure vanilla extract
2 cups dates, chop
½ cup raw honey
¼ tsp baking powder
1 Tbsp soy milk
1 cup nuts or seeds, chop

Add honey to Egg Replacer. Add sifted dry ingredients, dates and nuts or seeds, then soy milk and vanilla extract. Spread a thin layer in an oiled 9x9-inch pan. Bake at 250°F for 35 minutes. Cool and break into small pieces. Pile pieces alternately with whipped soy, nut, or rice cream, or soy yogurt in chilled sherbet glasses. Serves 4.

STRAWBERRY OR BERRY CUSTARD

4 Tbsps whole-grain pastry flour
Egg Replacer equal to 2 eggs
1 tsp almond or vanilla extract
4 Tbsps raw honey
8 cups strawberries
2 cups soy milk

You can prepare the custard sauce the day before so it will be thoroughly chilled. Mix honey and whole-grain pastry flour in the top of a double boiler. Stir in unbeaten Egg Replacer until well blended. Gradually stir in the soy milk. Cook over boiling water, stirring constantly, until smooth and thickened (about 5 minutes). Cool. Add pure almond or vanilla extract. Cover and chill. Pour chilled custard sauce over berries and serve. For variety, instead of strawberries, try blueberries, blackberries, or raspberries. All berries are nutritious and delicious. Serves 8.

There are many mental illnesses and diseases that are related to the consumption of meat. Depression, anxiety and schizophrenia can all be connected to meat. – American Alzheimer Association, www.alz.org

---

It is now known that such inexpensive foods as greens and fresh vegetables not only contain more iron than does the expensive beefsteaks, but better food iron than found in meats of any sort! – John Harvey Kellogg, M.D.

BAKED BANANAS

6 ripe bananas
3 Tbsps raw honey
1 tsp vanilla extract
1 Tbsp arrowroot powder
1 cup fresh squeezed orange juice
½ cup walnuts or almonds, finely chop

Dissolve arrowroot in orange juice and then combine this mixture with honey and vanilla. Place whole or halved bananas into this mixture and bake at 300°F for 15-20 minutes, or until bananas are medium soft. When serving, spoon sauce from bottom of pan and pour over bananas. *Optional:* top bananas with chopped nuts and coconut flakes. Serves 6.

APPLE SAUCE

4 cups organic apples, quarter
3 Tbsps raw honey (optional)

Cook organic apples until soft, adding a little distilled water to keep them from sticking to the pan. When done, if sweetening is desired, stir in honey or Stevia (4 drops). Sweet apples usually need no additional sweetening. Serves 6.

RF FRESH FRUIT FROZEN MOCK ICE CREAM

You can make your own delicious fresh fruit frozen *mock* ice cream with no sugar or cream. It's easy to prepare. Just freeze the fruit the night before and put it through the food processor, blender or juicer. Serve immediately. (See recommended juicers and blenders on page 51).

APPLE MUESLI

Juice of ½ lemon
¾ cup soy yogurt
2 apples, grate
2 Tbsps raw honey
2 Tbsps old-fashioned oatmeal
2 ½ Tbsps raw wheat germ
3 Tbsps walnuts or other nuts or seeds, chop
1 Tbsp sun-dried raisins

Soak oatmeal overnight in 4 teaspoons distilled water. In the morning, add lemon juice and soy yogurt. Mix well. Grate apples (unpeeled if organically grown) into mixture. Add remaining ingredients, mix well and eat immediately. Serves 2-4.

BAKED APPLES

4 baked apples, core
1 tsp cinnamon
¼ cup nuts, chop
¼ cup raisins

Mix nuts, raisins (or currants) and cinnamon. Stuff ¼ of mixture into core of each apple. Bake in glass, 1 cup water in bottom, cover, 350°F for 20 minutes or until done. Serves 4.

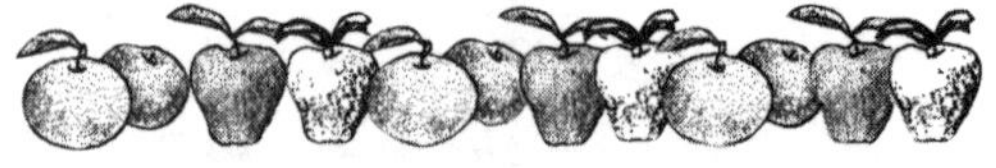

If a man earnestly seeks a righteous life,
his first act of abstinence is from animal food. – Leo Tolstoy

PINEAPPLE SHERBET

1 Tbsp raw honey
2 Tbsps fresh lemon juice
½ cup soy yogurt
1 sliced banana
1 cup pineapple (or fruit of choice) fresh or can (unsweetened)

Blend ingredients, pour into ice tray, freeze in freezer. When ready to serve, put in blender again until mixture is a creamy sherbert. (Delicious for most fruits.) Serves 2.

HONEYED APPLES AND RAW WHEAT GERM

2 pounds tart organic apples
1 cup raw honey
½ cup raw wheat germ
½ cup grated coconut

Wash and core apples. Cut in quarters. In stewing pan, allow honey to boil. Drop in one piece of apple at a time. Continue cooking until fruit is soft. When serving, sprinkle on raw wheat germ, Braggberry and grated coconut. Serve in bowls. Serves 5.

DRIED FRUIT AND NUT DESSERTS

WHEAT GERM - BRAN FRUIT BARS

RF

¼ lb pitted dried prunes
¼ lb natural dates
¼ lb natural figs
¼ lb organic raisins
1 Tbsp organic orange rind, grate
¼ cup raw honey
3 Tbsps lemon juice
1 cup bran
½ cup raw wheat germ

Grind fruit in food chopper, using the coarse grinder. Mix it with the other ingredients you desire. Mold the mixture in a pan. Refrigerate 1 hour. Cut into small bars.

ZESTY PROTEIN CONFECTION

½ cup raw carob powder
⅔ cup soy powder
2 Tbsps Bragg Olive Oil
¼ cup raw peanut butter
¼ cup rice bran
2 Tbsps nutritional yeast
2 Tbsps raw wheat germ
chopped nuts of choice

Place all ingredients in a bowl. Add enough raw honey to make consistency to knead. Spread into a square pan. Press chopped nuts over the top. Chill and cut into pieces.

Behind the nutty loaf is the mill wheel; behind the mill is the wheat field; on the wheat field rests the sunlight; above the sun is God. – James Russell Lowell

---

Exercise experts walk and run daily to maintain their health and fitness. A study on leading exercise experts revealed that most did daily walking, some did walking and running, and some played tennis, walked and ran. They all stressed at least 30 minutes a day, six days a week or two to three times a week for an hour each time. – Sports Medicine Digest

---

Wheat germ is rich in Vitamin E. It is also a good source of folic acid, thiamin, vitamin B6 and minerals like magnesium, manganese and zinc.

FRUIT AND NUT BALLS

1 cup natural dates, seeded
1 cup sun-dried natural raisins
¾ cup coconut, grated
raw honey to taste
1 cup raw wheat germ
1 cup sunflower seeds, coarsely chopped
1 cup sun-dried natural figs

Put all ingredients except grated coconut, through food processor. Place in pan. Add enough honey to make consistency kneadable. Spread in square dish. Sprinkle on natural unsweetened, unprocessed grated coconut and now roll into 2-inch balls. Refrigerate until served.

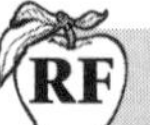

SESAME SEED PROTEIN DELIGHTS

½ cup sunflower seed meal
¾ cup tahini (sesame seed butter)
½ cup finely ground natural unsweetened unprocessed coconut

Mix all ingredients together. Separate into 2 portions. Place each on a piece of wax paper and form into a 1-inch roll. Wrap in the wax paper and store in the refrigerator. When ready to serve, slice into 1½-inch pieces.

SOY – CAROB BROWNIES

Have three sizes of mixing bowls ready. Mix as follows. In a large bowl mix:

½ cup raw honey
2 Tbsps blackstrap molasses
¼ cup sunflower seed oil
Egg Replacer equal to 2 eggs

In a small bowl: beat Egg Replacer and set aside.

In medium bowl mix :

½ cup soybean powder
½ cup sunflower seed meal
½ cup carob powder
½ tsp allspice (optional)
½ tsp ginger (optional)
1 tsp cinnamon (optional)
1 tsp pure vanilla extract can be used in place of spices

Now add this mixture to large bowl, a little at a time. This will be very stiff. Now add: ½ cup chopped raisins or dates; mix well. Add the Egg Replacer. Pour into an oiled 9-inch square pan. Bake in 350°F pre-heated oven for 25 minutes. Cool; cut into small squares.

FRESH BANANAS WITH NUT BUTTERS

Cut bananas in half and spread on raw cashew butter, raw almond butter, raw tahini or raw peanut butter or mix.

When we kill animals to eat them, they end up killing us because their flesh, which contains cholesterol and saturated fat, was never intended for human beings, who are natural plant herbivores. – William Clifford Roberts, M.D., Editor-in-Chief of The American Journal of Cardiology

---

Tahini is a thick paste made from ground-up sesame seeds and contains B Vitamins B1, B2, B3, B5 and B15. Tahini contains almost 35% of your recommended daily calcium intake. – www.NaturalNews.com

HI-PROTEIN YOGURT, NUT, WHEAT GERM MIX

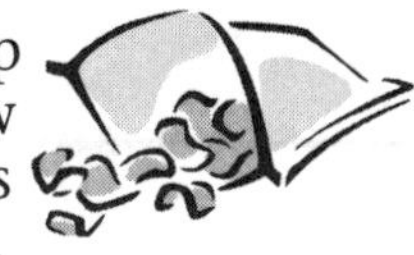

Place 3 tablespoons soy yogurt in deep dish. Sprinkle generously with raw wheat germ. Add chopped cashew nuts or cashew nut meal and honey to taste.

QUICK PICK-UP PROTEIN SWEETS

¾ lb natural sun-dried raisins
¾ lb natural sun-dried figs
½ lb walnut meats
½ cup sesame seeds
1 tsp Bragg Nutritional Yeast
¾ lb cashew nuts
¾ lb pitted dates
¾ cup raw wheat germ

Prepare the fruit by removing the seeds and stem ends. Put the fruit and nuts through a food grinder with the coarsest cutter. Roll the mixture out on a board until it is about ½-inch thick. Roll it with sesame seeds, cut into squares.

HI-PROTEIN RAW NUT ICE CREAM

½ cup raw sunflower seed kernels
½ cup raw sesame seeds
½ cup raw honey
¼ cup Bragg Organic Olive Oil
2 cups soy milk
1 cup raw almonds
1 cup raw pecans

Mix all the ingredients together and blend in an electric blender in batches until it has a smooth consistency. Pour this mixture into ice cube trays, freeze until needed. Serves 6-8.

PUDDINGS & OTHER DESSERTS

RAISIN PUDDING

1 cup whole-grain pastry flour
1 tsp baking powder
1 cup distilled water
½ cup raisins or currants
½ cup raw honey
½ cup soy milk
4 tsps Bragg Olive Oil
soy or rice cream

Sift whole-grain flour, baking powder and ¼ cup honey into a mixing bowl. Stir in raisins and soy milk. Spread batter in oiled baking pan. Combine remaining honey, water and olive oil in saucepan; heat until honey is dissolved. Pour syrup over batter. Bake at 350°F for 45 minutes or until done. As pudding bakes, batter rises to top of syrup. Serve warm with syrup from pudding and plain or whipped soy or rice cream. Serves 6-8.

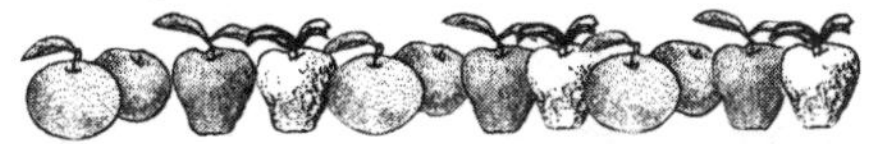

There is strong medical evidence that complete freedom from not eating animal flesh and cow's milk products is a gateway to optimal nutritional health. – Dr. Michael Klaper, M.D.

INDIVIDUAL FRUIT PUDDINGS

¾ cup whole-grain bread crumbs
¾ cup soy milk, scald
Egg Replacer equal to 3 eggs
3 Tbsps whole-grain pastry flour
3 oz Bragg Organic Olive Oil
⅓ tsp clove powder
1 cup sun-dried raisins, chop
4½ Tbsps lemon, chop
1½ cups bran
½ cup raw honey
1 tsp nutmeg
1½ tsps baking powder
⅜ tsp mace
½ tsp cinnamon powder
1 cup dates, chop
3 Tbsps grape juice

Combine dates, raisins, and citron. Set aside. Soak bran and bread crumbs in soy milk for 5 minutes. Add honey, beaten Egg Replacer and olive oil. Mix dry ingredients and stir into fruit mixture. Add grape juice. Fill 8 thin, ovenproof glass custard cups ⅔ full. Place custard cups in large pan, fill to almost top of cups and cover pan. Steam 2 hours, replenishing with water as needed. Cool puddings in cups. Serves 8.

PASKHA

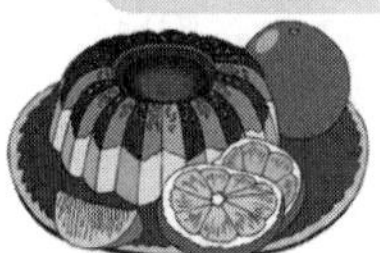

½ lb firm tofu, crumble
⅛ cup Bragg Olive Oil
¼ cup sun-dried raisins
⅛ tsp vanilla extract
¼ cup raw honey
½ Tbsp orange rind, grate
1 Tbsp soy sour cream

Purée tofu, putting through sieve twice. Mix thoroughly with olive oil, honey, vanilla extract, raisins, orange rind and sour soy or rice cream. Press firmly into mold, using press with weight to hold in place. Chill in refrigerator for at least 12 hours before serving. Serve in small portions. Serves 4.

YELLOW CORN PUDDING

1 cup molasses
5 cups soy or rice milk
½ cup Bragg Organic Olive Oil
1 cup fresh corn kernels, chop
½ cup yellow cornmeal
½ tsp cinnamon powder
½ tsp nutmeg powder
½ tsp vanilla extract

Scald 4 cups of soy or rice milk; mix with all other ingredients. Place in double boiler for 20 minutes, stirring frequently. Place in oiled baking dish and top with the remaining cup of milk. Bake at 225°F for 2 hours. Cut recipe in half for a smaller family. Serves 8-10.

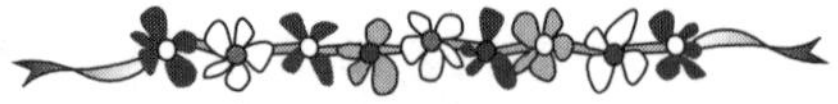

Before there was medicine, there was food. – Howard Murad, M.D.

He is the best physician that knows the worthlessness of most medicines.
– Benjamin Franklin, Inventor and author

True wisdom consists in not departing from nature, but molding our conduct according to her wise laws. – Seneca

If you love Mother Nature, you will see Beauty everywhere. – Van Gogh

SWEET-POTATO PUDDING

2 cups sweet potatoes, grated
Egg Replacer equal to 2 eggs
2 cups soy or rice milk
4 Tbsps Bragg Organic Olive Oil
½ cup softened dried apricots
½ cup walnut meats, chop
½ cup raw honey
dash of anise seed
½ tsp nutmeg
½ tsp cinnamon
¼ tsp fresh ginger, grate

Mix all ingredients; turn into oiled baking dish and bake at 300°F for about 45 minutes. Stir occasionally. Serves 6.

FAVORITE CAROB CUSTARD

4 cups soy milk
Egg Replacer equal to 6 eggs
2 Tbsps raw honey
1 tsp vanilla extract
1 cup carob powder

Scald milk. Add small amount of soy milk to carob and blend to smooth paste; add hot soy milk. Add honey and vanilla extract to slightly beaten Egg Replacer. Stir soy milk and carob mixture into Egg Replacer and bake at 350°F for about 30 minutes. Serves 6-8.

DATE AND BROWN RICE PUDDING

¾ cup dates or raisins, chop
3 cups warm soy or rice milk
1 cup cooked brown rice
Egg Replacer equal to 4 eggs
3½ Tbsps raw honey

Mix all ingredients well and pour into custard cups. Place cups in pan of hot water and bake at 350°F for 30-45 minutes.

CARROT PUDDING

1 cup pitted dates
½ cup Bragg Organic Olive Oil
3½ cups raw carrots, grate
½ cup raw honey
1 cup raisins
1 cup walnuts

Put carrots, raisins (or currants), dates and nuts through food processor. Add honey and olive oil, and pack in a glass casserole dish. Bake 30 minutes at 350°F. Serves 6.

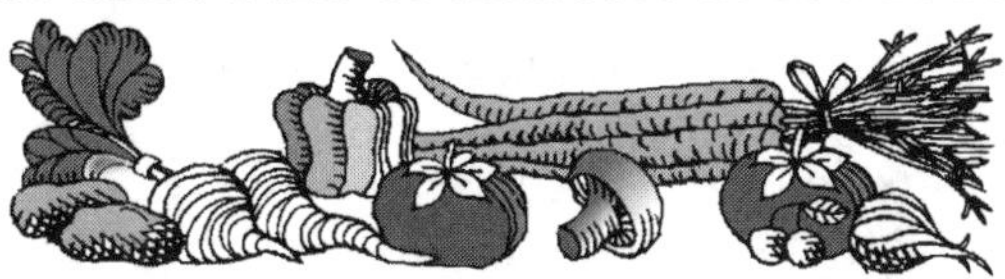

When you live the Bragg Healthy Lifestyle, you can help activate your own powerful, internal defense arsenal and maintain it at top efficiency. However, bad, unhealthy eating habits make it harder for your body to fight off illness!
– Paul C. Bragg, N.D., Ph.D., Originator of Health Food Stores

Living healthy, simple, natural and justly are all one thing. – Socrates

The fat in meat, particularly its saturated fat, comes up time and again as a contributor to heart disease, the nation's number-one-killer.
– Tufts University Health & Nutrition Letter

THE MIRACLES OF APPLE CIDER VINEGAR FOR A STRONGER, LONGER, HEALTHIER LIFE

The old adage is true:
"An apple a day keeps the doctor away."

- Helps promote a youthful skin and vibrant healthy body
- Helps remove artery plaque and body toxins
- Helps fight germs, viruses, bacteria and mold naturally
- Helps retard old age onset in humans, pets and farm animals
- Helps regulate calcium metabolism
- Helps keep blood the right consistency
- Helps regulate women's menstruation, relieves PMS, and UTI
- Helps normalize urine pH, relieving frequent urge to urinate
- Helps digestion, assimilation and balances the pH
- Helps relieve sore throats, laryngitis and throat tickles and cleans out throat and gum toxins
- Helps protect against food poisoning and brings relief if you get it
- Helps detox the body so sinus, asthma and flu sufferers can breathe easier and more normally
- Helps banish acne, athlete's foot, soothes burns, sunburns
- Helps prevent itching scalp, baldness, dry hair and helps banish dandruff, rashes, and shingles
- Helps fight arthritis and helps remove crystals and toxins from joints, tissues, organs and entire body
- Helps control and normalize body weight

– Paul C. Bragg, Health Crusader,
Originator of Health Stores

Our sincere blessings to you, dear friends, who make our lives so worthwhile and fulfilled by reading our teachings on natural living as our Creator laid down for us to follow. He wants us to follow the simple path of natural living. This is what we teach in our books and health crusades worldwide. Our prayers reach out to you and your loved ones for the best in health and happiness. We must follow the laws He has laid down for us, so we can reap this precious health physically, mentally, emotionally and spiritually!

With Love, Patricia

HAVE AN APPLE HEALTHY LIFE!

Bragg's Organic Raw Apple Cider Vinegar with the "Mother" is the #1 food I recommend to relieve Gerds and maintain the body's vital acid-alkaline balance.

– Gabriel Cousens, M.D., Author, Conscious Eating

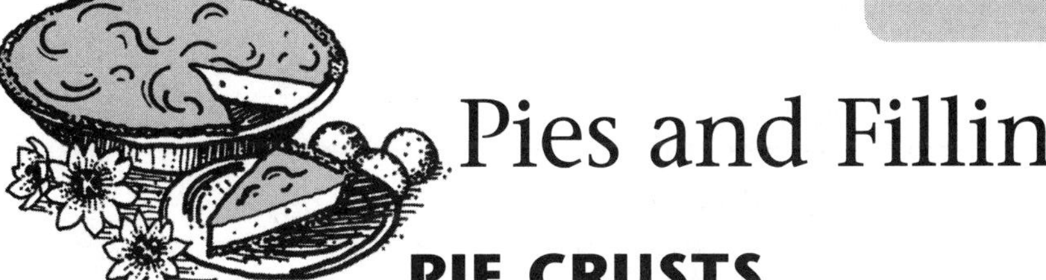

Chapter 19

Pies and Fillings

PIE CRUSTS

WHOLE-GRAIN PIE CRUST (1)

2 cups whole-grain pastry flour
½ tsp brown rice syrup, raw honey or barley malt sweetener
distilled ice water
½ cup Bragg Olive Oil

Add oil to flour and sweetener. Add ice water as needed to form soft dough. Wrap in wax paper and refrigerate for about 2 hours before rolling out on floured board. Makes 2 crusts.

WHOLE-GRAIN PIE CRUST (2)

2¼ cups whole-grain pastry flour
about 5 Tbsps distilled ice water
½ cup Bragg Organic Olive Oil

Mix oil into whole-grain pastry flour. Add water and mix slowly to form a soft dough. Roll on floured board to desired shape and thickness. Makes 2 crusts.

WHOLE-GRAIN & SOY PIE CRUST

1½ cups whole-grain flour
½ cup Bragg Organic Olive Oil
½ tsp raw honey, barley malt or brown rice syrup
½ cup soy flour
distilled ice water

Mix olive oil into flours. Add water and sweetener and mix to a soft dough. Wrap in wax paper and refrigerate about 2 hours before rolling out on floured board. Makes 2 crusts.

GRAHAM CRACKER PIE CRUST

18 graham crackers, finely roll
¼ cup Bragg Organic Olive Oil

Mix graham cracker crumbs and olive oil thoroughly. Press mixture firmly and evenly against sides and bottom of an oiled pie tin. Bake at 400°F for 10 minutes. Cool and fill.

RAW PIE CRUST

RF

2 cups bran
2 cups wheat germ
1 cup coconut, grate
1 tsp lemon juice
2 cups pitted dates, mash
4 Tbsps raw honey

Combine ingredients and mix well. Press evenly into an oiled 9-inch pie plate. Pour in filling, chill and serve.

Stressed spelled backwards is desserts.
Coincidence? I think not! – Author Unknown

LUSCIOUS ORANGE PASTRY "PIE CRUST"

1 cup whole-grain pastry flour
1 cup Bragg Organic Olive Oil
3 to 4 Tbsps fresh orange juice
2 cups soy flour
1 Tbsps orange rind, grate

Sift flours. Add in olive oil. Add organic orange rind, mix well; add juice, mix lightly. Roll out ⅔ of dough on lightly floured board. Place loosely in pie pan. Trim edges. Add desired pie filling. Top with ½-inch twisted crisscrossed strips cut from remaining dough. Bake at 425°F for 20 minutes until crust is golden brown. Makes one 8-inch pie.

PIE FILLINGS

PUMPKIN PIE FILLING

2 cups pumpkin, strain
½ cup raw honey
½ tsp ginger powder
½ tsp allspice powder
½ cup soy milk
Egg Replacer equal to 2 eggs
1½ tsps cinnamon powder

Add soy milk, sweetener, Egg Replacer and spices to pumpkin. Stir for 2 minutes. Pour into pie tin lined with whole-grain or whole-grain/soy pie crust (see recipe page 203). Bake at 425°F about 45 minutes or until filling is firm. Serves 6.

TASTY APRICOT FILLING

1½ cups dried apricots
½ cup raw honey
1 cup raisins or currants
2 Tbsps Bragg Organic Olive Oil
1½ Tbsps arrowroot
1 cup distilled water
2 tsps organic lemon rind, grate

Hot wash and scrub apricots thoroughly. Cook in small amount of distilled water until tender. Mix all other ingredients in a separate pan and cook until mixture thickens. Add drained apricots. Cool mixture and place in baked whole-grain pie shell. (page 203) Chill. Serves 6-8.

PLUM PIE FILLING

1 cup organic apple juice
2 cups plum purée
1 stick agar-agar (½ cup flakes)
¼ cup pitted dates, chop

Break agar-agar into pieces and soak in fruit juice until agar softens. Bring to a boil and cook until agar dissolves. Blend pitted fresh plums in blender until smooth. Pour in cooked agar fruit juice and blend to mix thoroughly. Mix in pitted dates and pour into raw pie shell. (See page 203) Refrigerate until it sets.

Vegetables are a must on a diet. I suggest carrot cake, zucchini bread, and pumpkin pie. – Jim Davis, American Cartoonist, known for Garfield comic strip

FRESH FRUIT FILLING

1 cup strawberries, slice
¼ cup tahini or cashew butter
¼ cup hot distilled water
2 cups bananas, mash
1 stick agar-agar (½ cup flakes)
1 raw pie crust (page 203)

Mix banana and tahini together. Add strawberries. Set aside. Soak agar-agar in hot water for 15 minutes. Bring to boil and cook until agar dissolves. Gradually add agar to fruit mixture, stirring well. Pour into raw pie crust and chill for 2 hours. (*Optional:* delicious served with soy whip cream.) Serves 6-8.

PRUNE AND BANANA ROLL FILLING

1⅔ cups pitted prunes, cooked
1 Tbsp raw honey
1⅓ cups banana, slice

Cut prunes into small pieces. Add the banana and honey; mix thoroughly. Place in pastry shell (recipe follows). Vary by mixing cooked apricots and chopped walnuts with the prunes, or by adding a few finely chopped dates or pecans.

PASTRY SHELL FOR ROLL

Egg Replacer equal to 4 eggs
2 tsps baking powder
2 cups whole-grain flour
1⅓ tsps lemon extract
⅓ cup raw honey
⅔ cup soy flour
6⅔ Tbsps cold distilled water
½ tsp vanilla extract (optional)

To make the pastry, beat Egg Replacer until very light. Mix in honey; add water alternately with the whole-grain and soy flour sifted with baking powder. Add lemon extract and mix thoroughly. Pour into an oiled shallow pan and bake 15-20 minutes at 425°F. Turn out on damp cloth and roll, then unroll and spread with filling. Roll again and remove from the damp cloth. Spread top with any frosting on page 218. Serves 8-10.

PIES

PECAN PIE

Egg Replacer equal to 3 eggs
1 cup pure 100% maple syrup
¼ cup Bragg Organic Olive Oil
1 cup pecans
½ cup raw honey
1 tsp vanilla extract
1 whole-grain pie crust (page 203)

Add honey, maple syrup, vanilla and olive oil to Egg Replacer. Layer pecans in a pie pan lined with whole-grain pastry shell (page 203). Add honey mixture. Bake at 350°F for 50-60 minutes. The nuts usually will rise to form a topping. Serves 6.

Prevent breads, pastries and cakes from sticking to pans by shake of Bragg Organic Olive Oil and spread it around pan.

DELICIOUS GRAHAM CRACKER APPLE PIE

18 graham crackers
4 Tbsps Bragg Organic Olive Oil
½ cup organic raisins
½ tsp nutmeg, grate
½ cup walnut meats, chop
6 organic apples
⅓ cup raw honey
1 tsp cinnamon
soy yogurt (optional)
Egg Replacer equal to 1 egg

Roll crackers fine. Add Egg Replacer and olive oil and mix. Line a glass pie dish with mixture, pressing it down tightly with back of a spoon. Save ¼ cup of mixture for the top. If this is not left over from crust lining, roll more crumbs to make ¼ cup. Wash, peel, core and halve apples. Cook with raisins, honey, and spices (in 1 cup of hot distilled water) until apples are soft, but not mushy. Amount of water used in cooking apples should be increased or decreased according to juiciness of fruit. If apples are too juicy for the pie, press juice out after cooking. Pour into pie pan, sprinkle top with nuts and remaining crumbs. Bake at 350°F for 20 minutes. Top with soy yogurt if desired. Serves 6.

TWO-CRUST BLUEBERRY PIE

whole-grain pie crust
⅔ cup raw honey
¼ tsp nutmeg
2 Tbsps lemon juice
4 cups berries, fresh or frozen
1½ Tbsps arrowroot powder
¼ tsp cinnamon powder
½ lemon, slice paper-thin

Line a 9-inch pie plate with whole-grain pie crust (page 203). Trim edge even with plate. To make filling, mix honey and arrowroot. Add berries, spices, lemon and lemon juice. Pour in pie shell. Moisten edge of crust with water. Cover with crust of whole-grain pastry leaving ½-inch overhanging edges. Fold edge of upper crust under lower crust all the way around. Press edges together with tines of fork dipped in flour. Bake at 400°F for 50 minutes. Serves 6.

GLAZED APRICOT PIE

2 lbs very ripe apricots
1 Tbsp lemon juice
1 baked whole-grain pie crust
nondairy whipped cream
½ cup raw honey
1½ Tbsps arrowroot or instant tapioca powder

Bake a whole-grain pastry pie crust (see page 203) and cool. Wash, halve and remove pits from apricots. Place half of apricot halves, uncooked, in the pie crust, cut-side up and slightly overlapping. Cook remaining apricots with 3 cups distilled water until soft. Mix thickener and honey, add to cooked apricots and cook until sauce is transparent. Remove from heat. Stir in lemon juice. While still hot, pour over apricot halves in pie shell. Cool, then chill. Serve plain or top with nondairy whipped cream, soy ice cream or soy yogurt. Serves 6-8.

BANANA-COCONUT CREAM PIE

4 cups soy milk
1 cup fresh coconut, grate
7 Tbsps arrowroot powder
1 cup raw honey
1 tsp vanilla
1 baked pie shell
1 cup mashed banana and banana slices

Combine soy milk, honey, coconut, vanilla, and arrowroot powder in blender until smooth. Pour into saucepan, stir constantly over medium heat until thick (about 15 minutes) Remove from heat and add mashed banana. Mix well, pour into baked pie shell. Top with banana slices. Chill one hour.

MOCK MINCE MEAT PIE

2 organic apples, core, chop
1½ cups raisins or currants
1 Tbsp Bragg Liquid Aminos
¼ tsp allspice
⅓ cup distilled water
½ unpeeled lemon
¼ cup raw honey
½ tsp cinnamon
¼ tsp clove powder
½ cup unsulphured molasses
whole-grain pie crust (page 203)

Chop apples. Put lemon and raisins (less ¼ cup) through food processor. Then combine all ingredients, except pie crust, but including the ¼ cup whole raisins. Bring to a boil, simmer 30 minutes, stirring often. Cool slightly. Roll out bottom pie crust and fill with "mincemeat". Cut ½-inch strips of dough and arrange in crisscross pattern. Bake at 450°F for 10 minutes; reduce heat to 350°F. Bake for 30-40 more minutes. Serves 6.

TARTS

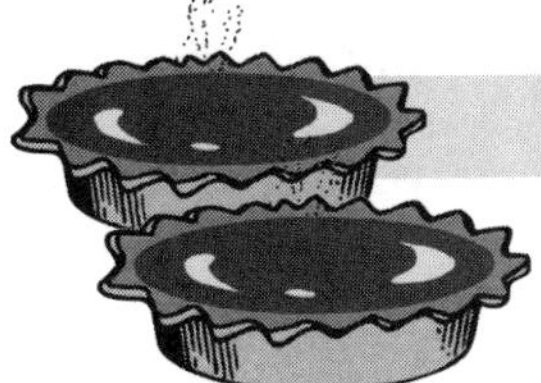

DATE TARTS

2⅔ cups dates, chop
4 Tbsps lemon juice
1 Tbsp raw honey
8 unbaked tart shells
2⅔ tsp lemon rind, grate
2⅔ Tbsps soy milk
1⅓ Tbsps Bragg Olive Oil
whole-grain flour

Mix chopped dates with lemon rind, lemon juice, honey, and soy milk. Fill tart shells, sprinkle each with a little flour and brush generously with olive oil. Bake at 400°F for 25 minutes. Serve plain, or top with soy yogurt or soy cream. Serves 8.

FIG TARTS

⅔ lb dried figs
⅔ Tbsp raw honey
⅔ tsp lemon rind, grate
1⅓ cups boiling distilled water
1⅓ Tbsps orange rind, grate
8 unbaked tart shells

Wash figs and cut off any stems. Cover with boiling water and simmer for 30 minutes. Drain; reserve juice. Chop figs. Boil the juice until it is cooked down to one half (about 5 minutes). Add orange and lemon rinds, honey and figs. Mix thoroughly. Fill the tart shells. Bake at 400°F for 30 minutes. Serves 8.

Take Time for 12 Things

1. Take time to **Work** –
   it is the price of success.
2. Take time to **Think** –
   it is the source of power.
3. Take time to **Play** –
   it is the secret of youth.
4. Take time to **Read** –
   it is the foundation of knowledge.
5. Take time to **Worship** –
   it is the highway of reverence and
   washes the dust of earth from our eyes.
6. Take time to **Help and Enjoy Friends** –
   it is the source of happiness.
7. Take time to **Love and Share** –
   it is the one sacrament of life.
8. Take time to **Dream** –
   it hitches the soul to the stars.
9. Take time to **Laugh** –
   it is the laughing that helps life's loads.
10. Take time for **Beauty** –
    it is everywhere in nature.
11. Take time for **Health** –
    it is the true wealth and treasure of life.
12. Take time to **Plan** –
    it is the secret of being able to have time
    for the first 11 things.

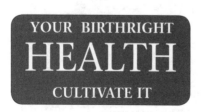

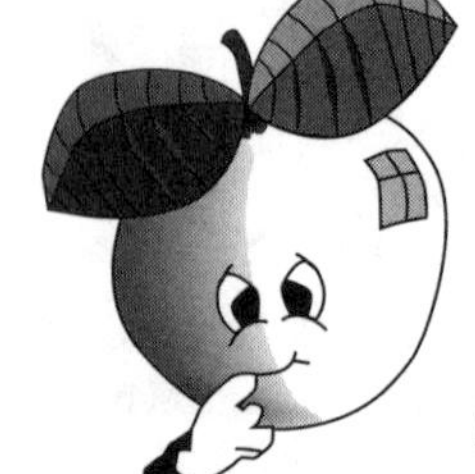

Have an Apple Healthy Life!

Teach me Thy way O Lord, and lead me in a simple plain path. – Psalms 27:11

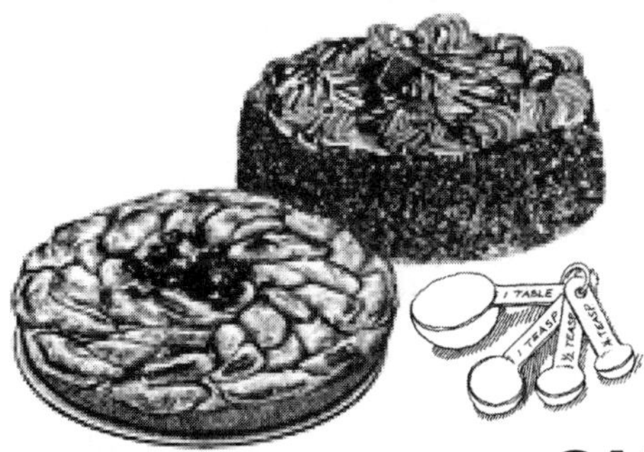

Chapter 20

Cakes and Frostings

CAKES

Always use 100% organic whole-grain pastry flour for all cakes. For lighter cakes be sure to sift flour before measuring and again several times before using.

Egg Replacer by Ener-G Foods, Inc. is a culinary egg substitute containing no eggs or animal products (see pg. 3). For 1 egg add: 1½ tsp Ener-G Egg Replacer plus 2 Tbsps warm water.

NEVER-FAIL SPICE CAKE

Egg Replacer equal to 1 egg
½ cup raw honey
1 Tbsp Bragg Olive Oil
1 cup soy milk
1½ cups whole-grain pastry flour
1 tsp baking powder
1 tsp cinnamon, powder
½ tsp clove powder
½ tsp nutmeg powder
1 cup raisins or currants
½ cup nuts (optional)

To Egg Replacer beat in honey and olive oil. Add milk. Sift flour, baking powder, cinnamon, cloves and nutmeg; add to the mixture. Stir in raisins or currants and nuts (optional). Turn into well-oiled cake pan, bake 40 minutes at 350°F. Use your favorite frosting (see page 218). Serves about 8-10.

FRUITED SPICE CAKE

1 tsp cinnamon powder
3 cups whole-grain pastry flour
¾ cup distilled water
½ cup Bragg Organic Olive Oil
Egg Replacer equal to 3 eggs
1 cup dried figs, dates or prunes (or mix)
1 cup soy milk
1 tsp clove powder
½ cup raw honey
1 tsp vanilla extract
1 tsp ginger powder
2 tsps baking powder

Wash dried fruit; dry and chop. Add cinnamon, ginger, cloves and water; boil 3 minutes, stirring constantly. Cool. Mix olive oil and honey together. Add Egg Replacer slowly, beating well after each addition. Sift remainder of dry ingredients together and add alternately with the soy milk to the creamed mixture. Do not overbeat; beat only until smooth. Fold in fruit mixture and vanilla. Turn into three oiled 9-inch layer pans and bake at 350°F for 25 minutes; or, if baked in tube pan, bake 70-80 minutes. Serves about 8.

TOASTED SPICE CAKE

CAKE:

1 cup raw honey
Egg Replacer equal to 3 eggs
1 tsp cinnamon powder
1 tsp vanilla extract
1½ cups soy milk, sour
1½ tsps baking powder
1 cup Bragg Organic Olive Oil
1 tsp clove powder
1 tsp nutmeg powder
½ tsp lemon extract
2½ cups whole-grain flour

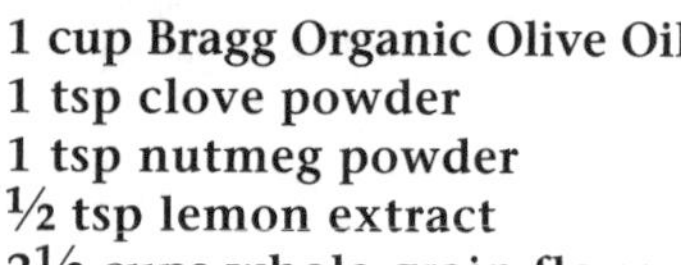

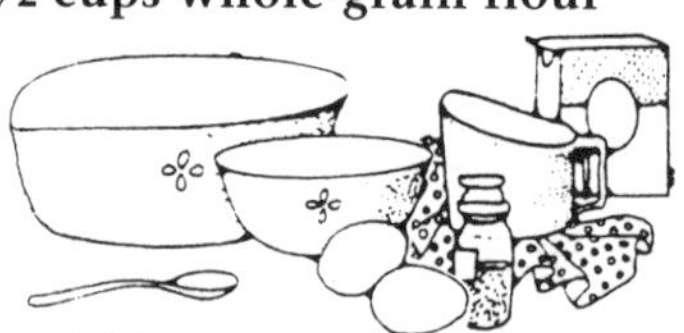

TOPPING:

Egg Replacer equal to 3 egg whites
1 cup nut meats
½ cup raw honey

Mix olive oil and honey together. Add Egg Replacer, cloves, cinnamon, nutmeg, vanilla and lemon extract. Add soy milk. Sift flour and baking powder; combine. Pour batter into an oiled pan. To make topping, beat Egg Replacer and blend in sweetener. Spread mixture over Spice Cake batter. Sprinkle nut meats over top. Bake 350°F for 40-50 minutes. Serves 10.

TEMPTATION SPICE CAKE

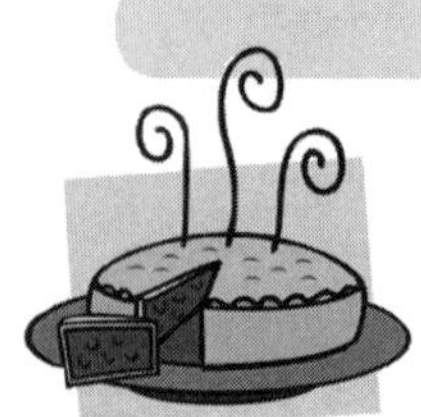

1½ cups whole-grain pastry flour
3½ tsps baking powder
1 tsp cinnamon powder
½ tsp nutmeg powder
¼ tsp clove powder
½ cup Bragg Olive Oil
⅓ cup raw honey
1 cup soy milk
1 tsp vanilla extract
Egg Replacer equal to 2 eggs

Sift all dry ingredients together. Add olive oil, honey, soy milk and vanilla. Beat mixture vigorously with a spoon for 2 minutes. Count number of strokes (about 150 per minute). If beaten by hand and it is necessary to rest a moment, the actual number of strokes will be assured. If an electric mixer is used, beat 2 minutes on medium speed. Scrape sides of bowl frequently to assure an even mix. Add Egg Replacer and beat for 2 more minutes. Turn into oiled layer pans. Bake at 350°F for 35-40 minutes. Cover with the desired frosting of choice (we suggest Creamy Vanilla Icing, page 218). Serves 8-10.

VEGAN CAROB "CHOCOLITE" CAKE

3 cups whole-grain flour
2 tsps baking soda
2 Tbsps Bragg Apple Cider Vinegar
2 tsps vanilla extract
1 tsp Stevia powder
6 Tbsps carob powder
¾ cup Bragg Olive Oil
2 cups distilled water

Add all ingredients together and stir until well blended. Pour into oiled cake pans and bake at 350°F for 30 minutes. Carob Frosting or Creamy Vanilla Icing (pg. 218) are both delicious.

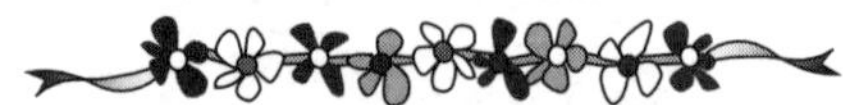

A house is no home unless it contains food for the soul, as well as the body.
– HeartWarmers.com – Free inspirational email publications that enrich your life

UPSIDE-DOWN CAKE

1 cup raw honey
½ cup Bragg Olive Oil
1 tsp baking powder
Egg Replacer equal to 3 eggs
¾ cup whole-grain pastry flour
5 Tbsps juice from fruit used in cake
pineapple rings, cherries or desired fruit

Add ½ cup honey to olive oil warmed in a large iron frying pan. Spread evenly over bottom of pan. Arrange fruit attractively on top of oil and honey mixture; over it, pour the dough, which is mixed as follows: Add ½ cup honey and fruit juice to beaten Egg Replacers. Mix and sift in flour and baking powder. Bake at 350°F for 45-60 minutes. Turn out upside-down on plate. Serves 6-8.

UPSIDE-DOWN GINGERBREAD CAKE

SIFT:

1 cup whole-grain pastry flour
1 tsp cinnamon powder
¼ tsp clove powder
1 tsp baking powder
1 tsp ginger powder
¼ tsp nutmeg powder

Add these ingredients to above mixture. Mix until well blended:

¼ cup raw honey
½ cup soured soy milk
⅓ cup Bragg Organic Olive Oil
⅓ cup unsulphured molasses
Egg Replacer equal to 1 egg

TOPPING INGREDIENTS:

2 Tbsp Bragg Organic Olive Oil
¼ cup 100% pure maple syrup

Prepare topping by combining ingredients in a round 10-inch cake pan. Heat and stir until melted. Remove from heat and arrange the following attractively in bottom of pan:

1 orange, in sections
½ cup nut meats
2 tsps orange rind, grate
¼ cup raisins or currants

Turn gingerbread batter into pan on top of the fruit and nuts. Bake for 30-35 minutes at 325°F. Turn out cake upside down on a large cake plate. Serves 8-10.

The Body is The Hero

"It is the body that is the hero, not science, not antibiotics, not machines, drugs or new devices. The task of the physician today is what it has always been, to help the body do what it has learned so well to do on it's own during its unending struggle for survival to heal itself!

It is the body, not medicine, that is the hero!

– Ronald J. Glasser, M.D., Author, *"The Body Is The Hero" (amazon.com)*

Too often we underestimate the power of a touch, a smile, a kind word, a listening ear, an honest compliment or the smallest act of caring, all of which have the potential to turn a life around.
– Leo Buscaglia, author, who praised Bragg teaching

The natural healing force within us is the greatest force in getting well.
– Hippocrates, Father of Medicine

Nature, time and patience are the 3 greatest physicians. – Irish Proverb

CAROB AND SOY MILK CAKE

½ cup Bragg Organic Olive Oil
Egg Replacer equal to 2 eggs
1 cup sour soy milk
1 Tbsp lemon juice
2 cups whole-grain pastry flour
½ cup raw honey
2 squares carob (melted)
1 tsp vanilla extract
1 tsp baking soda

Add honey gradually to olive oil and beat until creamy. Beat in Egg Replacer slowly, beating 2 minutes after each addition. Add vanilla, soy milk and melted carob. Add sifted flour. Lastly, add soda dissolved in lemon juice. Beat again. Pour into oiled pan and bake for 30-35 minutes at 375°F. Serves 8.

TOPSY-TURVY PINEAPPLE CAKE

1 cup whole-grain pastry flour
Egg Replacer equal to 3 eggs
1½ tsps baking powder
1 can unsweetened sliced pineapple
4 Tbsps Bragg Organic Olive Oil
1 cup raw honey
⅓ cup hot pineapple juice
½ tsp lemon extract

Add ½ cup honey to oil in a 9-inch skillet. Stir until blended. Arrange pineapple slices attractively over olive oil and honey mixture. Beat Egg Replacer with ½ cup honey until very light. Slowly add hot pineapple juice and continue to beat. Fold in remaining dry, sifted ingredients. Stir in lemon extract. Pour batter over pineapple slices and bake at 350°F for 45 minutes. Turn cake out upside down. Serves 6-8.

VANILLA CAKE

½ cup Bragg Organic Olive Oil
Egg Replacer equal to 3 eggs
½ cup raw honey
¾ cup soy milk
1¾ cups whole-grain pastry flour, sift
1 tsp vanilla extract
2 tsps baking powder

Blend olive oil, raw honey and vanilla extract. Add sifted dry ingredients, gradually alternating with soy milk. Beat Egg Replacer. Fold into dry ingredients. Turn batter into two oiled 8-inch layer cake pans. Bake at 350°F for 30-35 minutes. Remove from pans and cool. Delicious topped with Creamy Vanilla Icing (page 218). Serves 8-10.

HONEY CAKE - BALLS

1 cup raw honey
Egg Replacer equal to 2 eggs
3½ cups whole-grain pastry flour
½ cup walnut oil
2 tsps baking soda
1 tsp vanilla extract

Cream oil and Egg Replacer, add other ingredients. Mix well. Set in refrigerator overnight. Roll dough into 24 small balls; place them 2-inches apart on oiled cookie sheet. Bake at 300°F until brown. Spread with honey while still warm. Makes 24.

Think about words with honey, notice that when they are mentioned, it usually has to do with something sweet, good or positive. – benefits-of-honey.com

BLUEBERRY SQUARES

1½ cups whole-grain pastry flour
¼ cup Bragg Organic Olive Oil
4 tsps whole-grain pastry flour
Egg Replacer equal to 1 egg
2 tsps baking powder
¾ cup raw honey
½ cup soy milk
1 tsp vanilla extract
1G cups blueberries, fresh or frozen

Sift 1½ cups of whole-grain flour and baking powder together three times. Gradually add honey to olive oil and beat until light. Add Egg Replacer and mix well. Add flour mixture alternately with soy milk and vanilla, beating after each addition until smooth. Lightly toss blueberries with four teaspoons of whole-grain flour and fold into batter. Bake in an oiled and floured 8-inch square pan at 350°F for 60 minutes or until done. Cut in squares. Makes 16 squares.

Enjoy Healthy Fiber for Super Health

- KEEP BEANS HANDY, probably the best fiber sources. Cook dried beans and freeze in portions. Use canned beans for faster meals.
- EAT BERRIES, surprisingly good sources of fiber.
- INSTEAD OF ICEBERG LETTUCE, choose deep green lettuces, romaine, bib, butter, etc., spinach or cabbage for variety salads.
- LOOK FOR "100% WHOLE WHEAT" or whole grain breads. A dark color isn't proof; check labels, compare fibers, grains, etc.
- WHOLE GRAIN CEREALS. Hot, also cold granola with sliced fruit.
- GO FOR BROWN RICE. It's better for you and so delicious.
- EAT THE SKINS of potatoes and other organic fruits and vegetables.
- LOOK FOR HEALTH CRACKERS with at least 2 grams of fiber per ounce.
- SERVE HUMMUS, made from chickpeas, instead of sour-cream dips.
- USE WHOLE WHEAT FLOUR for baking breads, muffins, pastries, pancakes, waffles and for variety try other whole grain flours.
- ADD OAT BRAN, WHEAT BRAN AND WHEATGERM to baked goods, cookies, etc.; whole grain cereals, casseroles, loafs, etc.
- SNACK ON SUN-DRIED FRUIT, such as apricots, dates, prunes, raisins, etc., which are concentrated sources of nutrients and fiber.
- INSTEAD OF DRINKING JUICE, eat the fruit: orange, grapefruit, etc.; and vegetables: tomato, carrot, etc. – UC Berkeley Wellness Letter

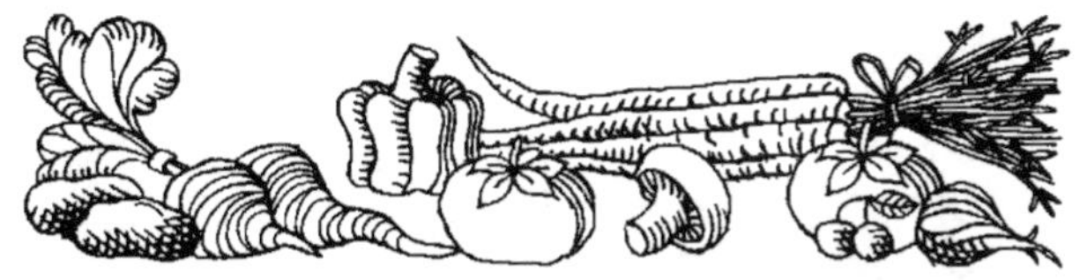

There is a great deal of truth in the saying that man becomes what he eats. – Gandhi

---

Kindness should be a frame of mind in which we are alert to every opportunity: to do, to give, to share and to cheer. – Patricia Bragg, ND, PhD.

FRESH FRUIT CAKE

1¼ cups whole-grain flour
¼ cup Bragg Organic Olive Oil
2 cups any fresh fruit or berries desired
¼ tsp baking powder
½ cup raw honey
Egg Replacer equal to 1 egg

CUSTARD (if needed):
Egg Replacer equal to 1 egg and ⅓ cup soy cream

Mix olive oil into dry ingredients and add Egg Replacer last. Then, press crust into coffee-cake pan. You may use any fruit or berries desired. Pour ½ cup of honey over fruit. If you used juicy fruit such as raspberries, strawberries or blueberries, make a custard blending the Egg Replacer and soy cream together; add this about 10 minutes before removing it from oven. Bake at 375°F for about 1 hour. Serves 6.

RAISIN NUT CAKE

Egg Replacer equal to 3 eggs
2½ cups whole-grain pastry flour
½ cup raw honey
1½ cups raisins or currants
1 tsp lemon extract
⅓ cup walnut oil
1 cup nut meats, chop
½ cup soy milk
1 Tbsp baking powder
1 tsp almond extract

Mix olive oil and honey until creamy. Add Egg Replacer ⅓ at a time, beating thoroughly after each addition. Add extracts. Sift 2 cups whole-grain flour, and re-sift, adding baking powder. Add to batter. Add raisins and nuts that have been floured with ½ cup of flour, alternately with soy milk and sifted ingredients. Pour into well-oiled loaf tin and bake at 275°F for about 1 hour. This delicious healthy cake keeps well. Serves 8.

PRUNE - NUT BARS

Egg Replacer equal to 4 eggs
1⅓ cups whole-grain pastry flour
1⅓ tsps baking powder
1 cup nuts, chop of choice
1⅓ tsps lemon rind, grate
2 cups uncooked prunes, chop
1 cup raw honey

Beat Egg Replacer until thick; add honey and lemon rind. Beat well. Sift whole-grain flour and baking powder and add to Egg Replacer mixture. Fold in chopped prunes and nuts of choice. Pour into 8 x 12-inch pan that has been oiled. Bake at 375°F for 40-45 minutes. Turn out on cooling rack and cut when cool. Optional: Frost with your favorite health icing. Makes 36 bars.

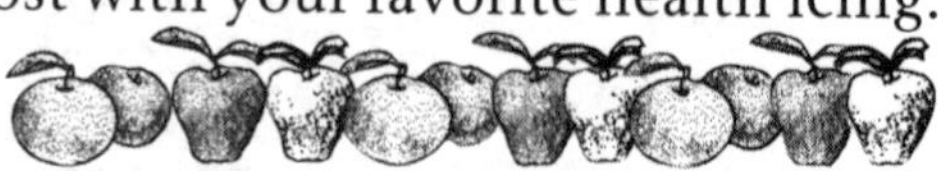

Raw honey has been proven to improve performance and power during endurance cycling trials when used as a source of carbohydrates.
– Edmund R. Burke, Ph.D., Professor, University of Colorado & Sports Physiologist

APRICOT ALMOND DELITE

Bragg Organic Olive Oil
½ cup apricots, slice
½ tsp baking powder
1¼ cups whole-grain pastry flour
1 cup granulated barley malt
½ cup plus 2 Tbsps lite silken tofu
⅛ tsp Bragg Liquid Aminos
½ tsp cinnamon powder
¼ cup almond pieces
¼ cup prune purée*
½ cup soy milk
½ tsp almond extract
¼ cup distilled water
½ tsp baking soda

Preheat oven to 350°F. Lightly oil an 8-inch square pan with olive oil. Place apricots in a small saucepan. Cook over low heat until water is absorbed, stirring frequently. Set aside. In a large bowl, stir together flour with the next 5 dry ingredients. Set aside. Place tofu in the food processor and blend. Blend prune purée*, Bragg Aminos and cinnamon. Add soy milk and almond extract. Blend smooth. Add tofu mixture to dry ingredients. Fold in apricots and almonds. Pour batter into prepared pan. Bake 25 minutes or until toothpick inserted into center comes out clean. Serve with Tofu Cream (page 218).

VEGAN TOFU CHEESECAKE

CRUST:
5 cups ground granola
¼ cup Bragg Olive Oil

TOPPING:
¾ cup apple juice concentrate
6 cups fresh strawberries
3 Tbsps arrowroot powder

FILLING:
1 cup soy milk
20 oz firm tofu
1 tsp almond extract
1 Tbsp vanilla extract
½ cup Bragg Olive Oil
2 tsps arrowroot powder
2 tsps Stevia powder

For crust, blend granola and olive oil. Spread in an oiled pie plate and bake at 350°F for 5 minutes. Blend filling ingredients in blender until smooth. Pour into pie crust. Bake at 350°F for 20 minutes. To make topping, mix ½ cup juice concentrate with arrowroot. Simmer strawberries with ¼ cup of juice concentrate. Add arrowroot mixture, simmer 15 minutes. Cool. Apply the topping, chill cheesecake overnight. Serves 8.

PEANUT BUTTER CUPCAKES

½ cup Bragg Olive Oil
2¼ cups whole-grain pastry flour
1 cup raw honey (split in half)
¾ cup natural peanut butter
Egg Replacer equal to 3 eggs, beat
¾ cup peanut oil
1⅛ cups soy milk
3¾ tsps baking powder
1½ tsps vanilla extract

Cream olive oil, peanut oil and ½ cup of honey. Add peanut butter and mix well. Mix beaten Egg Replacer with ½ cup honey. Add sifted dry ingredients with soy milk and vanilla. Fill oiled cupcake pans ½ full. Bake in a 350°F oven for 25 minutes. Frost with Creamy Vanilla Icing (page 218). Makes 12-14 cupcakes.

---

* *See page 112 on how to make Prune Pureé (under Pumpkin Ravioli)*

CALIFORNIA CHEESECAKE

2 cups whole-grain crackers, finely crush
1½ tsps cinnamon powder
Egg Replacer equal to 4 eggs
3 cups soft tofu
2 tsps lemon rind, grate
¼ cup whole-grain pastry flour
1 cup light soy cream
1½ Tbsps lemon juice
¼ cup walnuts, chop
½ cup Bragg Olive Oil
1 cup raw honey

Combine all but ¾ cup of crumbs with cinnamon, olive oil and ½ cup honey. Press crumb mixture to bottom and sides of 9-inch spring-form pan. Beat Egg Replacer lightly, then beat in ½ cup honey gradually. Add lemon juice, soy cream, tofu and whole-grain flour. Beat until thoroughly blended. Strain through fine sieve. Add lemon rind and stir well. Pour into pan and sprinkle top with remainder of crumbs and nuts. Bake at 350°F for 1 hour. Turn off heat, open oven door and let cake cool in oven for 1 hour. Chill and remove from pan. Serves 10-12.

BANANA GINGERBREAD

¼ cup Bragg Organic Olive Oil
Egg Replacer equal to 1 egg
1⅓ cups whole-grain pastry flour
½ cup unsulphured molasses
¾ cup whipped rice or soy cream
¼ cup raw honey
½ tsp fresh ginger, grate
½ tsp baking soda
½ cup hot distilled water
2 bananas, slice

Cream olive oil and honey; add Egg Replacer, ginger and molasses. Beat in mixed dry ingredients and water alternately in small amounts. Bake in two oiled pans 25 minutes at 350°F. Cool. Slice one banana on bottom layer and cover with whipped soy cream. Top with other cake and cover with remaining sliced banana and rice or soy cream. Serves 8.

APPLE SAUCE CAKE

2 Tbsps Bragg Organic Olive Oil
½ cup raw honey
¼ tsp nutmeg
2 cups whole-grain pastry flour
Egg Replacer equal to 2 eggs
1 cup apple sauce
¼ tsp cinnamon
¾ cup raisins
½ tsp baking soda

Add Egg Replacer to creamed olive oil and honey. Add apple sauce and spices. Sift flour with baking soda and mix with other ingredients. Dust raisins with a little whole grain flour and add to mixture. Bake at 350°F for 40 minutes. Serve plain or with Creamy Vanilla Icing (page 218). Serves 8.

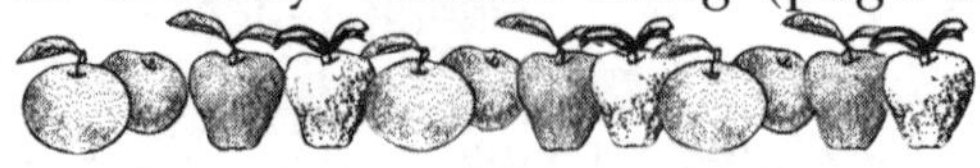

I have the wisdom of my years and the youthfulness of The Bragg Healthy Lifestyle and I never act or feel my calendar years! I feel ageless! Then why shouldn't you? Start living the Bragg Healthy Way today! – Patricia Bragg

SPICE CRUMB BREAKFAST CAKE

⅓ cup plus 3 Tbsps Bragg Organic Olive Oil
2½ cups whole-grain pastry flour
2½ tsps baking powder
1½ tsps ginger powder
Egg Replacer equal to 1 egg
1 cup raw honey
¾ cup soy milk
1 tsp nutmeg
½ tsp cloves powder
1 tsp vanilla extract
1 cup raisins or currants

Blend 3 tablespoons olive oil, ¼ cup honey and ½ cup flour to crumb-like consistency. Sprinkle these crumbs in bottom of an oiled and floured 8 x 8 x 2-inch cake pan. Combine ⅓ cup olive oil and ¾ cup honey and mix until light. Add Egg Replacer and beat thoroughly. Sift together remaining 2 cups of whole-grain pastry flour with baking powder, nutmeg, ginger and cloves. Add dry ingredients alternately in thirds with the soy milk, beating smooth after each addition. Stir in raisins and vanilla and pour into pan. Bake at 350°F for 50 minutes. Serves 6-8.

STRAWBERRY SHORTCAKE

2 cups whole-grain pastry flour
Egg Replacer equal to 2 eggs
6 Tbsps Bragg Olive Oil
1 cup whipped soy cream
1 tsp baking powder
2 Tbsps raw honey
⅔ cup soy milk
1 quart organic strawberries

Sift and measure flour. Add the baking powder and sift twice. Mix olive oil and honey into flour. Beat Egg Replacer and soy milk; pour into the flour mixture. Mix well. It will be a soft dough. Place in an oiled cake pan and bake at 450°F for 20 minutes. Remove from the pan, split, then oil the split sides. Cover the bottom half with strawberries. Put top half over it (cut-side up) and cover with the rest of the berries. Top with whipped soy cream or vanilla soy yogurt. Serves 8.

BANANA CUPCAKES

2¼ cups whole-grain pastry flour
Egg Replacer equal to 3 eggs
¾ cup Bragg Organic Olive Oil
1½ cups banana mash & sieve
½ cup raw honey
1½ tsps baking powder
⅜ cup sour soy milk
1½ tsps vanilla extract

Cream olive oil and honey together. Add Egg Replacer and beat well. Add sifted dry ingredients with soy milk, banana and vanilla. Fill oiled cupcake pans ½ full. Bake at 350°F for 25 minutes. Cover with Creamy Vanilla Icing (page 218). Makes 12-14 cupcakes.

Among healthiest of fruits, bananas are higher in vitamins and minerals.
– www.banana.com

How good it is to be well-fed, healthy and kind, all at the same time.
– Henry Heimlich, vegetarian physician & inventor of Heimlich Maneuver

---

Unhealthy, bad cooking diminishes happiness and shortens the lifespan. – Wisdom of Ages

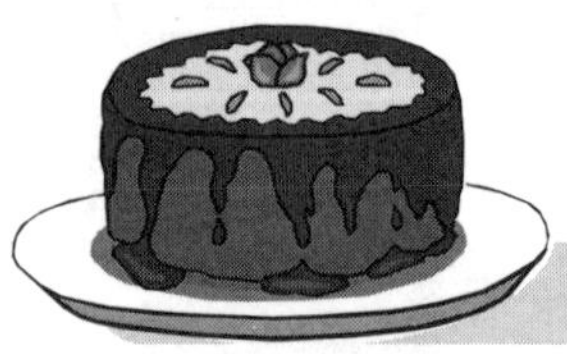

FROSTINGS

TOFU CREAM

½ cup plus 2 Tbsps firm tofu, drain
¼ cup fruit-sweetened apricot jam
3 Tbsps pure 100% maple syrup
1 tsp lemon peel, grate
1 tsp vanilla extract
¼ cup orange juice

Place drained tofu in food processor and blend. Add remaining ingredients and blend until smooth. Makes about 1½ cups.

NATURAL FRUIT FILLING

1 cup raisins, chop
2 tsp arrowroot powder
1 cup hot distilled water
2 tsps orange peel, grate
¾ cup dried figs, apples or prunes, chop
1 cup raw honey or juice concentrate

Mix fruit, sweetener and arrowroot powder. Pour hot water over mixture. Add grated orange peel and cook until thick, stirring constantly. Chill before spreading. Makes enough filling for one cake. (*Optional:* Add mixed chopped nuts or seeds and mashed bananas before spreading.)

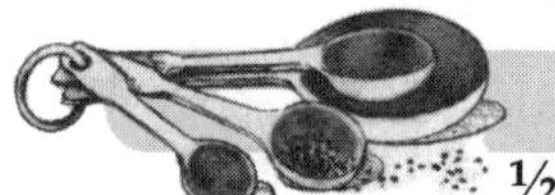

CAROB FROSTING

½ cup raw honey
1 cup carob powder
Egg Replacer equal to 2 eggs
1 tsp Bragg Organic Olive Oil
2 Tbsps soy milk
½ tsp pure vanilla extract

Combine Egg Replacer with honey; mix well. Add powdered carob and cook in double boiler until mixture thickens. Add the soy milk gradually and cook 2 minutes longer, stirring constantly. Remove from heat; add Bragg Olive Oil and pure vanilla extract. Blend well until spreadable.

CREAMY VANILLA ICING

½ cup frozen apple juice concentrate
3 Tbsps agar flakes
1 Tbsp lemon juice
1 tsp lemon peel, grate
⅓ cup raw honey
1½ tsps vanilla extract
1¼ cups tofu (firm or extra firm), drain

Place juice concentrate in a small saucepan; add agar flakes, and bring to a boil over medium heat, stirring until dissolved. Reduce heat and simmer, stirring frequently until thickened, about 5 minutes. Place tofu in food processor, and blend until smooth. Add grated lemon peel, lemon juice, vanilla extract and honey. Process until smooth, scraping down once or twice. Add thickened juice concentrate, and blend until smooth. Frost cake and decorate with sliced organic strawberries, saving a berry with greens intact for the center.

Vanilla was once so rare and expensive that only royalty had access to it. – www.joyofbaking.com

Chapter 21

Healthy Cookies

Egg Replacer by Ener-G Foods, Inc. is a culinary egg substitute containing no eggs or animal products (see page 3). For 1 egg add: 1½ tsp Ener-G Egg Replacer plus 2 Tbsps warm water.

GOLDEN BLOSSOM BARS

½ cup Bragg Organic Olive Oil
Egg Replacer equal to 2 eggs
1 cup nut or seed meats, chop
2½ cups sifted whole-grain pastry flour
½ cup raw honey
1 tsp baking powder
1 tsp vanilla extract
2 Tbsps lemon juice

Cream olive oil with honey and Egg Replacer, gradually. Beat until fluffy. Sift flour. Measure. Add baking powder and sift again. Add gradually to the oil mixture, beating thoroughly. Add nut or seed meats (walnuts, almonds, hazelnuts or sunflower, sesame, pumpkin seeds, etc.), and vanilla extract and lemon juice. Spread batter in oiled 8x8-inch baking pan and bake at 400°F for about 12 minutes or until golden brown. Cool and cut in strips. Makes 16-20 bars.

MOLASSES FRUIT BARS

½ cup Bragg Olive Oil
½ cup raw honey
½ tsp baking soda
1 tsp baking powder
2 cups raw nuts, chop
1 cup soy or rice milk
Egg Replacer equal to 2 eggs
1 cup molasses or 100% maple syrup
3 cups sifted whole-grain pastry flour
2 cups raisins or dates or mix, chop

Cream olive oil and honey gradually, until light and fluffy. Add Egg Replacer and molasses and blend thoroughly. Sift whole-grain pastry flour once. Measure; add baking soda and baking powder and sift again. Add to creamed mixture alternately with soy or rice milk, a small amount at a time. Beat thoroughly after each addition. Add chopped nuts and fruit. Spread very thin in several large shallow oiled pans. Bake at 350°F for 10-12 minutes. Cool and cut into 2-inch squares. Makes about 8 dozen bars.

The best exercise for the heart is to push yourself away from the table. In a recent study one group pursued weight loss without exercise, a second group exercised without dieting, while the third group neither exercised nor dieted. The dieting only group produced significant results, but those exercising with dieting produced the most significant results; those exercising without dieting, less dramatic results. Also, the study showed that exercise benefits lean people more than obese people – all the more reason to lose weight and exercise. – USA Today

BUTTERSCOTCH BRAN COOKIES

1 cup Bragg Organic Olive Oil
Egg Replacer equal to 1 egg
3 cups whole-grain pastry flour, sift
2 cups raw honey
1 cup bran
2 tsps baking powder

Cream olive oil and honey. Add Egg Replacer and beat well. Sift whole-grain flour. Measure, and sift again with baking powder. Add bran to creamed mixture, mixing well. Shape into long rolls, 2-inches in diameter. Wrap in waxed paper and chill 5 hours. Slice ⅛-inch thick and bake on un-greased cookie sheets in a 400°F oven for 10 minutes or until brown. This Butterscotch Bran recipe makes about 7 dozen cookies.

ALMOND STICKS

⅓ cup Bragg Organic Olive Oil
1⅓ cups whole-grain pastry flour
⅔ cup raw honey
1 organic lemon rind, grate
⅔ cup ground almonds
1⅓ tsps fresh lemon juice
4 tsps fresh orange juice
½ cup powdered coconut

Mix olive oil and almonds into whole-grain flour and honey. Add remaining ingredients except coconut. Shape into crescents. Bake in a 250°F oven for 30 minutes. Remove from pan and roll in powdered coconut. Makes 3 dozen sticks.

OATMEAL RAISIN COOKIES

Egg Replacer equal to 1 egg
2½ cups raw steel-cut oats
1 tsp organic lemon rind, grate
¾ cup whole-grain pastry flour
½ cup raw honey
2 Tbsps lemon juice
½ cup Bragg Olive Oil
1 cup raisins

Cream olive oil and honey. Add Egg Replacer and beat until fluffy. Add lemon rind and juice. Sift whole-grain flour and add oats to creamed mixture. Fold in raisins. Drop by spoonful on oiled baking sheet. Bake at 375°F for 12-15 minutes. Makes 36 cookies.

NUT OR SEED BUTTER CAROB BROWNIE

½ cup Bragg Organic Olive Oil
¾ cup raw honey
1⅓ cups whole-grain or pastry flour, sift
1 cup raw nuts and seeds, chop
½ cup peanut or nut butter
Egg Replacer equal to 3 eggs
4 Tbsps carob powder
½ tsp baking powder

Mix olive oil with nut or seed butter. Add honey gradually. Mix carob and Egg Replacer into nut butter mixture. Mix and sift dry ingredients; add to mixture. Add chopped raw nuts and seeds and mix well. Place in oiled, shallow pan. Bake 30-35 minutes at 350°F. Cut into squares while warm. Makes about 36 brownies.

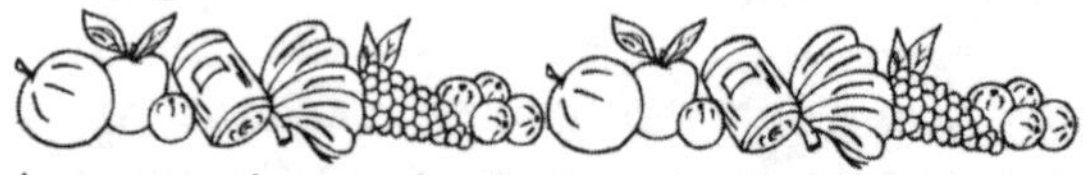

The future belongs to those who believe in the beauty of their dreams.
– Eleanor Roosevelt, wife of U.S. President Franklin D. Roosevelt, 1933-1945

BRAGG LIQUID AMINOS NUT DELIGHTS

Make a delicious finger food or crunchy topping for salads, fruits, vegetables, sandwiches, casseroles, and baked potatoes using raw seeds, nut meats (sunflower, sesame, pumpkin, almond, cashew, pine, macadamia, etc.). In heavy, warm skillet over medium heat, dry-cook mixture of raw nuts and seeds for 2-4 minutes; remove from heat, lightly spray with Bragg Liquid Aminos.

CRANBERRY OATMEAL COOKIES

2½ cups whole-grain pastry flour
1 Tbsp vanilla extract
¼ cup soy milk
2 cups rolled oats
1 tsp baking soda
1 cup dried cranberries
1 Tbsp Egg Replacer
1½ cups granulated barley malt
1 tsp baking powder
1 tsp cinnamon powder
1¼ cups soft tofu, drain
1 Tbsp Bragg Olive Oil
¼ cup distilled water
⅓ cup raw honey
⅓ cup soy grits

Preheat oven to 350°F. Lightly rub cookie sheets with a dash of olive oil. Mix flour, oats, barley malt, baking soda, baking powder and cinnamon in a large bowl. Set aside. Place tofu in food processor and blend. Add honey. Pulse, then blend. Whisk Egg Replacer with water in a small bowl until foamy. Add to tofu mixture along with vanilla, soy milk and the remainder of the olive oil. Blend until smooth. Fold the liquid ingredients into the dry. Add cranberries and soy grits. Mix thoroughly. Drop by rounded tablespoons onto cookie sheets. Bake 10 minutes or until lightly browned. Cool 1 minute on pan, then finish cooling on racks. Makes 5½ dozen cookies.

OATMEAL CRISPS

2½ cups organic rolled oats
1 cup Bragg Organic Olive Oil
3 tsps pure vanilla
2 tsps baking powder
½ cup oat bran
1 cup raw honey
Egg Replacer equal to 2 eggs
1½ cups whole-grain pastry flour
¼ cup soy or rice milk
raisins or nuts for topping

Mix oats, bran, honey, Egg Replacer and olive oil. Sift together whole-grain flour and baking powder. Add vanilla to milk and add dry ingredients and milk mixture alternately to first mixture. Drop level teaspoonsful of dough 2-inches apart on oiled cookie sheet. Flatten to ⅛-inch and decorate top with raisins or nuts. Bake in a 400°F oven for 10 minutes. Remove at once from pan. Makes 5-6 dozen cookies.

Oatmeal has been scientifically recognized for its heart health benefits, and the latest research shows this evidence endures the test of time and should be embraced as a lifestyle option for millions of Americans at-risk for heart disease.

– Dr. James W. Anderson, Professor of Medicine and Clinical Nutrition at the University of Kentucky College of Medicine

ORANGE-BLOSSOM HONEY CHIPS

7 Tbsps Bragg Olive Oil
Egg Replacer equal to 1 egg
1 cup whole-grain pastry flour
½ cup carob, grate
½ cup orange-blossom honey
½ tsp pure vanilla
1 tsp baking powder
¼ cup nuts, chop

Blend oil and honey. Add the Egg Replacer and beat. Add vanilla. Sift dry ingredients and stir. Mix in nuts and carob. Cover bowl and chill for 40 minutes. Drop dough by teaspoons on oiled cookie sheet. Bake at 350°F for 10-12 minutes. Remove at once from pan and cool. Makes about 2 dozen honey chips.

GINGERBREAD BOYS

1½ cups unsulphured molasses
5¼ cups whole-grain pastry flour
1 cup Bragg Organic Olive Oil
2¼ tsps ginger powder
¾ tsp baking soda
3 tsps baking powder
¾ tsp allspice

Heat molasses slowly to bubbling and add olive oil. Cool and add sifted dry ingredients. Mix to a smooth dough. Chill. Roll out on floured board to ¼-inch thickness and cut with cookie-cutter; or, make paper pattern of gingerbread man and cut out with sharp point of paring knife. Bake at 350°F for 10-12 minutes. Makes about 6 dozen cookies.

RAISIN-FILLED COOKIES

½ cup Bragg Olive Oil
Egg Replacer equal to 1 egg
1 tsp vanilla extract
2 cups whole-grain pastry flour
½ cup raw honey
1 tsp baking powder
¼ tsp nutmeg
½ cup raisins

Cream olive oil and honey; add Egg Replacer and vanilla and beat well. Sift together dry ingredients and add to wet mixture. On dough board, roll out mixture to about ¼-inch thick and cut with cookie-cutter. Cover cookies with the raisins and top with another cutout cookie. Press the edges together and bake at 350°F 10-15 minutes until brown. Makes 1 dozen cookies.

RAISIN COOKIES

1 cup Bragg Organic Olive Oil
Egg Replacer equal to 2 eggs
2 tsps baking powder
⅔ cup soy or rice milk
2 cups raisins, softened
½ cup raw honey or rice syrup
4 cups whole-grain pastry flour
1 tsp cinnamon
2 tsps vanilla extract
1 cup walnuts, chop

Blend the olive oil with the honey or rice syrup. Add the Egg Replacer and beat well. Sift flour before measuring and sift three times with the other dry ingredients. Add to the first mixture alternately with the milk. Add vanilla, raisins and nuts. Mix and drop by spoonfuls on an oiled cookie sheet or shallow pan. Bake at 375°F for about 15 minutes. Makes 5-6 dozen cookies.

SOFT MOLASSES HERMITS

3 cups sifted whole-grain pastry flour
1 cup unsulphured molasses
½ cup raw honey (or rice syrup)
Egg Replacer equal to 2 eggs
½ cup sour rice or soy milk
2 tsps baking powder
½ tsp ground cloves
1 cup raisins
1 tsp cinnamon powder
1 cup Bragg Olive Oil

Mix and sift dry ingredients. Mix olive oil and honey. Add Egg Replacer and beat well. Add molasses. Add flour mixture and soy milk alternately. Mix in raisins (softened in hot water). Drop dough by teaspoons 2-inches apart on an oiled baking sheet. Bake at 400°F for about 10 minutes. Makes about 7 dozen cookies.

CAROB - BAR COOKIES

3 carob squares
3 cups rolled oats
2 tsps pure vanilla
½ cup Bragg Organic Olive Oil
½ cup raw honey or rice syrup
⅓ cup chopped nut meats

Melt carob and olive oil in top of double boiler. Add remaining ingredients and blend well. Pack firmly into an oiled square pan. Bake at 425°F for 12 minutes. Chill. Cut into bars. Makes 2-3 dozen cookies, depending on bar size.

ICEBOX COOKIES

1 cup Bragg Organic Olive Oil
2 tsps baking powder
Egg Replacer equal to 2 eggs
3½ cups whole-grain pastry flour
1 cup raw honey
1 Tbsp vanilla extract
½ tsp cinnamon powder
½ cup nuts, chop

Cream honey with olive oil together. Add other ingredients in this order: vanilla, Egg Replacer, sifted dry ingredients and nuts. Place on waxed paper, shape into roll. Wrap in waxed paper and place in refrigerator overnight (or until ready for use). Slice thin. Bake on an oiled cookie sheet at 400°F for 10-15 minutes until delicately browned. Makes about 5 dozen.

MOLASSES STRIPS

3 cups whole-grain pastry flour
1 tsp cinnamon
½ cup unsulphured molasses
½ cup raw honey or rice syrup
⅓ cup pecans, chop
½ tsp baking powder
a dash clove powder
⅓ cup Bragg Organic Olive Oil
¼ cup distilled boiling water
½ cup raisins (optional)

Mix honey or rice syrup and olive oil. Blend molasses and raisins (optional) with boiling water. Add to mixture, fold in sifted dry ingredients. Allow to cool. When at room temperature, place in refrigerator for 30 minutes. Then turn out on a floured board and roll. Cut into the desired shape, sprinkle with nuts and bake at 350°F. Makes 4 dozen cookies.

Carob is a health substitute for chocolate. Carob has great chocolate flavor but not health risks or additives that chocolate has. – gilead.net/health/carob

NATURAL SWEETENERS

Stevia the Natural Herbal Sweetener

Stevia is from a family of 150 species of herbs in the sunflower family, native to subtropical and tropical South America and the Central Americas. *Stevia rebaudiana* is commonly known as sweetleaf, sugarleaf, or simply Stevia. It is widely grown for its sweet leaves. It has been used as a sweetening ingredient in foods and drinks by South American natives for many centuries. In its unprocessed form it is 30 times sweeter than sugar. Extracts of Stevia on the market today are up to 300 times the sweetness of sugar. Stevia and its extracts have been successfully used in a number of food products in Japan since the mid 1970's. It is very safe when used as a natural sweetener and natural alternative to sugar substitutes, especially for diabetics!

Stevia extracts are sold in health food stores and the demand for this sweet natural herbal ingredient is increasing. It is a low carbohydrate, low-sugar food alternative. Stevia shows promise for treating such conditions as obesity and high blood pressure. It does not effect blood sugar and it even enhances glucose tolerance. This makes Stevia a safe, delicious, health sweetener for diabetics, also for others on carbohydrate-controlled diets. Children can use Stevia without concerns, does not cause cavities. It can easily blend with other natural sweeteners, such as honey.

Stevia is heat stable and could be used in cooking and baking. However, this requires some experimentation as it seems to work better in some recipes than others. It works very easily in beverages and in liquid recipes. Stevia is available in health food stores in both liquid and powder (our favorite) forms. The FDA has now approved several Stevia Herb Extracts for use in foods and beverages. At Bragg we use Stevia Extract in some of our drinks and salad dressings.

Agave Cactus Nectar

Agave is a honey-like nectar with a low glycemic index, which makes it ideal for diabetics and others who are controlling their carbohydrate intake. It is made from Mexico's Blue Agave cactus. This is the same plant from which tequila is made. Agave sweetens naturally without spiking blood sugar and is a great alternative to honey for vegans who desire plant-derived sweeteners. Agave requires some experimentation when using it in various recipes. It works well in liquids, beverages, and over cereals, pancakes, and waffles.

Honey

Honey has been the natural sweetener for thousands of years. We recommend using natural organic raw honey in your recipes as an alternative to refined white sugar. It can be used successfully in many recipes including cooking and baking. Because honey is a concentrated natural carbohydrate, it is best to use in moderation.

High sugar consumption can overstimulate and harm your whole body system, and can lead to many serious health problems, ranging from obesity, cancer, and heart trouble, to high blood sugar levels and diabetes.

Chapter 22

Healthy Candies

RAISIN - NUT BALLS

¾ cup granulated barley malt
¾ cup raisins
⅓ cup distilled water
⅓ cup nuts, chopped

Boil barley malt and water until they form a firm ball when tested in cold water. Chop the raisins and nuts and add them to the syrup. Cook until stiff enough not to run. Drop by teaspoon on an oiled pan 2-inches apart to cool.

CALIFORNIA CAROB DATES

¾ lb dates
⅓ cup honey
1½ Tbsps boiling distilled water
4 squares carob
½ tsp pure vanilla extract

Wipe the dates and remove the pits through a small lengthwise slit. Grate the carob into a small saucepan; add honey, boiling water and vanilla. Heat without boiling until smooth, keeping mixture fluid by setting saucepan in a pan of boiling water. Fill dates with the carob mixture, gently pressing the edges together. Let stand to harden.

PERSIAN BONBONS

1 lb dates
1 lb nut meats
1 lb raisins
1 cup shredded, dried, unsweetened coconut

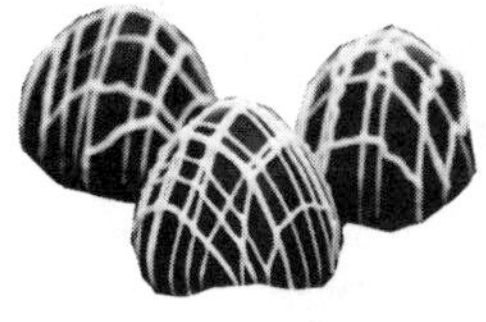

Use fresh, moist fruit. Run all ingredients through a grinder and knead as for a dough. Pat out on a coconut-covered board, cut with small cookie cutter, and then roll in shredded coconut. Wrap in waxed paper when dry.

TOASTED ALMONDS & NUTS

1½ cups almonds, blanched or nuts of choice
⅓ cup Bragg Organic Olive Oil
spray Bragg Liquid Aminos

Cover almonds with boiling water. Let stand 2 minutes. Drain. Cover with cold water. Rub off skins and dry on a towel. Heat olive oil in a large, heavy skillet and add enough nuts to cover bottom of skillet. Spray with Bragg Aminos. Stir until lightly browned. Remove oil from nuts on absorbent paper towel. You can use this recipe with walnuts, cashews, pecans, etc. and they have no skins to peel off. These make a delicious, crunchy snack.

RAISIN - PEANUT CLUSTERS

2/3 cup unsulphured molasses
1 1/3 cups organic raisins or currants
2 2/3 cups organic shelled peanuts
1/2 cup honey
1 1/3 tsps lemon juice
3 Tbsps Bragg Organic Olive Oil

Combine molasses, honey and lemon juice in a saucepan. Cook to 250°F ("hard ball" stage when tested in cold water). Remove from heat, add olive oil, stir until oil combines with syrup. Stir in peanuts and raisins. Drop by teaspoonsful on waxed paper. If candy hardens, reheat and then stir until soft.

DRIED FRUIT BALLS

3 cups of dried fruit (pitted dates, dried apricots, raisins, or dried fruit of choice)
shredded coconut or finely chopped raw nuts

In food grinder, grind dried fruit until fine. Shape into small balls. Roll balls in shredded coconut, chopped nuts or both.

Dried Fruits – Nature's Anti-Ageing Candy

Dried fruit is fruit that has been dried, either naturally (such as natural sunlight) or through use of a machine, such as a food dehydrator. Raisins, currants, plums (also known as prunes) and dates are examples of the most popular dried fruits. Other nutritious fruits that may be dried include apples, apricots, bananas, cranberries, figs, goji berries, mangoes, pears, papaya, and pineapples.

Dried fruit has a long shelf life and can provide a good alternate to fresh fruit, allowing out of season fruits to be available. Dried fruits are very sweet and delicious and are a much healthier alternative to unhealthy candies and they contain great flavor and nutrition and satisfy the craving for sweets.

Dried fruits are rich in vitamins (A, B1, B2, B3, B6, and pantothenic acid) and minerals (calcium, iron, magnesium, phosphorous, potassium, copper, manganese). They are also abundant in many anti-ageing and health protective phytochemcials. Due to the drying process they do lose some of their vitamin C content compared to fresh fruits.

Dried fruits are energy foods as they are a rich source of carbohydrates and natural sugars. They make great snacks for active children and athletes who need additional calories. Those on weight loss diets should eat dried fruits in moderation, depending on their activity level.

Most commercially prepared dried fruits may contain added sulfur dioxide which may trigger asthma and other respiratory problems in sensitive individuals! We recommend avoiding all dried fruits that have been prepared with sulfur dioxide! **Organic dried fruits are best and recommended for use in the recipes of this book.** We like naturally sundried fruits the best, as they meet the standards of a raw food diet. Also, fruits dried in dehydrators are fine and are simple and easy to use.

Chapter 23

BRAGG HEALTHY LIFESTYLE

The Bragg Blueprint for Physical, Mental and Spiritual Improvement – Healthy, Vital Living to 120 – Genesis 6:3

By Patricia Bragg, N.D., Ph.D.
Pioneer Life Extension Nutritionist

Just think – in 90 days you can build a new bloodstream! Not a thick, sluggish, toxin-saturated bloodstream, but a healthy bloodstream rich in all the vitamins, minerals and vital nutrients necessary for radiant and long-lasting health. First and foremost, we must increase the iron content in our bloodstream. This is one of the great secrets of life: the more iron in the bloodstream, the more *oxygen* is going to flood into your body, purifying every one of your cells. Oxygen is the greatest stimulant in the world. It stimulates, but does not depress. Unnatural stimulants cause an aftermath of depression. Tobacco, alcohol, coffee, tea, refined white sugar and drugs (prescribed and over-the-counter) have this negative effect on the body. Not God's own oxygen. It's the invisible staff of life!

In the Bragg Healthy Lifestyle, we reject these harmful, destructive stimulants. These are never going to enter your body! You will rely on the wonderful, natural stimulants to create a healthy vital force. First, you are going to follow the Bragg deep breathing program that is the key to the Bragg Healthy Lifestyle. You are going to use live foods such as fresh fruits & vegetables and freshly squeezed juices that help build vital blood sugar.

Before you eat or drink anything, I want you to ask yourself this important question: *"Is this going to build a healthy bloodstream or destroy it?"* Be on the alert to protect your river of life - your bloodstream! When the body demands liquids, give it pure distilled water or live fresh fruit and vegetable juices. Get yourself a juicer. Every day you can fortify your bloodstream with fresh orange, grapefruit or carrot and green drinks – combine juices such as celery, tomato, beet, carrot and parsley. Raw spinach and watercress juices are two of the best to add to your vegetable juice combinations. For a taste delight, add the juice of 1-2 garlic buds. Garlic is an excellent blood purifier.

Do not over consume these powerful live food juices. One to two pints a day is enough. Sometimes people get a juicer, and go overboard. Overloading your body with juices can upset your delicate blood sugar balance. Just because something is good for you, that does not mean that more is better. As with all things in life, moderation in your food intake is key for building supreme vitality!

Imagine: in just 11 months you will have an absolutely new you! The billions of soft cells that make up eyes, nose, skin, hands, feet, as well as all the vital organs of your body, will be renewed. You do not need to submit to the huge risk of a heart, kidney or any other dangerous organ transplant. You have it within your power, through the food you eat, the liquid you drink, and the air you breathe, to build a new vital body from the top of your head to the tip of your toes. You are what you eat and what you eat today will be walking and talking tomorrow! How wonderful our Creator has been, to give us the power every 90 days to build a new bloodstream and every 11 months an entirely new body.

Make Every Day A Healthy Day

The Creator gave us the intelligence and reasoning power to maintain a healthy body. But the flesh is dumb! You can stuff anything in your stomach and seem to get away with it! Most young people live this way, because they believe they are totally indestructible. What a sad, sad lesson they learn after 40 or 50 years of wrong living as the miseries and the aches and pains creep into their bodies, making life miserable and a lie of their myth and dream of indestructibility.

Live by the reason of mind rather than by the senses of the body. The dumb senses are constantly enticing you to do the very things that destroy your wonderful body. Look around you – look at the tragic human sights you see. Weak, mentally depressed people, and sickness everywhere. The average person's suffering is self-inflicted. For whatsoever a man soweth, shall he also reap (Gal. 6:7). We should know and observe the fact that everything in the universe is always governed by definite laws – we will sow the seeds of constructive healthy living!

Make every day a healthy day – and each day you will improve! You will feel new strength and energy flooding into your body. The feeling you will experience when you live a true natural healthy life is indescribable. What an incredibly powerful and joyful feeling it is to be fully alive, vigorous, with unlimited energy and powerful nerve force.

It's Never Too Late to Improve Your Health

Weak people find poor excuses to continue their bad habits of living. They will tell you they are too old to begin the Bragg Healthy Lifestyle Program. Age has no force nor is it toxic. Time is just a measure, nothing more, nothing less. Long ago the Bragg Family gave up living in calendar years. We only live in biological years. There are millions in their 30s and 40s who are prematurely old biologically. Yet there are many people in their 60s, 70s, 80s and 90s who are still biologically young!

In my opinion, if you are experiencing premature ageing you are suffering from a highly toxic condition and unnecessary nutritional deficiencies. This is the main cause of most human troubles. Our program will show you how to banish these two vicious enemies. From this moment on, stop living by calendar years! Just forget your birthdays, as I do. We are all reborn every second of the day as new body cells are being created. Cease this talk of getting old! From this minute on, you will have no age except your biological age and this you can control. Every day, repeat to yourself, "I Will Never Grow Old!" Burn it deeply in your conscious mind.

Most people have a dreadful fear of getting old. They picture themselves half-blind, hearing impaired, teeth gone, energy and vitality spent, senile. They see themselves as a burden to their family and friends. They envision themselves in the nursing home: alone, forsaken and forgotten. Despite the fear of old age and the train of ailments that go with getting old, you can prevent this human tragedy. You can change how you age by how you live from this day forward. Today is the day to begin preparing against senility. That is why I urge you to follow the wise, wonderful Laws of Mother Nature. You will grow younger as you live longer! That is what this program is all about: preservation of your youth through vibrant health!

Thousands of people every year pay thousands of dollars for state-of-the-art testing to learn their risk for heart disease. However, experts say that organic fruits and vegetables and a health club membership may be better buys than any lab test. People who eat a diet low in fat and cholesterol and rich in healthy plant foods, who don't smoke, who exercise regularly, and keep their weight and blood pressure in the normal range are less likely to have a heart attack than those who don't, despite any predisposition or genetic tendency toward heart disease. – Harvard Health Letter, www.health.harvard.edu

---

The unexamined life is not worth living. It is a time to re-evaluate your past as a guide for a bright future. – Socrates

---

It's never too late to be what you might have been. – George Elliot

Prevention Keeps You Healthy & Vigorous!

Lengthening life by special treatment of chronic illnesses often means merely adding years of ill-health and misery to a person's life – what is often called the living death. Who wants to extend life just to suffer? In my opinion, the true function of the Healer today is to prevent sickness & disease.

No man is able to heal you! The body heals itself when it is given the right conditions! It is essential for you to know how to live in order to always be well. *An ounce of prevention is worth a pound of cure!*

Diet for health and youthfulness – Compose your diet of 65% organic raw fruits and vegetables, and some properly cooked (steamed, baked or wokked) vegetables. With this lifestyle, conditions as stomach upsets, constipation, etc. often occurring in children and adults, can be avoided!

Our greatest enemy to health is constipation – which can easily be eliminated with a diet that gives you sufficient bulk moisture, lubrication and vigorous exercise of the entire abdominal cavity. Outgo should equal intake. You should have a bowel movement upon arising and after each meal. In the remote parts of the world where we have traveled beyond the influence of so-called modern civilization, mankind indulges in the normal habit of defecation after every meal. Children can be taught this habit from infancy. With the Bragg Healthy Lifestyle, constipation vanishes.

Constipation creates toxins in the body – Studies reveal the presence of toxic poison in cases of constipation. When these toxins are absorbed into the general circulation, the liver, which is one of your detoxifying organs, is unable to cope. These toxins make their way back in the bloodstream and cause trouble and sickness. *Toxemia is our real enemy!*

My father and I firmly believe diet plays a major role in health maintenance and the prevention of illness. We found in research that fast/junk food diets composed of refined white flour and sugar, preserved meats (hot dogs, deli meats, etc.), white rice, coffee, tea, cola drinks, alcohol, margarine, overcooked vegetables, and salted foods can bring on serious body illnesses, especially respiratory and stomach problems. None of these refined, processed, embalmed, dead, unhealthy foods should be eaten by you! See Foods to Avoid list, page 236.

To increase your dietary intake of vitamin E, eat more nuts, seeds and whole grains. In supplement form, take 200 to 400 IU of natural vitamin E daily.

More than 95% of food poisoning cases are derived from fish, meat, poultry and their products. – Professor Richard Lacey, University of Leeds

Energy Is Your Body's Spark Plug

Your energy comes from the spark of life which is maintained by the atomic energy contained within every cell of the human body. It embodies electrons, protons, neutrons, positrons and alpha particles. They are constantly discharging their ionic compounds as energy is expended in work – whether mental or physical – in accordance with natural laws. This energy loss must be replaced. Every cell in your body is like a battery, that when run down must be recharged. Primarily this is done through the intake of food. Proper breathing and exercise also helps recharge the cells.

There are two kinds of foods. The first kind is in a low rate of physical vibration, such as the foods we mentioned just above: processed, chemicalized non-foods, like refined white flour and sugars, etc. It is impossible to have a youthful, energized dynamic body when year after year you feed it foods and drinks with low rates of vibration (see page 236).

The Bragg Healthy Lifestyle Program consists only of: **The second kind of foods that are in a high rate of physical vibration.** Many people have the preconceived idea that protein has the highest rate of vibration. While protein is an important nutrient to the human body, fresh fruit has a higher rate of vibration. Fruit produces blood sugar which helps to feed the nerves of the body. Fruit has a twofold purpose in the body. First, it's rich in blood sugar; second, it's an important, needed detoxifier and destroyer of harmful obstructions, wastes and toxins that can do great bodily harm.

Often you will hear people say, *I am allergic to apples, grapefruit, peaches, strawberries, etc.* These people have no idea what these foods are doing in their bodies. To give you an example, when my father Paul C. Bragg was reared in the South many years ago, his typical Southern diet was rich in animal proteins and fats from the hogs, chickens, beef, sheep and fowl they raised. At meals they had a wide variety of these meat proteins. They also ate white flour biscuits, bread, mashed and fried potatoes and a heavy, sugary desserts.

When he ate strawberries, tomatoes, green peppers and many other fruits and vegetables, he would break out in painful, red, itching hives. While attending military school from age 12 on, his body became so saturated with toxic poisons, mucus and putrid food residues that when he ate any fresh fruits, he suffered not only hives, but colds, headaches, aches and pains. These symptoms were erroneously thought to be allergic reactions, but they were the body's natural response to a toxic system. The fruits were cleaning out his body by pushing out the toxins!

He refrained from eating these vital foods until he became a health advocate at the age of sixteen. Nearly dying from a severe case of tuberculosis was the outcome of the wrong foods he ate. Only after he had been cleansed and purified with healthy foods, apple cider vinegar and fasting one day a week, along with occasional longer fasts, could he eat fresh fruits and vegetables without a negative, allergic reaction.

For this reason, people living on a diet high in animal proteins, fats, starches, refined sugars and saturated fats cannot immediately include large amounts of fresh fruits and raw vegetables into their diet. It's best to ease into the Bragg Healthy Lifestyle and allow the body to gently start cleansing.

The Transition Diet – Everyone who wants to live the healthy life must understand just what is going on with their body chemistry. Organic, fresh raw fruit and fresh vegetables help flush toxins out of the body. However, the body cannot be rushed. It takes the average person a long time to saturate the body with toxic poisons and, likewise it is going to take time for this debris to be flushed out!

The more organic raw fruits and raw vegetables you have conditioned yourself to handle, the more cleansed your body will become! So, recognize foods which are in the highest rate of healthy physical vibration. But please, also respect their great cleansing, detoxifying action, that wants you healthy!

We often eat 100% raw meals of fruits, vegetables and salads for a few days, but usually our meals are 60% to 70% raw.

BREAKFAST Fresh raw juices (orange, grapefruit or carrot, celery, garlic, spinach, etc.) and later, raw fruit (melon, apple, banana, etc.) or the nutritious, delicious, and easy to prepare Bragg Healthy Energy Smoothie – see recipe on page 49.

LUNCH Large, raw combination salad with fresh organic greens, vegetables, sprouts and a few raw nuts or seeds (sunflower, sesame, pumpkin, almonds, pecans, walnuts, etc.).

DINNER Variety salad, followed by steamed, baked or wokked fresh vegetables and one of the following: cooked beans, lentils, brown rice, whole grain pasta, tofu, or baked potatoes.

Remember to get your daily Bragg Apple Cider Vinegar (ACV) into your diet with the ACV Cocktail and sprinkle ACV over steamed greens, kale, collards, cauliflower, squash, broccoli, cabbage, green beans, etc. It is also especially delicious on garden salads. See page 32 for healthy salad dressing recipes.

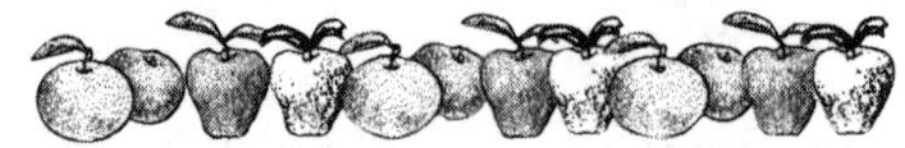

Happiness is not being pained in body or troubled in mind. – Thomas Jefferson

People are told that they should start the day with a big breakfast as this will give great energy in the morning hours when they need energy after fasting all night. Often, they heavily gorge themselves on processed cereal with cream and sugar; ham or bacon and eggs; hot cakes or stacks of buttered toast and jelly – all this washed down with coffee, milk or cocoa. You will note there is no fruit at this meal.

Only a person doing the most strenuous physical labor could possibly burn up a meal like this (and I doubt even that). All the vital energy of the body will be needed to digest these heavy animal proteins and fats, refined starch, and white sugar breakfasts. All too often they lie in the stomach like a ton of bricks and have to be dynamited out. Now you know why there is so much indigestion and constipation and why laxatives are one of the biggest selling items in drug stores.

How can a big meal like this give a person strength for their morning duties? It can't. This is how people are so brainwashed with TV fast food ads, etc. *big food interests who profit from the sale of commercial, unhealthy foods.*

You must change your ideas about food – learn to eat in moderation. It is important that you do not overfuel your body. If you overfeed your body you will clog it up. A diet rich in an abundance of healthy, raw foods with a high rate of vibration will keep your insides clean and vitalized.

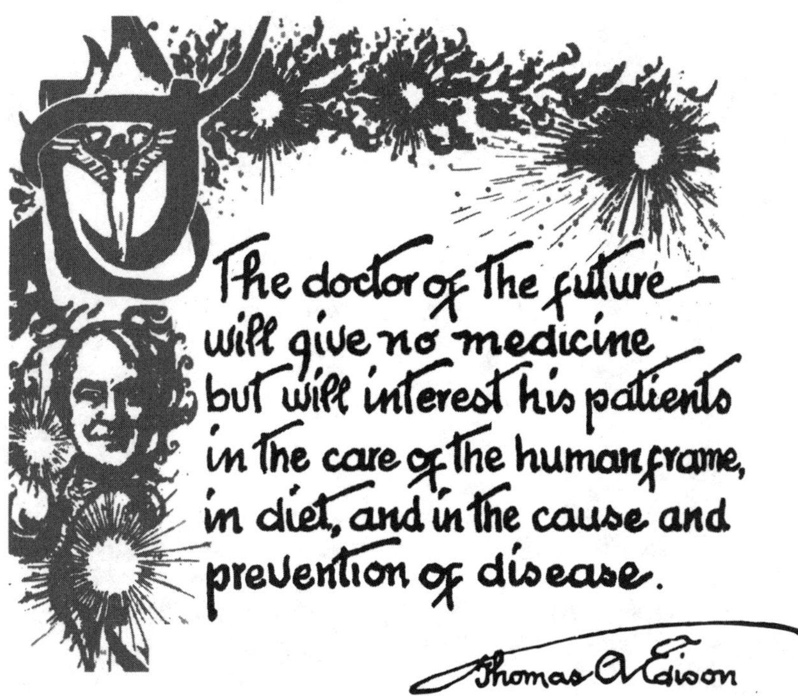
The doctor of the future
will give no medicine
but will interest his patients
in the care of the human frame,
in diet, and in the cause and
prevention of disease.
Thomas A Edison

Be brave as your fathers before you. Have faith & go forward.
– Thomas Edison, genius inventor of light bulb, telephone and phonograph

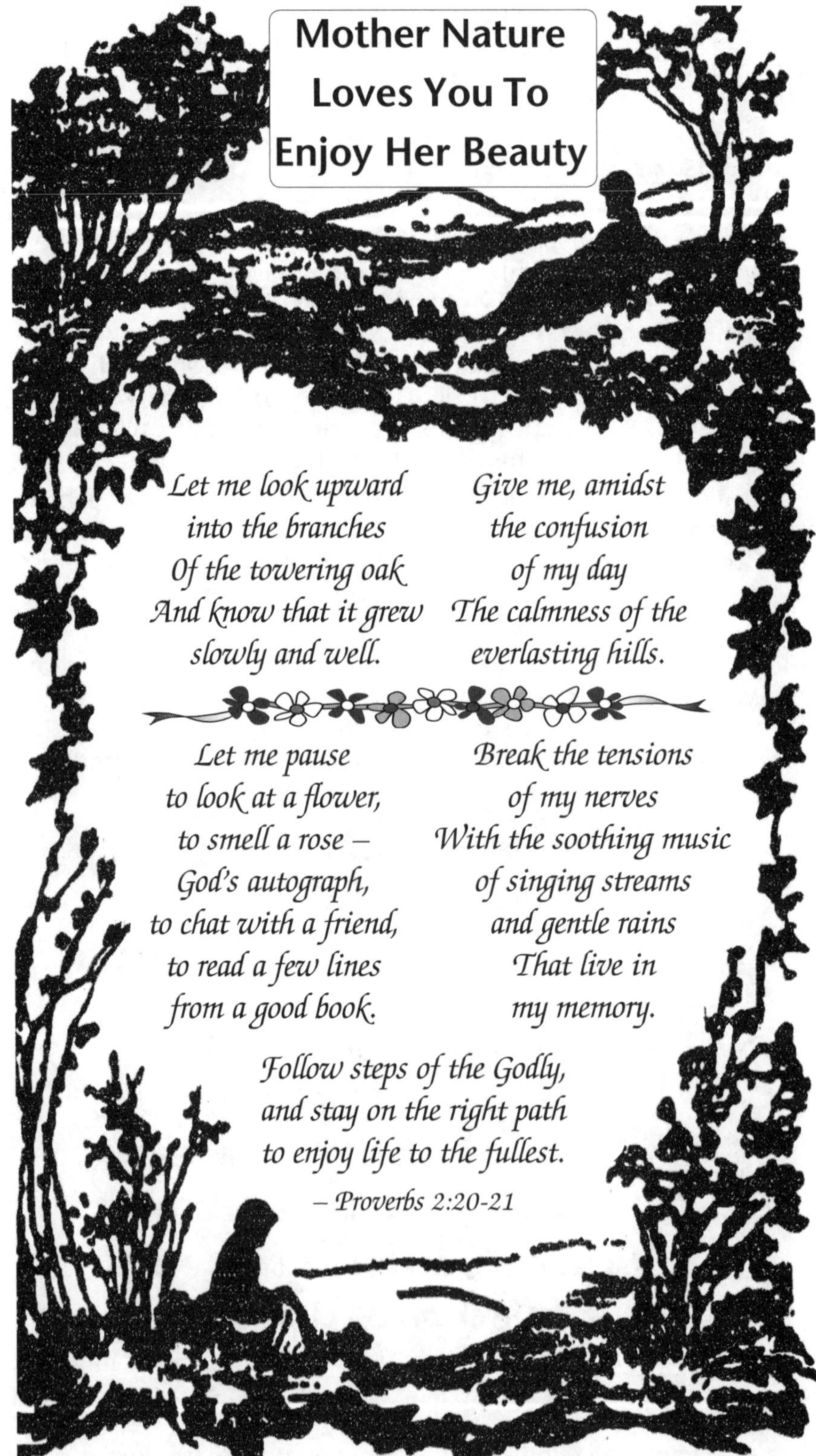

Mother Nature Loves You To Enjoy Her Beauty

Let me look upward
into the branches
Of the towering oak
And know that it grew
slowly and well.

Give me, amidst
the confusion
of my day
The calmness of the
everlasting hills.

Let me pause
to look at a flower,
to smell a rose –
God's autograph,
to chat with a friend,
to read a few lines
from a good book.

Break the tensions
of my nerves
With the soothing music
of singing streams
and gentle rains
That live in
my memory.

Follow steps of the Godly,
and stay on the right path
to enjoy life to the fullest.
– Proverbs 2:20-21

Mother Nature and friendships are cozy shelters for life's rainy days.

Healthy Heart Habits for a Long, Vital Life

Remember, *organic live foods make live people. You are what you eat, drink, breathe, think, say and do.* So eat a low-fat, low-sugar, high-fiber diet of organic whole grains, fresh salads, sprouts, greens, vegetables, fruits, raw seeds, nuts, fresh juices and chemical-free, purified or distilled water.

Earn your food with daily exercise, for regular exercise, brisk walking, etc. improves your health, stamina, go-power, flexibility, endurance and helps open the cardiovascular system. Only 45 minutes a day truly can do miracles for your heart, arteries, mind, nerves, soul and body! You become revitalized with new zest for living to accomplish your life goals!

We are made of tubes. To help keep them open, clean and to maintain good elimination, add 1 tsp psyllium husk powder or oat bran daily – hour after dinner to juices, herbal teas, even Bragg Vinegar Drink. Another way to guard against clogged tubes daily is to add 1-2 tsps soy lecithin granules (*fat emulsifier-melts like butter*) over potatoes, veggies, soups and to juices, etc. Also take one cayenne capsule (40,000 HU) daily with a meal. Take 50 to 100 mgs regular-released niacin (B3) with one meal daily to help cleanse and open the cardiovascular system, also improves memory. Skin flushing may occur, don't worry about this as it shows it's working! After cholesterol level reaches 180, then only take niacin twice weekly.

The heart needs healthy balanced nutrients, so take natural multi-vitamin-mineral food supplements, Omega-3 and extra heart helpers – vitamin E Tocotrienols, C, Ubiquinol CoQ10, D3, MSM, D-Ribose, garlic, turmeric, selenium, zinc, beta carotene and amino acids, L-Carnitine, L-Taurine, L-Lysine and Proline. Folic acid, CoQ10, B6 and B12 helps keep homocysteine level low. Magnesium Orotate, Hawthorn Berry Extract brings relief for palpitations, arrhythmia, senile hearts and coronary disease. Braggzyme contains systemic enzymes (nattokinase and serrapetase) to keep blood thin, preventing dangerous blood clots. Take bromelain (from pineapple) also found in Braggzyme, multi-digestive enzyme and probiotics with meals – aids digestion, assimilation and elimination.

For sleep problems try 5-HTP Tryptophan (an amino acid), melatonin, calcium, magnesium, valerian in caps, extract or tea, Bragg vinegar drink and sleepytime herb tea. For arthritis or joint pain/stiffness, try aloe juice or gel, Braggzyme, Glucosamine - Chondroitin - MSM combo caps and shots, help heal and regenerate. Capsaicin and DMSO lotion helps relieve pain.

Use amazing antioxidants – E Tocotrienols, C, Quercetin, grapeseed extract (OPCs), CoQ10, selenium, SOD, Resveratrol, Alpha-Lipoic Acid, etc. They improve immune system and help flush out dangerous free radicals that cause havoc with cardiovascular pipes and health. Research shows antioxidants promote longevity, slows ageing, fights toxins, helps prevent disease, cancer, cataracts, jet lag and exhaustion.

Recommended Heart Health Tests

- **Total Cholesterol:** **Adults:** 180 mg/dl is optimal; **Children:** 140 mg/dl or less
- **LDL Cholesterol:** 100 mg/dl or less is optimal
- **HDL Cholesterol:** **Men:** 50 mg/dl or more; **Women:** 65 mg/dl or more
- **Triglycerides:** 100 mg/dl or less (optimal 70-85)
- **HDL/Cholesterol Ratio:** 3.2 or less • **Triglycerides/HDL Ratio:** below 2
- **Homocysteine:** 6-8 micromoles/L
- **CRP** (**C-Reactive Protein high sensitivity**):
  lower than 1 mg/L low risk, 1-3 mg/L average risk, over 3 mg/L high risk
- **Diabetic Risk Tests:** • **Glucose:** 80-100 mg/dl • **Hemoglobin A1c:** 7% or less
- **Blood Pressure:** 120/70 mmHg is considered optimal for adults

Avoid These Processed, Refined, Harmful Foods

Once you realize the harm caused to your body by unhealthy refined, chemicalized, deficient foods, you'll want to eliminate these "killer" foods. Also avoid microwaved foods! Follow The Bragg Healthy Lifestyle to provide the basic, healthy nourishment to maintain your health.

- Refined sugar, artificial sweeteners (toxic aspartame, Splenda) & their products as jams, jellies, preserves, marmalades, yogurts, ice cream, sherbets, Jello, cake, candy, cookies, chewing gum, colas & diet drinks, pies, pastries, and all sugared fruit juices and fruits canned in sugar syrup. **(Health Stores have delicious healthy replacements, Stevia, etc, so seek and buy the best. Page 224)**
- White flour products such as white bread, wheat-white bread, enriched flours, rye bread that has white flour in it, dumplings, biscuits, buns, gravy, pasta, pancakes, waffles, soda crackers, pizza, ravioli, pies, pastries, cakes, cookies, prepared and commercial puddings and ready-mix bakery products. Most made with dangerous (oxy-cholesterol) powdered milk and powdered eggs. **(Health Stores have huge variety of 100% whole grain organic products, delicious breads, crackers, pastas, desserts, etc.)**
- Salted foods, such as corn chips, potato chips, pretzels, crackers and nuts.
- Refined white rices and pearled barley. • Fast fried foods. • Indian ghee.
- Refined, sugared (also, aspartame), dry processed cereals – cornflakes etc.
- Foods that contain olestra, palm and cottonseed oil. These additives are not fit for human consumption and should be totally avoided.
- Peanuts and peanut butter that contain hydrogenated, hardened oils and any peanut mold and all molds that can cause allergies.
- Margarine – combines heart-deadly trans-fatty acids and saturated fats.
- Saturated fats and hydrogenated oils – enemies that clog the arteries.
- Coffee, decaffeinated coffee, caffeinated black & caffeinated green teas. Also alcoholic beverages, caffeinated & sugared water-juices, cola & soft drinks.
- Fresh pork and products. • Fried, fatty greasy meats. • Irradiated GMO foods.
- Smoked meats, such as ham, bacon, sausage and smoked fish.
- Luncheon meats, hot dogs, salami, bologna, corned beef, pastrami and packaged meats containing dangerous sodium nitrate or nitrite.
- Dried fruits containing sulphur dioxide – a toxic preservative
- Don't eat chickens or turkeys that have been injected with hormones or fed with commercial poultry feed containing any drugs or toxins.
- Canned soups - read labels for sugar, salt, starch, flour and preservatives
- Foods containing benzoate of soda, salt, sugar, cream of tartar and any additives, drugs, preservatives; irradiated and genetically engineered foods.
- Day-old cooked vegetables, potatoes and pre-mixed, wilted lifeless salads.
- All commercial vinegars: pasteurized, filtered, distilled, white, malt and synthetic vinegars are the dead vinegars! *(We use only our Bragg Organic Raw, unfiltered Apple Cider Vinegar with "mother" as used in olden times.)*

The Miracle Health Power of Fruit

Always keep in mind that the most perfect food for man is fresh, ripe fruit. Nature, in her inimitable way, brings together in her fruits a marvelously balanced, living combination of vital nutrients, in a high rate of vibration, bio-magnetized, to release the living building blocks so necessary for all body functions.

Tinted by basking rays of vitalizing sun, breathing in droughts of magnetized air, drawing into itself vital minerals through its roots in the earth, delicious, organic fruit is God's perfection from His electrochemical miracle laboratory. Man can take all the chemicals of an apple out of a chemist's dish, but he cannot construct an apple! Man may analyze all the minerals in a cherry, but he does not even know what makes them red. He may take apart and try to reconstruct a grape, and find that the grape supports life and the broken-down chemicals do not!

Fruit contains certain bioelectric principles that give the electric spark of life! Fruit is the most perfect food of Nature and will support life indefinitely to a superior degree – when a body is cleansed and living in a natural environment.

Whose mouth has not watered when seeing a luscious dish of fruit – for instance, a couple of yellow pears with a dash of pink or a beautiful bunch of tapering grapes, green, red or purple? The sight of fruit and the taste of it, more so, bring an abundant secretion of digestive juices. I can safely say that fruit is designed particularly well for our digestive tracts. I have seen a sick person turn down all other food and drink a glass of freshly squeezed orange juice. His sick body craved the vital nutrients which are found in ripe, juicy oranges. I have seen children torn with fever ask for fruit juice. Why didn't they ask for a hot dog?

On the whole, diets which consist solely of fruits are inefficient and impractical for the average American, although they would be splendid in a tropical climate. While man has come so far from his natural state that he cannot maintain an efficient standard as a fruitarian, you still need *to eat more fresh fruit!* One of the many reasons we love Hawaii – the luscious tropical fruits! Plan a Hawaiian vacation and also enjoy free Bragg Exercise Classes (see page i or visit *bragg.com*).

I especially recommend ripe bananas. Bananas are not a fattening fruit as is commonly supposed. They are 70% water and are extremely high in potassium. Apples of all kinds make excellent eating, as do pears and grapes. In the fall, winter and spring, eat organically grown dates, sun-dried figs, raisins and apricots along with fresh fruit. When you eat fruit regularly, see how wonderful you look and feel!

The Miracle Food: The avocado stands high as a miracle food of nature. The avocado tree is strong and insects do not bother it. It requires no spraying with poisonous chemicals. The avocado has a perfect balance of life-giving nutrients. It has an unsaturated fat which the body can easily digest. They contain even more potassium than bananas!

I eat avocados 3-4 times a week from my Santa Barbara Farm, where I grow three varieties. When they're ripe, I cut them in half, spoon avocado out and mash and then add spray of Bragg Aminos and fresh crushed garlic (use a garlic press) and shake of Bragg Sprinkle. I slice tomatoes, celery, carrots, cabbage strips, radish, cucumber, green/red bell peppers for this **"delicious guacamole dip"** for lunch.

Enjoy Super Health with Natural Foods

1. **RAW FOODS:** Fresh fruits and raw vegetables organically grown are always best! Enjoy nutritious variety garden salads with raw vegetables, sprouts, raw nuts and seeds.
2. **VEGETABLES and PROTEINS:**
   a. Legumes, lentils, brown rice, soy beans, and all beans.
   b. Nuts and seeds, raw and unsalted.
   c. We prefer healthier vegetarian proteins. If you must have animal protein, then be sure it's hormone–free, and organically fed and no more than 1 or 2 times a week.
   d. Dairy products – fertile range-free eggs (*not over 4 weekly*), unprocessed hard cheese and feta goat's cheese. We choose not to use dairy products. Try healthier non-dairy soy, rice, nut, and almond milks and soy cheeses, delicious yogurt and soy and rice ice cream.
3. **FRUITS and VEGETABLES:** Organically grown is always best – grown without the use of poisonous sprays and toxic chemical fertilizers whenever possible; urge your market to stock organic produce! Steam, bake, sauté or wok vegetables as short a time as possible to retain the best nutritional content and flavor. Also enjoy fresh juices.
4. **100% WHOLE GRAIN CEREALS, BREADS and FLOURS.** They contain important B-complex vitamins, vitamin E, minerals, fiber and the important unsaturated fatty acids.
5. **COLD or EXPELLER-PRESSED VEGETABLE OILS:** Bragg Organic Extra Virgin Olive Oil (is best), soy, sunflower, flax and sesame oils are excellent sources of healthy, essential, unsaturated fatty acids. Use oils sparingly.

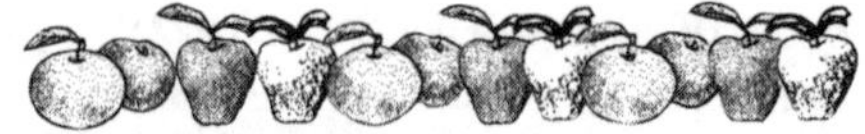

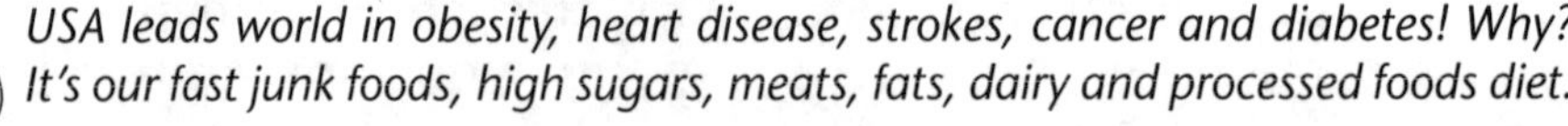

USA leads world in obesity, heart disease, strokes, cancer and diabetes! Why? It's our fast junk foods, high sugars, meats, fats, dairy and processed foods diet.

Enjoy a Tireless – Ageless – Painless Body With The Bragg Healthy Lifestyle

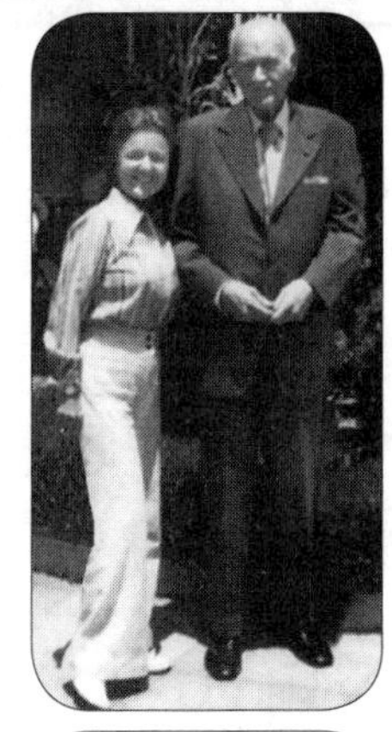
Conrad Hilton with Patricia

Don't despair in your golden years – enjoy them! My dad Paul C. Bragg, said *life's second half is the best* and can be the most healthy fruitful years. Linus Pauling, painter Grandma Moses and amazing Mother Teresa, have all proven that! These three famous Bragg health followers – Conrad Hilton, J.C. Penney and foot Dr. Scholl – all lived strong, productive, active lives to almost 100 years. Countless others have lived long, healthy fulfilled lives following The Bragg Healthy Lifestyle, you can too!

We teach you how to forget calendar years and to regain not only a youthful spirit, but much of the vigor of your youth. It's your duty to yourself to start to live The Bragg Healthy Lifestyle today – don't procrastinate! Square your shoulders and look life straight in the eye. Keep premature ageing out of your body by faithfully living this healthy lifestyle blueprint. You must eat foods that have a high health vibration rate (abundance of raw, organic fruits and vegetables) and do a water fast weekly.

Suggestions for a Daily Health Program

Be sure you sleep in a well ventilated room so you get a large amount of oxygen while sleeping. Make sure your mattress is firm and flat. Sleep in a spread-out position.

Oxygen is the invisible staff of life and the life of the blood, and blood is the life of the body. A person weighing 150 pounds contains 88 pounds of oxygen. Oxygen is the most important chemical of the body. Yet it is colorless, odorless and tasteless. Its main function is purification. Lack of oxygen in the body can lead to serious consequences! Most people are oxygen-starved because they are shallow breathers.

To have a youthful, vital life we need fresh air in abundance, pure distilled water and plenty of fresh vegetables and fruits. Oxygen is an unquestionable source of indispensable energy, necessary for higher vital activity in the human organism. It insures elimination, reconstruction and regeneration within the vital factors and metabolic activities of the physical body.

Organic whole grains, vegetables, fruits, raw nuts and seeds give needed vitamins and minerals to the body. – Patricia Bragg, ND, PhD., Health Crusader

Through the function of the lungs, oxygen is absorbed, transformed and assimilated into the blood, bringing with it unknown factors in the vital forces of the atmosphere.

Plants – through their roots in the ground – absorb all the vital elements in the soil necessary for life. If I cut or damage their roots, they die! Man's roots are his lungs.

We can only breathe adequately with sufficient physical movement. With the proper movements we are motivated to obtain the full elixir of life, the breath of air. The stronger and more vigorous our movements are, the more air we need and the greater is our rate of breath acceleration.

The oxygen in the air we breathe dissolves and eliminates waste and builds the continuum of our cellular structure, thus maintaining our body to the highest degree possible. Each breath should detoxify and regenerate our vital forces.

This must be supplemented completely by following the Bragg Healthy Lifestyle. I want it definitely understood that both exercise and conscious deep breathing must be fortified with proper nutrition to prevent the degenerative process of the cells.

This explains why there is a decline of top athletes in their late twenties and thirties, who haven't consumed a correct, nutritionally balanced diet. The average athlete reaches a peak at about 27 and then, sadly, begins to decline. I know this to be true, as my father was an active athlete for over 75 years and we saw the finest athletes reach their peak and then slowly decline, many of them dying young.

Other Factors Affecting Breathing: Our thoughts and emotions interfere with our breathing. That is why, if we have a headache, or some other sudden symptom, a few minutes of deep conscious breathing exercises in the open air will help us detoxify and reestablish our internal balance.

Upon waking in the morning, stretch your legs, arms and body as you do when yawning. Continue this stretching process until you feel that every muscle has been properly and thoroughly awakened. Good circulation and elimination are the master keys to good health! For this reason it is important to stretch and exercise your body. Do not do exercises only in the morning. Make time during the day to keep your circulation strong throughout your cardiovascular system. During your waking hours, do not sit longer than 1-2 hours at a time. Get up and move around. *To rest is to rust and rust is destruction!* Don't sit in a car for more than 1-2 hours – stop the car and get out and stretch. Exercise your legs, body and do some deep breathing exercises. Read the Bragg Breathing Book for our super Breathing Exercises.

Water is Key to Health & All Body Functions:

- Elimination
- Circulation
- Digestion
- Bones & Joints
- Assimilation
- Metabolism
- Muscles
- Heart
- Nerves
- Energy
- Sex
- Glands

Cocktail of Toxic Chemicals

Chlorine, fluoride, calcium carbonate, cadmium, aluminum, trihalomethanes, chloroform, arsenic, copper, lead and unpleasant taste.

Tap-Water Average Contents

Pure Water is Important for Health

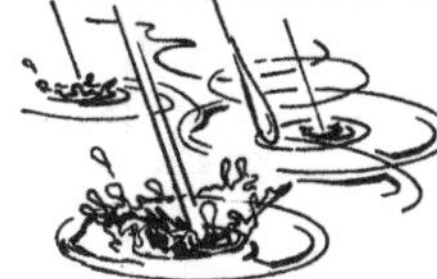

To the days of the aged it addeth length;
To the might of the strong it addeth strength;
It freshens the heart, it brightens the sight;
It's like drinking a goblet of morning light.

The body is 70% water and purified, steam-distilled (chemical-free) water is important for total health. You should drink 8-10 glasses of water a day. Read our revealing book, *Water – The Shocking Truth That Can Save Your Life,* for more info on importance of distilled, purified water.

Your Waistline is Your Life-Line, Date-Line and Health-Line!

Get a tape measure and measure your waist. Write down the measurement. If you pursue vigorous abdominal and posture exercises combined with correct eating and a weekly 24 hour fast (and later on longer 3, 5 or 7 day fasts) in a short time you'll see a more trim and youthful waistline. Trim waistlines can make people appear years younger! Now, let's get yours down to where it should be, if it's grown too big and fat. *It is a trim, lean horse for the long race of life.* I am sure we all want to be here for a long time! Living the Bragg Healthy Lifestyle is so wonderful. Each present day is a precious gift to enjoy, treasure and guard, for the healthy life is truly beautiful!

There is only one water that is clean and that is steam distilled water. No other substance on our planet does so much to keep us healthy and get us well as distilled water does! – James Balch, M.D., Co-Author, *Dietary Wellness*

Drinking 8 glasses daily of pure distilled water recharges and cleanses the human batteries! – **Paul C. Bragg, N.D., Ph.D.**

People abuse their abdomens abominably! You cannot eat dead, empty calorie foods and tell yourself that a tiny snack here and there won't show! You are completely wrong! Dead, devitalized foods create toxic poisons inside your body and this all helps add flabby inches onto the abdomen. Do not overeat even the correct healthy foods, for your body only needs enough food (fuel) to maintain energy. When you stuff too much fuel into it, you have over-fueled your body and are not burning up the excess. When you see overweight people walking around, make sure you do not become one of them!

You won't get away with this kind of cheating – it's just cheating (hurting) yourself! Bear in mind as we live longer, the internal abdominal structure and stomach muscles relax more. This is called visceroptosis, or droopy tummy, and it is a common condition among older people who don't exercise those waist muscles. It can be a contributing cause of constipation, sluggish liver and even hernias.

When the abdominal wall becomes lazy and the consequent droop is compounded by a few layers of flab, trouble starts inside the abdomen. By the time most people have reached 50 they have a completely prolapsed abdomen. Start looking at people and you will notice that what I'm saying is true! So, don't let your abdomen droop: make every effort to bring it back to firmness again . . . it's amazing how quickly it responds to exercises and especially good posture (see exercises on *bragg.com*).

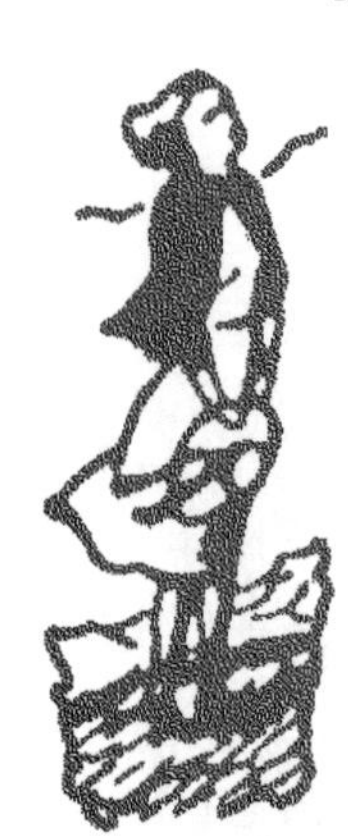

WE THANK THEE

For flowers that bloom about our feet;
For song of bird and hum of bee;
For all things fair we hear or see,
Father in heaven we thank Thee!
For blue of stream and blue of sky;
For pleasant shade of branches high;
For fragrant air and cooling breeze;
For beauty of the blooming trees;
Father in heaven we thank Thee!
For mother love and father care,
For brothers strong and sisters fair;
For love at home and here each day;
For guidance lest we go astray,
Father in heaven we thank Thee!
For this new morning with its light;
For rest and shelter of the night;
For health and food, for love and friends;
For every thing His goodness sends,
Father in heaven we thank Thee!

– Ralph Waldo Emerson

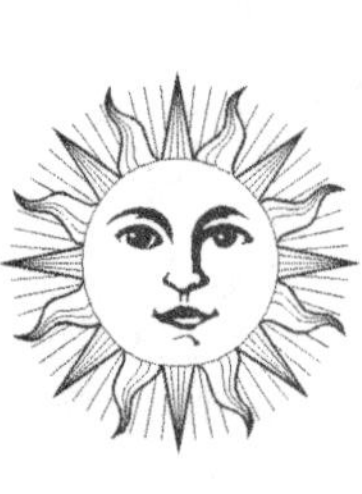

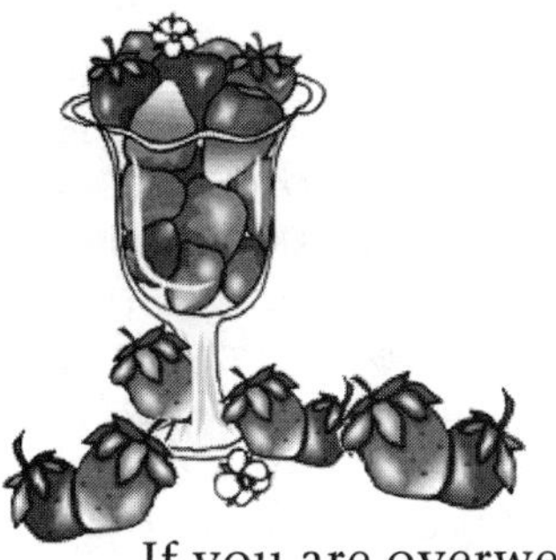

Chapter 24

Reducing

If you are overweight, don't start reducing today! Peculiar advice? No, just a lesson learned from my experience with thousand of would-be yo-yo reducers. Don't start your reducing program today. Think about it for three days. If you are still determined to do it, then by all means, begin. If you have weakened in this length of time, you would have weakened anyway and nothing is lost. However, if you are really determined to gain better health and desire a greater capacity for enjoying a long, fit life, you will be more likely to carry through with your reducing program. You will be more successful having planned it carefully than having proceeded impulsively.

The erratic reducer cannot be blamed. It is hard for the slender person to realize the real difficulty that confronts those who are overweight. Superhuman willpower is needed to control the appetite, and this is nearly always required at a time when the reducer is not feeling well, because no abnormally overweight person can feel completely well! So, we require the exhibition of strong character at a period of low vitality and often poor physical health. We pamper our invalids when they are bedridden, but the poor overweight person is no less an invalid because he or she is walking around. They receive no pampering and very little sympathy.

Whatever you do, don't try to reach normal weight within one week, or even one month. Reducing healthfully must be done gradually, with daily persistence, patience, and a sensible, consistent diet and exercise program. This is the only sure and safe way. Pills, powders, diets, "magic potions" and overly strenuous exercise programs can be dangerous.

If you have indulged in overeating, now is the time to repent and get busy cleaning and reducing the excesses off and out of your body. Remember, following the Bragg Healthy Lifestyle has helped millions to balance their weight and their life.

Counting calories can be very dull! Eating flat, tasteless foods is unpleasant and an ordeal! If the food the reducer eats is attractive, delicious and digestible, he or she will be much more inclined to be satisfied and happy with his or her diet, and more determined to stick to it. Yes, and less inclined to cheat even after the ideal, normal weight is achieved! For that reason, these menus have been carefully worked out to take into consideration lowered calorie intake and your taste satisfaction.

A great mistake made by many on a reducing programs is the elimination of all fats and starches. It is true, these are the weight-builders, but the human body is constituted so that it requires some of these food factors. Natural fats, starches and natural sugars should be limited, but not completely eliminated. The reducer should still have ample vitamins and minerals while on lowered food intake regimen. (See pyramid chart page 4) We suggest natural vitamin and mineral supplements; (see page 235) you may add green barley or spirulina powder to juices or pep drinks on food days, but none on fast days.

One-Day Juice Diet

This weekly, one-day juice diet is a super cleanser of body toxins. For more cleansing and reducing, then follow with a one-day water fast. Read Bragg *Miracle of Fasting* for more info.

two 8-oz glasses orange or grapefruit juice
(preferably fresh squeezed is best),

one 8-oz glass pineapple juice, unsweetened,

three 8-oz glasses Bragg Apple Cider Vinegar Drink (pg. 49)

two 8-oz glasses tomato juice, salt-free,

eight 8-oz glasses of the following:
juice of 8 lemons
distilled water to make eight glasses
2-3 Tbsps raw honey or Stevia to taste

This makes a total of 16 glasses of liquid, two to drink each hour. The quantities of the above liquids may be varied; that is, you may use three of orange juice and none of pineapple, etc., but the total liquid should be one gallon during the day. The results are amazing – you feel light and refreshed – so continue on juice or water another day, if desired. We suggest you drink daily the Bragg Healthy "Energy" Smoothie (page 49) after your juice-water diet.

Healthy, Organic, Fruits and Vegetables

Fresh, organically grown fruits and vegetables are best for reducing, as these will give you full nutritional value and none of the harmful pesticides and chemicals used in the growing of the commercial fruits and vegetables.

Low-Calorie Menu for Reducers

Eight full glasses of water must be taken daily. (Items on the menus preceded by an asterisk * are listed in index.)

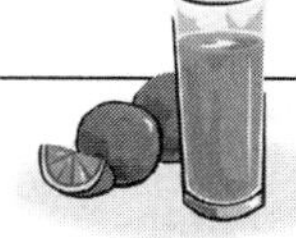

Upon Rising

(Drink any one of the following)

1 - 8 oz glass fresh citrus juice, orange or grapefruit
1 - 8 oz glass hot herb or mint tea with lemon juice
1 - 8 oz glass hot or cold distilled water with lemon juice or 2 tsps Bragg Apple Cider Vinegar with 1 tsp raw honey, maple syrup or pinch Stevia powder if diabetic (See drink recipe Page 49)

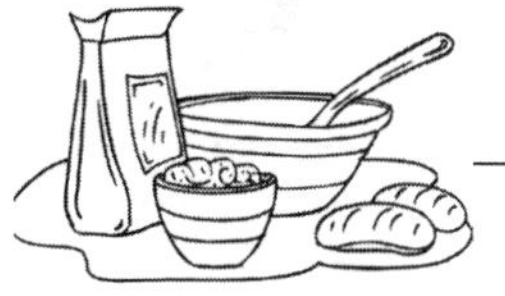

Breakfast

(Choice of any one)

1 serving fresh fruit
1 serving canned or frozen fruit, water packed or sugar free
1 - 8 oz glass of fruit or vegetable juice
1 serving dried fruit, cooked with raw honey

(Choice of any one)

1 serving of scrambled or steamed tofu with tomato
1 slice whole-grain toast
(Note: This means toast only– not the other foods listed plus toast.)
1 serving of scrambled or steamed tofu with capers
2 oz cooked whole-grain cereal with ½ tsp raw honey and ½ cup soy or rice milk

(Choice of any one)

1 - 8 oz glass fruit or vegetable juice
1 - 8 oz glass water with lemon juice
1 - 8 oz glass herb or mint tea

Lunch

(Choice of any one)

One 8 oz bowl of any of the following soups:

*Consommé
*Corn Chowder
*Veggie Soup
*Spring Broth Soup

(Choice of any one)

One medium-sized serving of any of the following salads:

*Nasturtium Salad
*Purslane Salad
*Summer Herb Salad
*Lamb's Lettuce Salad
*Skin-Beautiful Salad
*Cabbage Salad Bowl
*Healthy Grand Slam Salad
*Papaya Hawaiian Salad
*Spring Mixed Greens Salad
*Bragg Famous Raw Garden Salad

With any salad on the reducing program, you may use Bragg Healthy Vinaigrette, Ginger & Sesame, Braggberry or Hawaiian Dressings. Also try dressing recipes on pages 32-37 and page 247.

Choice of one: 1 slice whole-grain toast or 3 whole-grain wafers.

Dinner

(Choice of any one of the following)

One medium serving of any of the following salads:

*Dandelion Salad
*Gourmet Mixed-Green Salad
*Spring Mixed Greens Salad
*Buckwheat Tenderleaf Salad
*Summer Herb Salad
*Famous Vegetable Salad
*Sprouted Soybean Salad
*Tropical Hawaiian Delight

(Choice of any one)

One 8 oz+ serving of any of the following soups:

*Cream of Tomato Soup
*Veggie Soup
*French Onion Soup
*Spring Broth

(Choice of any one)

One medium serving of any of the following:

*Garlic Roasted Eggplant
*Mixed Nut Loaf
*Bean Loaf
*Vegetarian Loaf
*Lentil Loaf
*Vegetarian Mushroom Cutlets

(Choice of two small servings of the following)

Two small servings of any of the following vegetables:

*Baked Asparagus
*Beets en Orange
*Baked Cauliflower
*Baked Acorn Squash
*Green Beans with Herbs
*Glazed Carrots with Honey
*Scalloped Eggplant
*Peas in Onion Sauce

(Remember items on the menus preceded by an asterisk * are listed in index.)

Between Meals

To make up part of the 8 glasses of liquid per day, two glasses of fruit or vegetable juices may be taken. Use any of the above combinations, *tomato-herb drinks, or other combinations listed under the chapter "Drink Health the Juice Way" (pages 45-52). Hot vegetable bouillons are excellent, as Bragg Aminos (for broth ½ -1 tsp. in cup of hot distilled water).

Lemon, Lime or Orange Fresh Squeeze Squirter

Great for reducers! Roll a lemon, lime or orange on kitchen counter to break down the cells for more juice. Poke a small hole in the end with a toothpick or knife. Now, you have a super squirter for distilled water on fasting days at work or home; also great for salads, vegetables and herb teas.

Here's some Salad Dressings for those on reducing diets.

TOMATO-BASIL DRESSING FOR REDUCERS

⅓ cup fresh lemon juice
1 Tbsp raw honey or Stevia drops
½ Tbsp Bragg Liquid Aminos
shake of Bragg Sprinkle
½ cup soft tofu
1 cup tomato juice
1 clove garlic, mash
½ tsp sweet basil

Blend all ingredients well. (You may add 2 Stevia drops instead of honey.) Allow to stand for 2 hours before using. Serves 1.

TOMATO DRESSING FOR REDUCERS

½ cup tomato juice
¼ cup lemon juice
⅓ tsp Bragg Liquid Aminos
½ tsp onion juice
½ tsp chives
shake of Bragg Sprinkle

Combine ingredients. Beat vigorously and let stand for 1 hour to set flavors before serving. Serves 2.

GRAPEFRUIT FRENCH DRESSING FOR REDUCERS

2 Tbsps soft tofu
3 Tbsps grapefruit juice
½ Tbsp lemon juice
¼ tsp paprika
1 tsp soy Parmesan cheese, grate
½ tsp raw honey or Stevia

Combine ingredients. Beat vigorously. Allow to stand 2 hours to blend flavors before serving. Serves 2.

LIME DRESSING FOR REDUCERS

3 Tbsps soft tofu
4 Tbsps fresh lime juice
2 tsps raw honey or Stevia drops
⅛ tsp Bragg Liquid Aminos
1 tsp celery seed
1 tsp oregano

Combine ingredients. Beat vigorously and allow to stand one hour to set flavors before serving. Serves 2.

MUSTARD DRESSING FOR REDUCERS

⅓ cup lemon juice
½ cup soft tofu
1 tsp raw honey or Stevia drops
1 tsp mustard powder
½ tsp Bragg Liquid Aminos
shake of Bragg Sprinkle

Blend all ingredients thoroughly and allow to stand 1 hour to set flavors before serving. Serves 1.

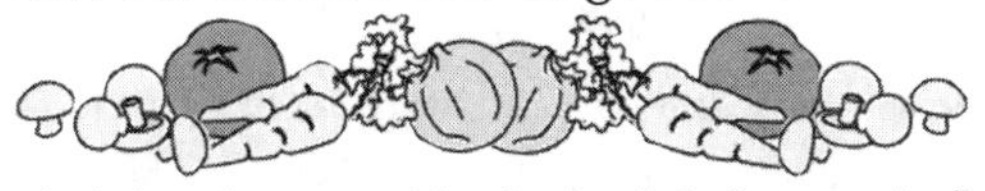

Studies have revealed that fat stored in the body's "spare tire" around the waist increases the risk for diabetes and heart disease and shortens the life-span!

I have no doubt that it is part of the destiny of the human race in its gradual improvement to leave off eating animals. – Henry David Thoreau, 1854

Lycopene is more readily available to the body from cooked tomatoes than from raw ones. Cook them in Bragg Olive Oil to aid in absorption. – Andrew Weil, M.D.

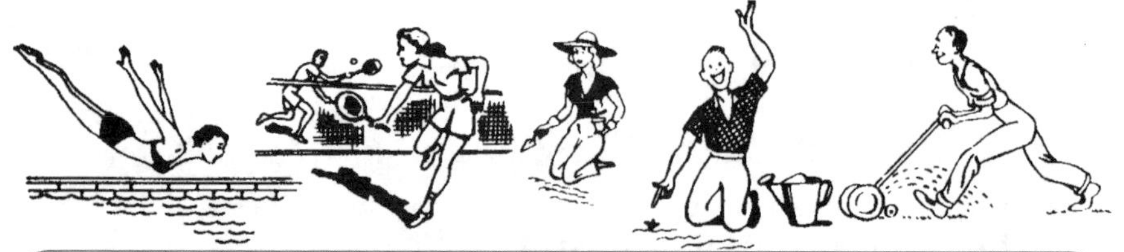

King of Exercise – Walking is Important

No reduction program is complete without a walking regimen. The first day of your diet, start stretching, deep breathing and walking. Begin with a short, brisk walk every day for a week, then each week increase the distance until you walk 2 to 5 miles. For a busy person, brisk walking is the king of exercise and, in conjunction with the diet, is absolutely necessary for successful reducing and maintaining of weight.

Most Americans Overeat

Overeating robs energy! Don't overeat, even healthy foods! Help your body detoxify by giving it cleansing time! When you eat, your body is forced to work on digesting food and has no energy for detoxification. So, in time the toxins and waste pile up and then you accumulate physical miseries and age prematurely. Don't over-burden your amazing human machinery and kill yourself prematurely! Life is precious and we want you alive, healthy and happy for a long time! A diet related death is an unnecessary tragedy!

Losing Weight Naturally

Moderation is the key to all weight loss regimes. Your body knows when and how much you should be eating, the key is to listen to what your body is saying. Keep in mind these few tips when striving for your weight loss:

- Start cutting your food quantities in half. You might be surprised to learn that most people are drastically overeating which is harmful to your body.
- Take your time when eating. Savor each bite of delicious, healthy food. Put your fork down between each bite and drink at least one 8-oz. glass of distilled water before each meal.
- Remember that leftovers can be a good, quick meal. When dining in restaurants, order wisely, don't over-indulge, eat only until you are satisfied. Ask for a carry out box and save the leftovers for another meal.
- Drink pure, distilled water between meals. Sugar in soda or other drinks will give you a false sense of being full. Thirst often masks itself with hunger.

Don't overburden and injure your digestive system by overfeeding it!

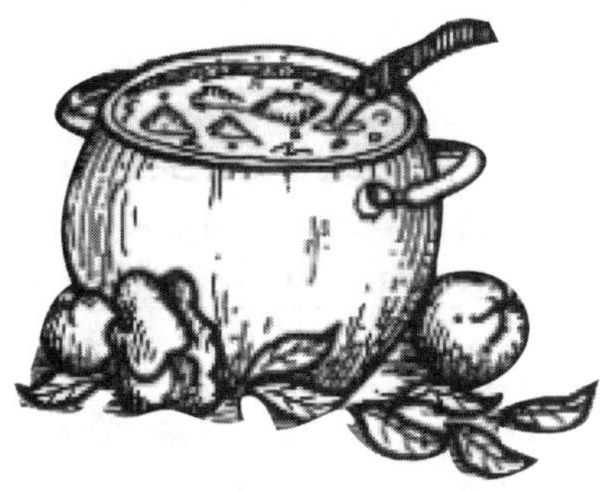

Chapter 25

Gaining Weight

No person who is underweight can enjoy the exuberance of positive health. Being excessively lean brings on a general rundown condition and a depleted nervous system. It is unfortunate that, unlike most overweight persons, the majority of the underweight cannot regulate their size entirely by the intake of food. It has been popular belief that gaining weight is simply a matter of stuffing food into the body. That is not true. I have seen thin people gorge for years and never gain a pound, often stuffing themselves on foods low in calories. The thin person who has nothing organically wrong with them may find the basic weight-gaining menus given below to be a source of the foods he or she needs.

Rest and Exercise

Rest and exercise are important. The ordinary person requires eight hours of sleep per night; but a thin person should have a minimum of nine, and ten hours are preferable. By ten hours of sleep, I mean actual sleeping time. If it takes you 30 minutes to relax and go to sleep after you go to bed, that time is well spent, but it is not sleeping time.

The Richness of Whole Foods

Whole-grains are nature's richest offering among all her tremendous stores of bounty. The cereals, breads and other baked foods made from 100% whole-grain offers the person who is trying to gain weight, not only delicious flavors, but the protective value of the little golden flakes of germs found in the grains. This germ contains oily substances that add flavor and nutrition to the diet. Be sure to get whole-grains in a wide variety. When you use only one whole-grain, even though it may be one of nature's finest foods, you are not getting the benefit of the wide variety of nutritional forces found in the various whole-grains. Vary your whole-grain

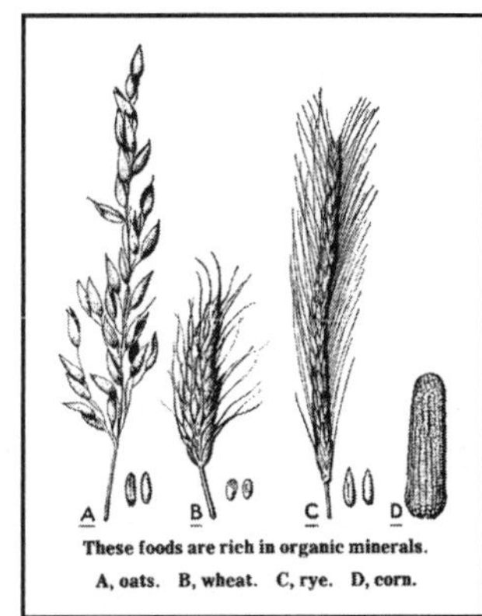

These foods are rich in organic minerals.
A, oats. B, wheat. C, rye. D, corn.

diet by using the variety of whole-grains listed throughout this book. Many grains can be blended into one delicious cereal, and a variety can be obtained each day by using this selection.

A complete set of weight-gaining menus follows, but there are a few important points to remember. The underweight person can use a great variety of dried legumes, beans, lentils, peas, lima beans, garbanzos and soybeans. These can be enjoyed throughout the week in soups, casseroles, entrées and also are delicious cold in a variety of salads.

Organic brown rice is one of our main staples. It is high in nutrition and is non-allergenic and gluten-free, as well as easy to digest by sensitive stomachs (and is great blended, for babies). It should be eaten four to six times per week, and is a healthy, ideal entrée or side dish.

Tofu from soybeans is one of the best protein foods, ideal for normalizing and building strong bodies. Broiled, baked or blended, tofu is great. You can even have tofu ice cream!

Unsulphured dried fruits, unsulphured blackstrap molasses, raw nuts and seeds, raw honey and fresh fruits – bananas, apples, pears and avocados – as well as Bragg Organic Extra Virgin Olive Oil, safflower and soy oils are wonderful additions to help normalize the body weight.

Healthy Foods to Normalize Weight

The average underweight person, whose thinness is due to malnutrition and not organic disturbance, does not usually have enough of the right wholesome foods. They may have even more total food intake than their overweight neighbor, but it may not be food designed to give them healthy weight. Here is a set of healthful, easy-to-follow menus starting on page 251.

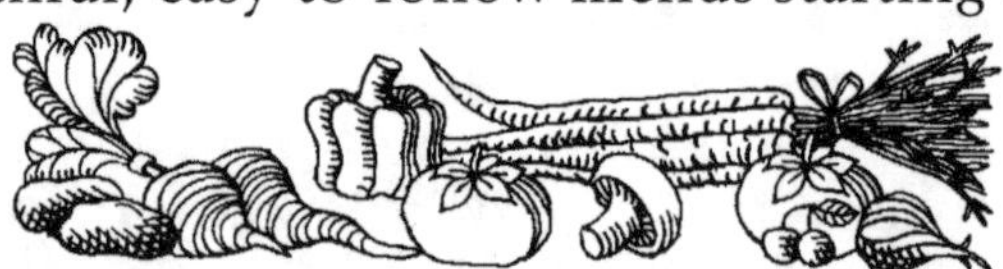

Think of yourself as a "battery" – you discharge energy and you must recharge yourself with proper food, rest and constructive emotions.

There is more hunger for love and appreciation in this world than for bread. – Mother Teresa

---

Half the costs of illness are wasted on conditions that could be prevented. – Dr. Joseph Pizzorno, author *Total Wellness*

True friendship is like sound health, the value of it is seldom known until it is lost. – Charles Caleb Colton

---

How beautiful a day can be when kindness touches it. – George Elliston (1883-1946); news reporter & poet

Menu for Gaining Weight

Eight to ten full glasses of healthful liquid must be taken daily: distilled water, a hot cup of distilled water with 1-2 tablespoons blackstrap molasses, herbal teas or freshly squeezed fruit juices. See pages 45-52 for juices, page 49 for the Bragg Healthy "Energy" Smoothie. (Recipes indicated with asterisk * are listed in the index).

Upon Rising

Have the Bragg Vinegar Drink (1-2 tsps Bragg Apple Cider Vinegar with 1-2 tsps raw honey (optional) in 8-oz glass of distilled water) and then do some stretching, deep breathing and exercise. Then you are ready for the Bragg Health "Energy" Smoothie (page 49).

Breakfast

Remember to earn your breakfast first with exercise and activity. Take vitamin/mineral supplements with a multiple enzyme with your meals. The Bragg Health "Energy" Smoothie (page 49) can be substituted any morning instead of breakfast.

(Choice of 1 large portion of any of the following)

Fresh fruit in season
Any dried, unsulphured, cooked or soaked fruit
A combination of dried figs, apricots, peaches and pears

(1 large portion of the following)

***My Favorite Health Meal (recipe on page 168) with choice of:**
- **sliced figs, pecans, raw honey and soy cream**
- **fresh fruit, raw honey and soy cream**
- **dried or soaked apricots, chopped walnuts, raw honey & soy cream**

(Choose 1 portion of any of the following)

***Fresh fruit waffles**
***Soy flour waffles**
***Whole/multi-grain pancakes**
***Buckwheat waffles**

(Choice of one 8-oz serving of any of the following)

Any herbal tea
Grain coffee substitute

(Choice of one of the following)

2 slices whole-grain toast
***breakfast muffin or roll**

At 10:00 a.m.

(Choice of one 8-oz. glass of any of the following)

citrus fruit juice
pineapple juice
grape or berry juice

Recipes indicated with asterisk * are listed in the index

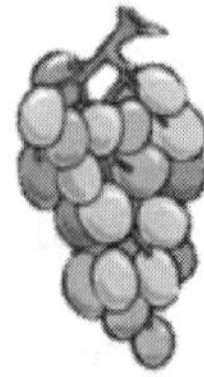

Lunch

(Choice of 1 large serving of the following)

*Fresh mushroom salad
*Carrot and mint salad
*Pear and grape salad
*Avocado and tomato salad bowl
*Bragg Famous Raw Garden Salad
*Ambrosia

(Choice of 1 medium portion of any of the following)

*Corn chowder
*Cincinnati's famous split pea soup
*Sweet potato soup
*Black soybean soup
*Barley, tomato and bean soup
*Creamed carrot soup
*Golden soup
*Bragg lentil soup

(Choice of 1 medium portion of any of the following)

*Baked Asparagus
*Stuffed artichoke hearts
*Beet greens
*Broccoli with soy cheese
*Spinach with pepper
*Any of the basic greens recipes
*Baby limas marjoram
*Green beans with mint or herbs
*Leeks au gratin
*Sauerkraut-stuffed peppers
*Spinach stuffed tomatoes
*Zucchini with herbs

(Choice of 1 medium portion of any of the following)

*Beets en orange
*Spiced carrots en casserole
*Caramelized carrots
*Glazed carrots with honey
*Baked cauliflower
*Squash and lima beans
*Eggplant with herbs & soy cheese
*Eggplant in okra
*Tomato okra
*Parsnip patties
*Braised celery
*Onion tomato bake

(Choice of 1 large portion of the following)

*Mushroom lentil burgers
*Soybean casserole
*Stuffed baked potatoes
*Bean squash casserole
*Cornbread stuffed tomatoes
*Vegetarian sausages
*Cincinnati mock turkey
*Lentil loaf
*Celery and pecan loaf
*Mushroom loaf
*Vegetable and soybean stew
*Soybean loaf
*Moroccan stew
*Vegetable Pot Pie
*Chestnut croquettes
*Mixed nut loaf

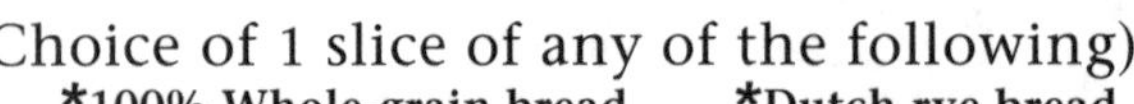

(Choice of 1 slice of any of the following)

*100% Whole-grain bread
*Oatmeal bread
*Dutch rye bread
*Barley bread

(Choice of 2 of any of the following)

*Corn bread
*Whole-grain rolls
*Dinner rolls or Fluff rolls
*Speedy pan rolls

(Choice of 3 of any of the following)

*Rye muffins
*Banana raisin muffins
*Apple-corn muffins
*Date bran muffins

(Choice of one 8-oz. cup of any of the following)

mint tea
herb tea

(Choice of 1 of any of the following)

*Fresh strawberry sponge
*Raisin pudding
*Favorite carob custard
*Individual fruit puddings
*Date and brown rice pudding
*Strawberry or berry custard

Recipes indicated with asterisk * are listed in the index

At 3:00 p.m.

(Choice of one 8-oz glass of any of the following)

Tomato juice with herbs

Tomato juice with celery juice

Dinner

(Choice of 1 large portion of any of the following)

*Dandelion Salad
*Gourmet Mixed-Green Salad
*Spring Mixed Greens Salad
*Buckwheat Tenderleaf Salad
*Summer Herb Salad
*Bragg Famous Raw Garden Salad
*Sprouted Soybean Salad
*Tropical Hawaiian Delight

(Choice of 1 medium serving of any of the following)

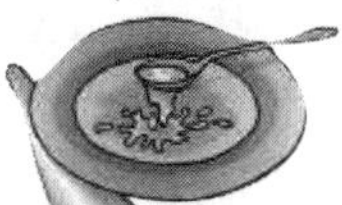

*Consomme
*Chestnut
*Ripe-olive soup
*Veggie soup
*Spring broth
*Royal Soup

(Choose any vegetable in the first Luncheon Vegetable section that you did not use on your luncheon menu.)

(Choose any vegetable in the second Luncheon Vegetable section that you did not use on your luncheon menu.)

(Choose any item on the Luncheon Entree section that you did not use on your luncheon menu.)

(Choice of 1 large serving of any of the following)

Baked potato with
*Mushroom Stuffing
*Potatoes au gratin
*Zesty potato casserole
*Soy cheese stuffed potatoes

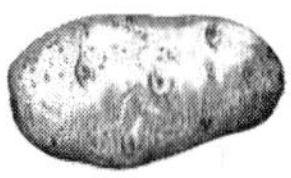

(Choice of 1 of any of the breads listed in the Luncheon Bread Section – bottom page 252.)

(Choice of any of the desserts listed in the Luncheon Dessert section that have not been used for lunch or 1 serving of any of the following)

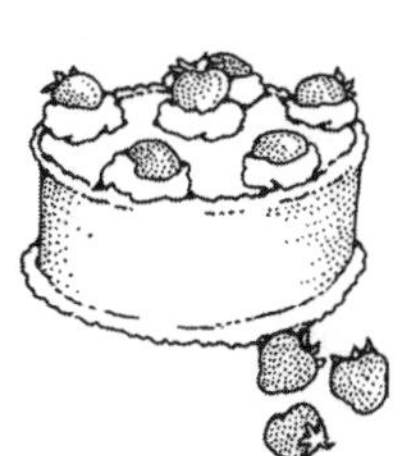

*Upside-down cake
*Strawberry shortcake
*Blueberry squares
*Fruited spice cake
*California cheesecake
*Banana cupcakes
*Banana gingerbread
*Apple sauce Cake
*Pittsburgh pumpkin pie
*Pecan pie
*Banana-coconut cream pie
*Glazed apricot pie
*Delicious graham cracker apple pie
*Strawberry or berry custard
*Baked bananas
*Sweet-potato pudding

(Choice of one 8-oz glass of any of the following)

Mint or other herb tea

Fruit or vegetable juice

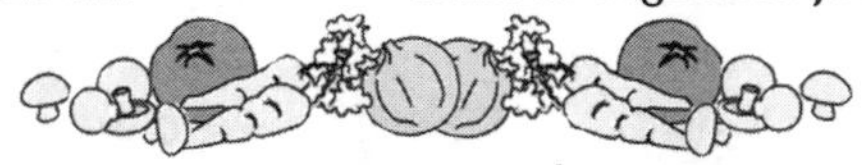

Recipes indicated with asterisk * are listed in the index

Patricia's Delicious Health Popcorn

For more healthy fiber in your diet, enjoy fresh home-popped organic popcorn. My favorite method is air (non-oil) popper. Melt desired amount of trans-fat free soy butter or use Bragg Organic Extra Virgin Olive Oil. Blend soy butter and oil, add 3-5 fresh crushed garlic cloves and several sprays or dashes of Bragg Aminos to mixture and pour over popcorn. Then sprinkle with Bragg Nutritional Yeast and for variety, add shake of delicious Bragg Sprinkle (24 herbs & spices), mustard powder or cayenne pepper to liquid mixture. This is a tasty bread substitute served with soups, salads and almost any meal. Keep warm in oven until serving

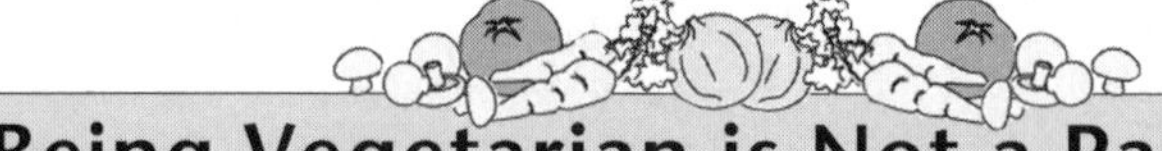

Being Vegetarian is Not a Passing Fad

Some of the greatest known people in world history were vegetarians. And today many of the great minds, influential leaders, athletes and popular celebrities follow the healthy vegetarian diet, even President Bill Clinton does (pg 260).

FAMOUS HISTORICAL VEGETARIANS

Adam & Eve	Sir Isaac Newton	Sylvester Graham
Clara Barton	Pythagoras	John Harvey Kellogg
Leo Tolstoy	Albert Schweitzer	Ellen G. White
Thomas Edison	George Bernard Shaw	Leonardo da Vinci
Albert Einstein	Upton Sinclair	Mahatma Gandhi
John Wesley	John Milton	Henry David Thoreau

FAMOUS MODERN DAY VEGETARIANS

Dr. Henry Heimlich, *physician and inventor of Heimlich Maneuver*
Dr. Dean Ornish, *physician and author*
Tony Robbins, *motivational speaker and author*
Dr. John McDougall, *physician and author*
Dr. T. Collin Campbell, *nutrition scientist and researcher*

Bob Barker, *TV personality*	Kim Bassinger, *actress*
Cindy Blum, *opera singer*	Christie Brinkley, *model*
Marilu Henner, *actress/author*	Elliot Gould, *actor*
Dustin Hoffman, *actor*	Elton John, *rock musician*
Casey Kasem, *radio personality*	Billy Jean King, *tennis champion*
Cloris Leachman, *actress*	Carl Lewis, *Olympic runner*
Madonna, *singer, actress*	Paul McCartney, *singer, musician*
Olivia Newton-John, *singer*	Bill Pearl, *four-time Mr. Universe*

The American Dietetic Association has affirmed that a vegetarian diet can meet all known nutrient needs. The key to a healthy vegetarian diet is to eat a wide variety of foods, including fruits, vegetables, plenty of leafy greens, whole grain products, nuts, seeds and legumes. Limit your intake of sweets and fatty foods.

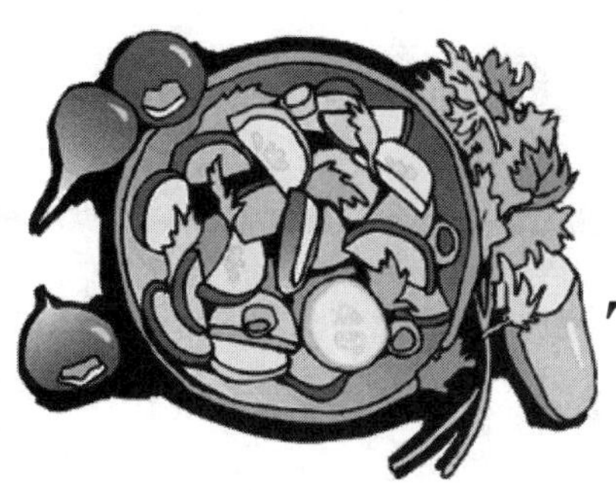

Chapter 26

Modified & Transition Diets

Not everyone is fortunate enough to get off to a good start by eating healthy foods. People with ulcers, acid reflex (Gerds), colitis, irritable bowel syndrome, and who are recovering from surgery or illness often require soft, bland foods. However, a diet composed of these foods is not always nutritionally perfect. During the brief transition back to health, compromises often are needed.

Slowly introduce healthy fiber plant foods into your diet: grated and minced salads, fresh sprouts, fresh fruits and the whole grains, especially the oat bran and psyllium husk powder mixture for healthy elimination (see page 235).

These recipes are created to make the soft diet more appetizing and nutritionally correct as possible. People on recovery diets require ample vitamin/mineral supplements, especially vitamin C, green barley and spirulina powders and live juices (see pages 45-52). For any stomach, ulcer and colon problems, drink this healing combination twice daily: fresh squeezed juice containing ⅔ cabbage juice, ⅓ fresh celery and apple juice (remove seeds) and 1 Tbsp aloe vera gel or juice.

People recovering from illness no longer need adhere to a boring lifeless diet, composed of over-cooked, nutritionally depleted foods. Appetizing flavors may be introduced without harm in the soft diet. Keep in mind that although the patient's appetite may be tempted, foods with strong or spicy flavors can be distasteful to those in poor health. Judgment should be used in the use of the seasonings in these recipes to the individual. Very often, seasonings of any kind are not allowed and must be eliminated from these recipes. This may also be true of other foods. The following are general diets adaptable to most people and may need to be individualized according to possible food intolerances and immediate health requirements. Your daily journal helps monitor food reactions.

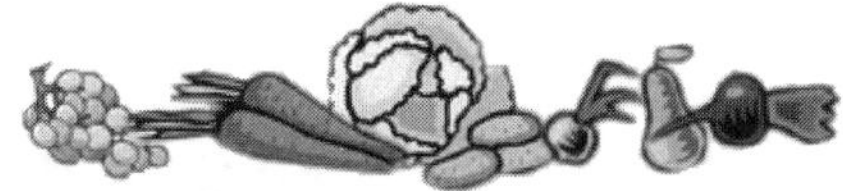

Dr. Dean Ornish has been able to reverse heart disease in more than 80% of his patients who follow, among other things, a low-fat vegetarian diet.

A bland diet usually consists of foods that are easy to digest.

Puréed and Juiced Foods

Many foods that ordinarily could not be used in gentle diets can be adapted by juicing, puréeing, blending or straining the foods. Puréeing is easily done with blenders, strainers, food processors or juicers.

Liquefied and Freshly Juiced Foods

The juicer, food processor and blender are great for preparing foods for gentle or bland diets and baby foods. Fibers of fresh fruits and vegetables, juiced, can be tolerated on most gentle diets. Any raw or cooked fruit or vegetable can be liquefied and added to non-dairy (nut, rice, oat or soy) milk, broth or soup. Live, fresh juices supercharge your energy level and immune system, and maximize your body's health power. You may fortify your liquid meal with green barley or spirulina powder for extra nutrition (see page 51 for blender recommendations).

We recommend using the Jack LaLanne HealthMaster 100 and the Jack LaLanne Power Juicer in making healthy fruit and vegetable juices, see web: *www.jacklalanne.com.*

Suggestions for Bland and Gentle Diets

There are many recipes throughout this book that can be used as they are, or adapted to the bland, gentle diet. Also, most of the recipes for fruit and vegetable juices under the Drink Health, the 'Live Juice Way' section are excellent for anyone on a bland, gentle diet (see pg. 45)

Bragg Healthy Lifestyle For Super Health

Bragg Healthy Living consists of eating 60-80% of your diet from fresh, live, organically-grown healthy foods: raw vegetables, salads, fresh fruits and juices, sprouts, raw seeds, nuts and some cooked all-natural 100% whole-grain breads, pastas and cereals; and nutritious beans and legumes. This is the reason people become revitalized and reborn into a fresh new life filled with joy, health, vitality, youthfulness and longevity! There are millions of healthy Bragg followers world-wide who prove that Bragg Healthy Lifestyle works miracles!

Our mental and emotional diets determine our overall energy levels, health and well-being more than we realize. Every thought and feeling, no matter how big or small, impacts our inner energy reserves.

I cannot stress enough the benefits of juicing. You are the most important person on this earth, be kind to that person! – Jack LaLanne, Bragg follower, since 15

Puréed Vegetable Soup in 8 Minutes!

Puréed soups provide an excellent means of introducing vegetables into the restricted diet. Use one or more vegetables of choice: sliced carrots, onions, potatoes, zucchini, etc. Steam 8 minutes in steamer basket using distilled water. For seasoning variety, add, as desired, fresh garlic, Bragg Sprinkle (24 herbs & spices) or salad herbs, Bragg Aminos, frozen stock cubes, etc. to water. Blend steamed vegetables and liquid in blender. Add more hot distilled water if needed; serve. Garnish with crumbled tofu, minced parsley and a sprinkle of Bragg Nutritional Yeast.

PURÉE OF MUSHROOM SOUP

½ lb mushrooms & stems, slice
2 cups distilled water
3 Tbsps potato flour
2 Tbsps Bragg Olive Oil
3 Tbsps soft tofu (optional)
½ cup soy milk
½ tsp Bragg Liquid Aminos
shake of Bragg Sprinkle

Slice mushrooms, sauté in olive oil for 4 minutes. In blender add flour and tofu to soy milk and water; add seasonings if desired. Mix all ingredients until smooth. Heat again. Garnish with soy yogurt or soy sour cream if desired. Serves 2.

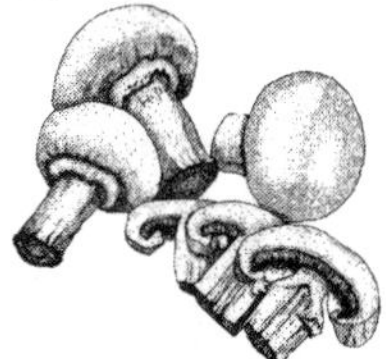

PURÉE OF SPINACH SOUP

Use above Mushroom Soup recipe replacing mushrooms with ¾ cup steamed spinach. *Variation*: any vegetable of your choice, carrots, squash, or mix. Makes delicious creamed soup.

CONSOMMÉ – COLD OR HOT

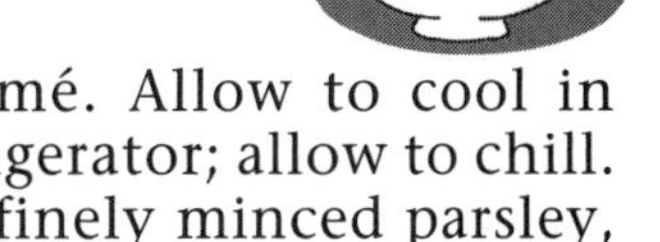

1 quart consommé
(recipe on page 54)
3 Tbsps arrowroot powder

Mix arrowroot powder with consommé. Allow to cool in shallow bowl. When cool, place in refrigerator; allow to chill. Cut into cubes and stir. Garnish with finely minced parsley, watercress and green onions. Delicious served cold or hot.

PURÉE OF STRING BEANS

2 lb green beans
2 tsps onion, mince
1 cup vegetable stock
2 Tbsps Bragg Organic Olive Oil
shake of Bragg Sprinkle
2 cups distilled water
1 tsp Bragg Liquid Aminos
2 Tbsps potato flour

Slice beans into small pieces. Steam beans 8-10 minutes in steamer basket with distilled water; add onions, vegetable stock, Sprinkle and Bragg Aminos. Purée beans and liquid with flour and Bragg Olive Oil in blender and serve. Serves 4-6.

PURÉE OF MINTED CARROTS

2 cups carrots, slice
1 Tbsp mint leaves, mince
2 tsps raw honey
2 Tbsps Bragg Olive Oil

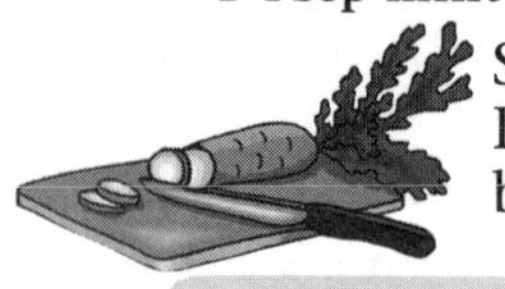

Steam carrots in steamer basket until lightly done. Purée carrots, with liquid, olive oil and honey in blender. Garnish with fresh mint leaves. Serves 2-4.

PURÉE OF OKRA AND TOMATOES

2 cups okra, slice
2 cups tomatoes, dice
1 tsp parsley, mince
grated Parmesan cheese and Bragg Nutritional Yeast (for garnish)
1 tsp chives
1 tsp Bragg Liquid Aminos
1 Tbsp Bragg Organic Olive Oil
a shake of Bragg Sprinkle

Cook okra in small amount of water until tender, then add remaining ingredients; simmer 10 minutes. Purée in blender and serve. *Optional:* garnish with grated soy Parmesan cheese and Bragg Nutritional Yeast Flakes. Serves 4-6.

PURÉE OF CELERY ROOT AND EGGPLANT

2 cups celery root, slice
2 cups unpeeled eggplant, dice
grated Parmesan cheese and Bragg Nutritional Yeast (for garnish)
1 tsp onion, minced
1 Tbsp Bragg Organic Olive Oil
1 tsp Bragg Liquid Aminos

Cook unpeeled celery root until tender, then peel and slice celery root and add to eggplant, onions, olive oil and Bragg Aminos. Simmer 15 minutes in small amount of distilled water. Purée in blender and serve. Garnish with grated soy Parmesan cheese and Bragg Nutritional Yeast. Serves 4.

PURÉE OF SQUASH

2 cups summer or winter squash, slice
grated Parmesan cheese and Bragg Nutritional Yeast
1 Tbsp Bragg Olive Oil
1 tsp Bragg Liquid Aminos
shake of Bragg Sprinkle

Slice summer or winter squash, remove seeds and pulp; steam until tender in distilled water, adding Sprinkle. Purée steamed squash with liquid in blender with olive oil and Bragg Aminos. Reheat. Garnish with grated soy Parmesan cheese and nutritional yeast large flakes. Serves 4.

PURÉE OF BEETS WITH SOY YOGURT

2 lbs beets
4 Tbsps soft tofu or soy yogurt
1 Tbsp Bragg Organic Olive Oil
1 tsp Bragg Liquid Aminos

Cook or steam beets with skins until tender in distilled water. Purée cooked beets with liquid, add olive oil and Bragg Aminos. This is delicious hot or cold and even as a soup. Top with soy vanilla yogurt or tofu sour cream. Serves 6.

PURÉE OF PEAS

2 cups peas, shell
1 tsp onion, mince
½ tsp Bragg Liquid Aminos
1 tsp Bragg Olive Oil

Cook peas and onion until tender. Purée peas, adding olive oil and Bragg Aminos. Garnish with grated soy Parmesan cheese or soy yogurt; serve. Serves 2-3.

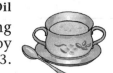

PURÉE OF CELERY WITH MUSHROOMS

2 cups celery, slice
½ cup mushrooms, button or shiitake
1 Tbsp Bragg Organic Olive Oil
shake of Bragg Sprinkle
1 Tbsp Bragg Nutritional Yeast

Cook celery, mushrooms and seasonings together until tender. Purée in blender with olive oil and Bragg Nutritional Yeast. If desired as soup, add more distilled water and one tablespoon of potato flour while cooking. Serves 3.

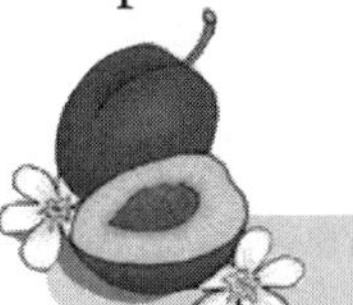

FRUIT COMPOTES

PRUNE – PLUM COMPOTE

1 cup prunes
6 Satsuma plums
1 Tbsp raw honey
¼ tsp cinnamon powder
3 Tbsps soy or nut cream

Add cinnamon powder to prunes and plums; cook in distilled water until tender. Pit and then purée blend with honey. Top with soy or nut cream. Serves 2.

PURÉE OF APRICOTS

1 dozen organic apricots, fresh or dried
1 tsp organic orange rind, grated
1 Tbsp raw honey

Cook ingredients in small amount of distilled water until tender. Purée. Serve plain or with soy or nut cream. Serves 4.

PURÉE OF PEARS

4 organic pears, halve, seeded
1 clove
1 cup pineapple juice, unsweetened

Cook pears in pineapple juice with clove for 10 minutes. Remove clove. Purée pears with liquid. Serve plain or top with soy yogurt or nut cream. Serves 2-3.

To consider yourself an environmentalist and still eat meat is like saying you're a philanthropist who doesn't give to charity. – Howard Lyman

---

A number of studies have found a connection between high red meat consumption and colon cancer. – Harvard Health Letter, *www.health.harvard.edu*

There are always flowers for those who want to see them.

PURÉE OF MINTED APPLES

2 cups organic apples, core and quarter (peel, optional)
1 Tbsp raw honey
4 Tbsps mint leaves, mince
½ cup raisins (optional)
3 Tbsps distilled water

Cook apples until tender. Add mint and raisins if desired during last 5 minutes of cooking. Purée in blender with liquid, add honey if desired. Top with soy or nut cream. Serves 2.

APRICOT AND BANANA COMPOTE

1 dozen apricots, fresh or dried
3 bananas, ripe
1 Tbsp raw honey
soy or nut cream

Cook apricots until tender in small amount of distilled water. Purée with honey, then cool. Before serving, add bananas (or fresh fruit of choice) and blend with the apricot purée. Top with soy or nut cream. Serves 3-4.

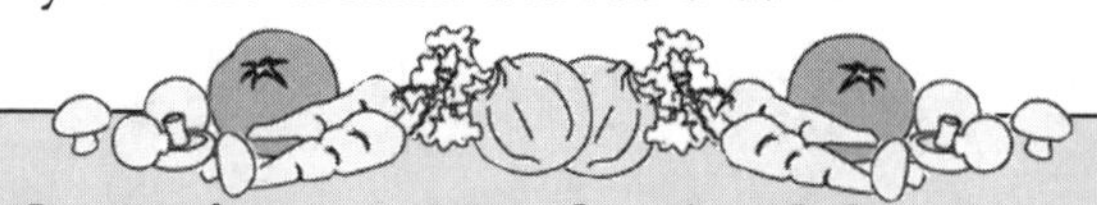

Meat is an Undesirable Food

Scientific studies conducted over the past two decades have established to the health science community that meat is an undesirable food for at least these six reasons:

1. Meat is a major contributor to the leading causes of death, such as cancer and heart disease.
2. Meat is deficient in two major food components: dietary fiber and complex carbohydrates.
3. Contrary to popular belief, it is actually more difficult to achieve optimal nutrition utilizing a meat-based diet.
4. The cost of meat is excessively high in relation to the nutritional value it provides.
5. The production of meat as a food is environmentally unsound as its production wastes energy, water and other natural resources. Meat production produces increased toxic contamination to our environment.
6. The best alternative diet, a vegetarian diet, has none of these above mentioned problems.

I have from an early age abstained from the use of meat, and the time will come when men such as I will look on the murder of animals as they now look on the murder of men. – Leonardo da Vinci

---

I live on legumes, vegetables & fruits. No dairy, no meat of any kind, no chicken, no turkey, & very little fish, once in a while. It changed my metabolism & I lost 24 pounds. I did research & found 82% of people who go on a plant-based diet begin to heal themselves, as I did. – U.S. President Bill Clinton, 1993-2001

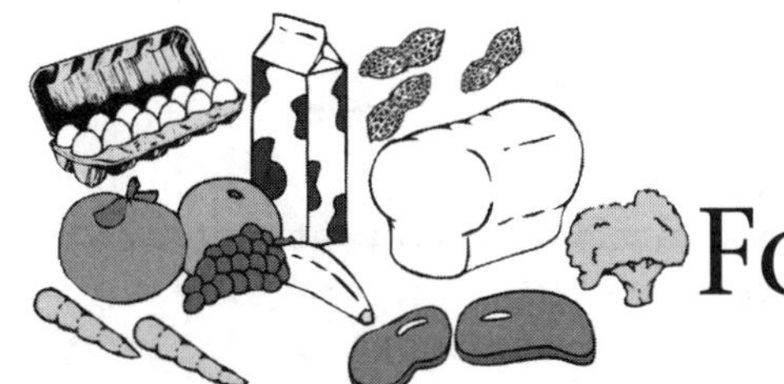

Chapter 27

Food Allergies

Most Common Food Allergens

Cereal grains: wheat, corn, oats, rye, buckwheat

Dairy: cheese, ice cream, butter, milk, yogurt, etc.

Eggs: cakes, pasta, dressings, custards, mayonnaise

Fish: shellfish, crab, lobster, shrimp

Meats: pork, bacon, sausage, veal, chicken, smoked meat or fish

Fruits: strawberries, citrus fruits, melons

Vegetables: cauliflower, brussels sprouts, onion, celery, spinach, legumes, as well as tomatoes, potatoes, eggplant and others of the nightshade family

Nuts: peanuts, walnuts, pecans, almonds, Brazil nuts, cashews, pistachios, all chemically dried, salted and preserved nuts

Others: chocolate, cocoa, coffee, China tea, spices, salt, monosodium glutamate (MSG), cottonseed oil, palm oil, honey and allergic reactions can be caused by toxic pesticides residue on salad greens, fruits, vegetables, and other produce.

Foods Rarely Causing Allergies Are Often Used in "Elimination" Diets

At times every known food may cause an allergic reaction. Thus, foods used in "elimination" diets may cause allergic reactions in some individuals. But since the incidence of reaction to these foods is generally low, they are widely used in test diets. By keeping your own daily Food Journal you will soon realize "problem" foods that must be eliminated from your diet.

- apricots
- asparagus
- beets
- carrots
- corn/corn oil
- grapefruit
- green beans
- olive oil
- pears
- peas
- pineapple
- rice
- rye
- soybeans
- squash

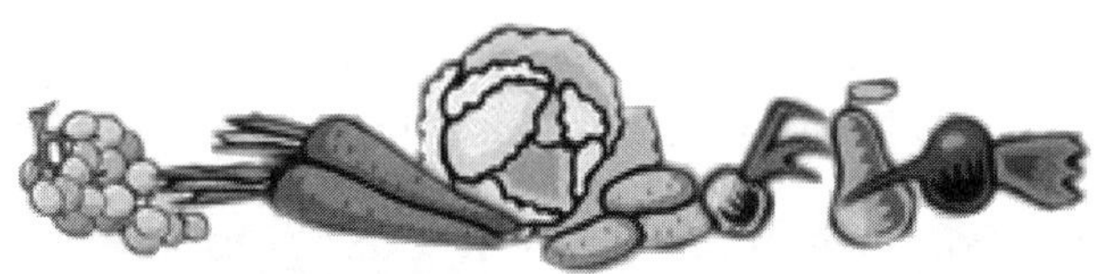

Food Allergies and Their Reactions

If your body has an adverse reaction after eating a particular type of food (especially if it happens each time you eat that food) chances are you have an allergy or sensitivity to it. The following symptoms can occur very quickly after a particular food has been eaten! If you wheeze, sneeze, develop a stuffy nose, nasal drip or mucus, dark circles or pouches under your eyes, headaches, lightheadedness, dizziness, stomach or chest pains, diarrhea, extreme thirst, break out in a rash or have a swelling of external or internal tissues (ankles, feet, hands or stomach bloating, etc.), you may have an allergy. Allergic reactions to foods can occur up to five days after consumption, and can take place in multiple locations in the body.

Consider yourself lucky if you know what your allergies are. If you don't know try to find out so you can eliminate those foods from your diet. To reevaluate your daily life as a guide to your future, start a daily journal (8½ x 11" notebook) of foods eaten and your reactions, moods, energy levels, weight, elimination and sleep patterns. You will soon discover the foods and situations that cause problems. By charting your activities, you will be amazed at the swings following eating certain foods. My father kept his journal faithfully for over 70 years.

If you are hypersensitive to certain foods, you must delete them from your diet! There are hundreds of allergies and it is impossible to discuss each one here. Many who suffer from this unpleasant affliction have allergies to seafood, milk or eggs, while some are allergic to all grains. Fruit allergies have been purposely omitted here, not because they are not as important as grain allergies, but because it's easier to secure a variety of replacement fruits than to replace grains. Most of our recipes have been designed to help those with grain allergies.

General Tips for People with Allergies

Milk – Milk and its by-products are the #1 allergy culprits, often clogging the respiratory and arterial systems. Since pasteurization and homogenization were developed, heart and respiratory ailments in America have soared! Non-dairy products are healthy and readily available. Soy, rice, nut milks and their products (non-dairy cheeses, creams, butters, yogurts, spreads, etc.) are delicious. Those who insist on using cow's and goat's milk should take enzyme lactase to better tolerate milk. (*www.notmilk.com*)

Wheat – There are many wonderful, healthy alternatives for this grain. Health food stores carry a wide variety of wheat-free flours: rye, corn, brown rice, millet, barley, oat, soybean, lima bean, potato flour, etc. You can use them alone or blended together for an assortment of delicious flavors.

Eggs – Fertile eggs, from healthy, free-range chickens, are best. Health stores have Egg Replacer made of potato, tapioca starch and leavening agents. It is designed for use in baking. For thickening in baking use arrowroot, instant tapioca, or agar agar. Use potato flour for gravies, soups, stews, casseroles, vegetable pies, etc. (See Egg Replacer, pg. 3)

Oil – Hydrogenated cottonseed, palm and palm-kernel oils should never be used, as they cause clogging of the arteries and other health problems and especially for the allergic person. You can often consume these oils without knowing it, as many shortenings, candies, dressings and commercially baked products use these unhealthy, cheap oils. Please read labels carefully to know what you are eating.

Raw food – Many persons suffering from allergies discover that they can tolerate cooked foods better than raw or fresh foods. After following the Bragg Healthy Lifestyle, people can tolerate more healthy raw fruits and vegetables, and their health begins to improve and thrive.

Special products – Most grocery and health food stores have wheat-free mixes, non-dairy products, cold (expeller) pressed vegetable oils, egg-free and salt-free mayonnaises and many other products for people with food allergies.

Food preparation – It is vital that a person with allergies understands the preparation of food. Many foods you can tolerate successfully become definitely irritating if prepared with an ingredient to which you are allergic. Take care not to be misled by creamed dishes, sauces or foods containing fillings, seasonings and additives that you may not be able to tolerate. With food preparation knowledge, health menus of the allergic person can be every bit as appetizing, attractive and nourishing as that of the unrestricted food person.

Recipes

Bread, muffins, etc., baked without grain flour are not as light and fine in texture, but can be just as delicious and nutritious. Experiment! At first, make a smaller version of the recipe, remembering that wheat-free mixtures often require longer and slower baking. Sift flours repeatedly and thoroughly beat the mixtures. The increase of air produced by sifting and mixing helps lighten the batter.

For centuries, Christians fasted during the Lenten season, which extended from Ash Wednesday to Easter Sunday. Many stopped eating meat during this time for religious reasons; however, modern science is now urging people to give meat up for health reasons. Meatless meals are nutritious and delicious: try these recipes to tantalize your taste buds and improve your health!

BREADS

APRICOT RYE BREAD

1 pkg quick-rise yeast
4 Tbsps lukewarm distilled water
4 tsps raw honey
2 Tbsps Bragg Organic Olive Oil
2 cups cooked apricots, purée
5½ cups 100% rye pastry flour or flour of choice

Dissolve the yeast in lukewarm water; beat in half the flour. Add honey, olive oil and puréed (sun-dried, unsulphured) apricots. Blend well; add second half of flour slowly. Mix again. Flour board and hands and knead well. Cover, let rise in a warm place until doubled in bulk. Flour board, shape into loaves and knead again for several minutes. Place in oiled pan (liquid lecithin is great). Let rise until light. Bake in a hot oven (375-400°F) for 20 minutes. Reduce heat to 350°F. Bake 40-50 minutes longer. This makes 2 large loaves.

GERMAN RYE BREAD

3 cups 100% rye pastry flour
1 tsp dry yeast
1 Tbsp Bragg Organic Olive Oil
2 Tbsps sauerkraut, drain (optional)
1¾ cups lukewarm distilled water
1 Tbsp raw honey

Dissolve yeast in lukewarm water; add olive oil, honey (to prevent sticking, oil measuring cup or spoon) and then the rye flour. Mix and knead to a dough on rye-floured board. Add two tablespoons drained sauerkraut (optional). Cover and let rise in a warm place until doubled in bulk. Shape into loaves. Place in oiled bread pan; let rise again and bake in hot oven (375-400°F) for 20 minutes. Reduce heat to moderate (about 350°F). Continue to bake 40-50 minutes. Makes 2 loaves.

100% CORN BREAD

2 cups corn meal, stone-ground
Egg Replacer equal to 2 eggs
2 Tbsps raw honey
½ cup soy or nut milk

FOR VARIETY ADD: grated zucchini, carrots and raisins or currants, sunflower seeds, or fresh garlic and a shake of Bragg Sprinkle.

Scald cornmeal with as much hot distilled water as it will absorb. Add soy milk and honey. Mix well. Add Egg Replacer and mix well. For variety, add one or more of grated zucchini, carrots, raisins, currants, sunflower seeds, fresh garlic or a shake of Bragg Sprinkle (24 herbs & spices). Bake in shallow, oiled pan (use liquid lecithin to prevent sticking) at 350°F for 35 minutes. Serve with honey. Serves 8.

Whole-grain breads are the staff of life world-wide!

The true cook is the perfect blend of artist & philosopher. He knows his worth: he holds in his palm the happiness & health of mankind. – Norman Douglas

FOUR - FLOUR BREAD

3 cups lukewarm distilled water or soy milk
1¼ cups brown rice flour
1¼ cups oat flour
2 pkgs quick-rise yeast
1½ cups soy flour
½ cup lima bean flour
2 Tbsps Bragg Organic Olive Oil
2 Tbsps raw honey or barley malt or brown rice syrup

Dissolve yeast in 1 cup lukewarm water or soy milk. Heat remaining milk; cool to lukewarm. Add olive oil, sweetener, yeast and flours. Flour board with one of the flours used in the recipe and knead dough until stiff. Cover and let rise in a warm place until doubled in bulk. Shape into loaves. Place in an oiled bread pan and let rise again. Bake at 400°F for 20 minutes. Reduce heat to 350°F and continue baking for 40-50 minutes. Makes 2 large loaves.

BROWN RICE AND LIMA BEAN FLOUR BREAD

1 cup brown rice flour
¾ cup soy or oat flour
¼ cup lima bean flour
⅛ cup warm water or warm soy milk
1 pkg quick-rise yeast
1 tsp raw honey
2 tsps Bragg Organic Olive Oil
1½ cups distilled water
shake of Bragg Sprinkle

Dissolve the yeast in warm soy milk; blend well with olive oil and honey and allow to stand. Sift all dry ingredients several times. Stir water into dry ingredients; add yeast and honey mixture and blend thoroughly. Let rise in a warm place until doubled in bulk. Flour board and hands with soy flour. Knead well and shape into loaves. Place in pan coated with liquid lecithin and let rise again. Bake at 300°F for 12 minutes. Increase heat to 375°F and continue baking 40 to 50 minutes longer. Makes 2 small loaves.

RYE ROLLS

2 cups warm soy milk
2 Tbsps Bragg Organic Olive Oil
2 Tbsps raw honey
1 pkg quick-rise yeast
4-5 cups rye pastry flour or mixed flours as desired

Dissolve yeast in ½ cup warm soy milk. Heat 1½ cups soy milk, add honey and olive oil. Cool. Combine liquids. Add unsifted flour. Mix well and cover and let rise to double in bulk. Make into rolls or loaf. Let rise again until bulk is doubled and bake 30 minutes at 425°F. The first setting of dough will be very soft, but easy to handle. If desired, add one tablespoon caraway, sesame, chia seeds or mix them. Makes 4 dozen rolls.

RYE MUFFINS

See recipe for Rye Muffins on page 183.

Enjoy healthy, organic foods for their wonderful abundance of life energy.

RYE FRUIT MUFFINS

See variation of Rye Fruit Muffins recipe on page 183.

RYE BISCUITS

2 cups rye flour
3 tsps baking powder
2 Tbsps Bragg Organic Olive Oil
¾ cup soy milk

Sift flour and baking powder. Cut in olive oil. Add soy milk and mix to a light dough. Roll out on a board floured with rye flour. Cut into biscuits and bake at 400°F for 15 minutes. Delicious served with hummus (page 69). Makes 12 biscuits.

PANCAKES & WAFFLES

WHEAT-FREE PANCAKES

1 cup potato flour
1½ cups soy milk
Egg Replacer equal to 2 eggs
4½ tsps Bragg Olive Oil
1 cup rice flour
2¼ tsps baking powder
4½ Tbsps raw honey
pure maple syrup

Combine and sift dry ingredients three times. Set aside. In another bowl beat Egg Replacer until light, adding olive oil slowly. Add soy milk and honey and beat again. Add dry ingredients. Mix. Bake on a hot griddle. Top with maple syrup. Makes 8-10 pancakes.

CORNMEAL WAFFLES

2 cups organic cornmeal
4 tsps baking powder
2 Tbsps raw honey
Egg Replacer equal to 3 eggs
1½ cups soy milk
⅓ cup Bragg Organic Olive Oil

Sift cornmeal and baking powder together. Set aside. Beat Egg Replacer and honey. Add Bragg Organic Olive Oil and soy milk. Combine with dry ingredients, stirring until smooth. Bake in a hot waffle iron. Top with maple syrup. Makes 6 waffles.

WHEAT-FREE WAFFLES

1 cup rice flour
½ cup yellow organic cornmeal
Egg Replacer equal to 2 eggs
2 Tbsps arrowroot powder
6 Tbsps Bragg Olive Oil
2 Tbsps raw honey
½ cup potato flour
1 cup soy milk
2 tsps baking powder
pure maple syrup (as topping)

Sift flours twice before measuring. Mix and sift all dry ingredients several times. Beat Egg Replacers; add olive oil and beat again. Add soy milk and honey; beat again. Add dry ingredients and mix until smooth. Bake in hot waffle iron. Makes 6 waffles.

Organic whole grains, vegetables, fruits, raw nuts and seeds give needed vitamins and minerals to the body. – Patricia Bragg, ND, PhD., Health Crusader

SOY FLOUR WAFFLES

2 cups soy flour
¼ coarse rye and oatmeal
1 Tbsp raw honey
Egg Replacer equal to 2 eggs
2 Tbsp Bragg Olive Oil
1 tsp baking powder
1 cup soy milk

Sift together flour and baking powder in a large mixing bowl. Set aside. Beat Egg Replacer and mix with sifted flour and other dry ingredients. Add milk and honey gradually and beat vigorously until the batter is thin. Bake in a hot waffle iron for 3-5 minutes. Serve with 100% maple syrup. Serves 2-4.

FRESH FRUIT WAFFLES

Add ½ cup mashed strawberries, raspberries, bananas (our favorite) or other fresh fruit to recipe for Soy Flour Waffles.

CAKES & COOKIES

PEANUT BUTTER CAKES

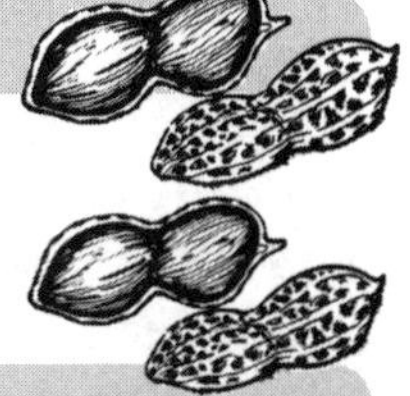

See recipe for Peanut Butter Cupcakes on page 215. Replace one cup rice flour and ½ cup potato flour for the 2¼ cups whole-wheat flour.

BANANA GINGERBREAD

See Banana Gingerbread recipe on page 216. Replace ⅔ cup rice flour and ⅔ cup potato flour for 1⅓ cups whole-wheat flour.

APPLE SAUCE CAKE

See recipe for Apple Sauce Cake on page 216. Replace one cup rice flour and one cup potato flour for the 2 cups of whole-wheat flour.

MOLASSES FRUIT BARS

See recipe Molasses Fruit Bars, page 219. Replace ¾ cup rye pastry flour and ¾ cup rice flour for 1½ cups whole-wheat flour.

OATMEAL RAISIN COOKIES

See recipe for delicious Oatmeal Raisin Cookies on page 220. Replace ¾ cup rice flour for ¾ cup whole-wheat flour.

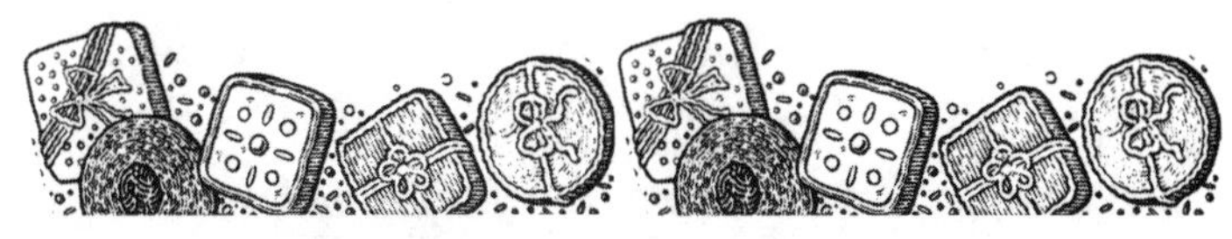

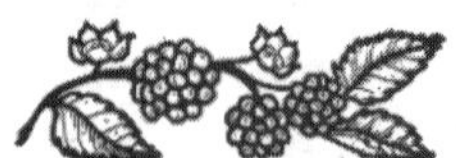

PIES AND FILLINGS

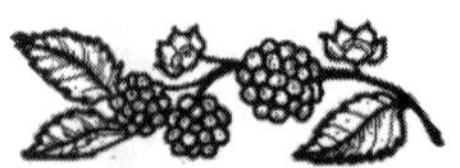

Use any filling that contains ingredients to which you are not allergic to; or, fill with healthy fresh fruit filling and sweetened with raw honey or Stevia herb powder (see page 224) to taste.

CORNMEAL PIE CRUST

(Ideal for pumpkin pie.)

Grease a pie pan with Bragg Organic Olive Oil using twice as much oil as you would using other oils. Pack about ¼ cup yellow organic cornmeal into the pan, entirely covering pan with cornmeal. Gently shake off any excess so as not to disturb that which clings to the sides of the pan. Pour in pumpkin-pie filling carefully filling the pan as full as possible. Bake as for any pumpkin pie.

WHEAT-FREE PIE CRUST

1 cup rye pastry flour
½ cup Bragg Olive Oil
distilled ice water
1 cup potato flour
½ tsp baking powder

Mix and sift dry ingredients. Cut in olive oil. Add as much ice water as needed to form a soft dough. Wrap with waxed paper and put in refrigerator for about 2 hours.

FRUIT FILLING

1 quart desired fruit
2 tsps Bragg Organic Olive Oil
¼ cup fruit juice
⅓ cup raw honey

Blend ingredients and fill pie.

Less Sodium & Sugar in Processed Foods: *New 2011 U.S. Government Nutrition Guidelines urging Americans to use less sodium and sugar in their diets; also places pressure on the food industry to reformulate processed foods; Walmart just announced a 5-year plan to reformulate its store-brand packaged foods and to drop the prices on fruits and vegetables. Kraft Foods, one of the largest food makers in the world, has vowed to reduce sodium by an average of 10% by 2012, and would eventually reformulate more than 1,000 products.*

Eating a diet high in refined foods can lead to fatigue, illness and weight gain.

Fruit bears the closest relation to light. The sun pours a continuous flood of light into the fruits, and they furnish the best potion of food a human being requires for the sustenance of mind and body. – Louisa May Alcott

---

You don't get to choose how you will die. Or when.
You can only decide how you are going to live – NOW! – Joan Baez

---

When a man has pity on all living creatures, then only is he noble. – Buddha

Chapter 28

How to Grow A Culinary Herb Garden

Savory herbs obtain a special flavoring quality from their characteristic essential oils, in their seeds, leaves or flowers. Herbs are at their best when fresh, and very satisfactory when dried.

Cultivation of savory herbs is not difficult. Even the novice can be successful at growing a herb garden by following a few simple directions. Many of the culinary herbs can be grown in cold frames during the winter, in mild climates. In the warm, southern sections of the country quite a few herbs can be grown year-round, outdoors. In the northern sections of this country, they must be carefully protected. Some, of course, will not stand extreme heat or direct exposure to sun, and these, when grown in warmer areas require shade and plenty of moisture.

It may not be practical for every gardener in every section of the country to grow a large, complete list of herbs for his or her kitchen, and yet even a limited number of herbs can contribute greatly to the enjoyment and creation of really fine cuisine.

Set aside a small section of the garden where the biennial and perennial herbs may be grown year after year without disturbing the pollen and cultivation of other plants in the garden. The location of the herb garden should be convenient for frequent watering during dry periods. The ideal location is close to the kitchen, where small quantities of fresh herbs can be gathered at the moment they are required during the preparation of a meal. A garden ranging from 6 x 8 feet to 8 x 10 feet will supply all the herbs the average family will want to use.

It is wise to plan your herb garden carefully, because certain herbs are annual and must be started from seeds each year, while the biennials and perennials can remain in their allotted space for more than one season. Order and neatness can be maintained in the herb garden by locating all of the biennials and perennials at one side of the plot of ground.

Because many of your plants will remain in the ground for more than one year, it is extremely important that the soil is well fertilized before the plants are started. Plow or spade the ground to a depth of 15-inches. Bone meal, cottonseed meal and well-rotted manure can be worked into the soil down to the full depth of plowing. For each 100 square feet, use at least 5 pounds of bone meal, 5 pounds cottonseed meal and one bag of rich manure. It is of utmost importance to mix in the fertilizer thoroughly

ROSEMARY

with the soil to the full depth so that the soil is broken. All lumps of soil should be broken so that it is pulverized and blended with the fertilizer. The soil must be cultivated, free from weeds and watered frequently.

Many of the herbs can be started by sowing the seeds where the plants are to be grown, then thinning them to their proper spacing after they have become established. Other plants do best when started in a cold frame, in the house, or in a hotbed, and transplanted later when conditions are favorable.

The culture of various culinary herbs does not differ greatly, but there are a few requirements that make for the better development of certain herbs.

HOW TO GROW HERBS

ANISE

Anise is an annual and can easily be grown from seed sown in the garden. Only very fresh seed should be used, as this plant does not develop well from older seed. The seeds should be planted in rows about 3 feet apart, with the plants 12-18 inches apart in the row, and about ¾-1 inch deep in mellow soil; if the soil is heavier, cover with less soil. Half a dozen plants will usually produce all of the seeds required for your kitchen.

BASIL

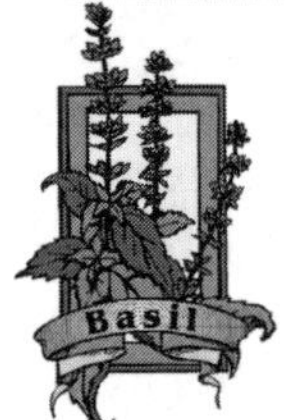

Basil is an annual and the seeds can be started by sowing in the open ground where the plants are to remain. Sow the seeds in a drill, cover about ½ of an inch, and then thin the plants so that they will be 12-14 inches apart. A few plants are all that are needed for kitchen use by the average family.

CARAWAY

Caraway grows best as a biennial. In cold climates, the plants need protection during the winter. Normally, caraway produces its seed after the second season. If the seed is sown during the spring and the plants carried through the winter with protection, they will produce a crop of seeds early the following spring. The seeds are saved by cutting off the seed heads before the ripening seeds begin to shatter, then spreading them on cloth in the shade to dry. When they are dry, they can be rubbed or shaken out of the heads, after which they should be thoroughly dried, and not washed until just before using for flavoring. Do not disregard the young shoots of tender leaves for use in salads. A dozen plants grown a foot apart in rows 3-feet apart will furnish a supply for the average kitchen.

CHIVES

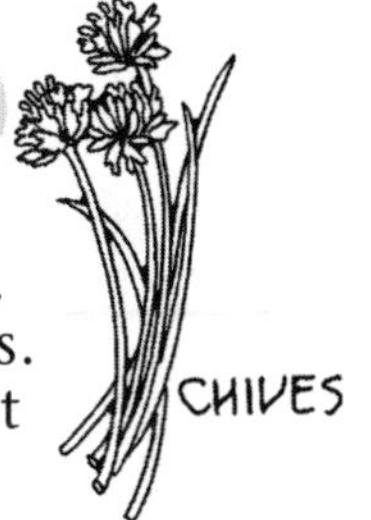

The clumps or bunches of bulbs should be divided either in the fall or in the spring and set in the soil. They should be divided at least once every 3 years. Aside from a fair amount of moisture and being kept free of weeds, they require very little cultivation.

CILANTRO / CORIANDER

Coriander is an annual. Plant a few seeds early in the spring, but do not allow them to become scattered or they will be a weed pest. They should be grown in 3-foot rows with the plants about 18-inches apart in the row. The seeds should be gathered when they are nearly ripe. Cut the seed heads off and spread on a tray to dry. When dry, shake out and clean.

DILL

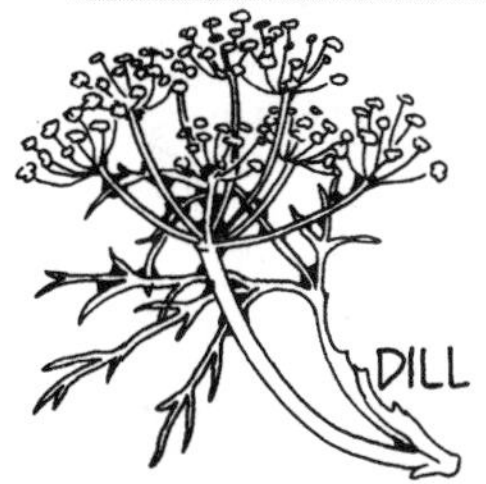

Normally, dill does not produce seeds until the second season. However, if plants are started very early, it is possible to grow them as an annual and mature the seeds the first season. If this is desired, plants should be started indoors and transplanted later to the garden. If you want them to grow as a biennial, sow the seed in the ground in rows 3-feet apart, with the plants 12-15 inches apart in the row. They require a rich soil and plenty of moisture.

SWEET MARJORAM

Sweet marjoram is a perennial and requires about 2 years to produce seed. It can be grown as an annual; this is desirable in cold climates because the plants require very thorough protection in the winter. The seeds are difficult to start, so they should be grown from cuttings, or the seeds grown indoors in the early spring. This is possible since sweet marjoram can be grown in flowerpots inside the house.

MINT

Both peppermint and spearmint are easy to grow; in fact, they spread wildly. But the true flavoring mints are not easy to grow and must be cultivated constantly and kept within bounds. Five mint plants occupying a space of 3′ x 3′ will provide ample flavoring for the average family. The mint bed should be constantly cut and watered and not allowed to grow too high if you are to have good flavored plants. When blooms start to form cut plants back heavily.

MINT

NASTURTIUMS

Although the nasturtium is also considered a flower, it is excellent to include with the savory herbs. Use plants of the dwarf nasturtium and thin them to stand 6-8 inches apart. They require rich soil and plenty of moisture. The first planting should be made as soon as the ground is warm in the spring, and other plantings should follow at intervals of 5 and 6 weeks.

PARSLEY

The moss-curled parsley is the best variety to grow for flavoring purposes. A half dozen plants are sufficient for the average family. The seeds should be very fresh, for they soon lose their vitality. They can be sown in a box in the house and the plants transplanted to a cold frame and then to the garden. They should be thinned to stand 6-8 inches apart. The plants will continue to produce fresh growth if the leaves are kept closely cut.

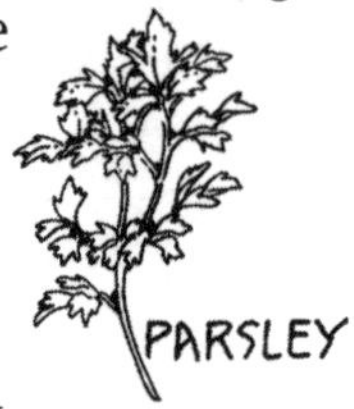

PARSLEY

SAGE

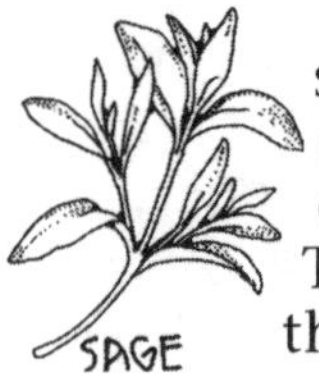

SAGE

Sage plants can be grown from seed and should stand about 2-feet apart. One or two plants will supply enough seasoning. The leaves of the best dried sage are picked before the blooming stage. The sage can be dried in the oven, and must be thoroughly dried before placing in airtight containers.

SAVORY

Summer savory is an annual. Sow the seeds in open ground in the early spring, thin the plants to stand 6-8 inches apart. The rows need not be more than 18-inches apart.

TARRAGON

Tarragon is a perennial. Cuttings should be rooted in a propagating bed and the roots divided. Whenever the flower stems appear, they should be cut out. The plants should be set about 1-foot apart. They require a moist (but not wet) soil. Tarragon plants are not very hardy, and in winter the stems should be cut down and the plants well covered with leaves. The tarragon bed should be relocated every three or four years to avoid disease.

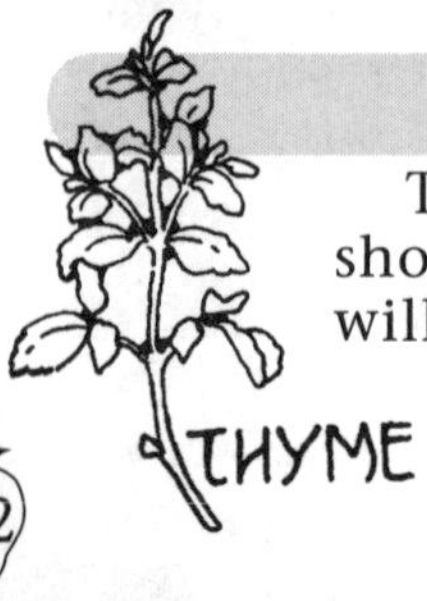

THYME

Thyme can be grown from seed, and new plants should be started every two or three years or they will not produce a good grade of tender leaves. They should be set about 18-inches apart, in rows wide enough to cultivate. They require a rich soil and plenty of moisture.

THYME

WATERCRESS

Watercress is the only herb mentioned here that will not grow practically in the herb garden. It grows best in shallow ponds of water, especially in localities where limestone springs occur. It can, however, be grown successfully on beds of rich soil if provided with an abundance of lime and kept moist. The watercress grown in this manner should be in a cold frame, or in a special framework of boards for protection, and it also requires considerable shade in hot weather. Either seeds or tips of stems will root quite readily if placed in water fortified by lime. The soil should be specially prepared for watercress, working it over, screening it and then adding enough lime to make the surface white. The lime must be worked thoroughly into soil, then moistened. Plants should be set 6-inches apart in each direction. Plants will not stand freezing, nor exposure to extreme heat.

Healthy Benefits from Eating Onions and Garlic

Ancient Egyptians and Romans prized the extraordinary healing powers of garlic and onions. Recent research supports these claims. According to studies done by the nutrition department at Pennsylvania State University, consuming one medium onion a day may lower your cholesterol by 15 percent. The sulfur compounds in onions help lower dangerous levels of blood fats and keeps plaque from adhering to artery walls. As for garlic's role in protecting your heart, the cloves contain natural anticoagulants that help thin the blood, and they protect against platelet stickiness - thus lowering the risk of clotting and even stroke! Also, garlic has potent immune-enhancing properties. It may eradicate many types of bacteria and fungi, including salmonella and candida, as well as inhibit gastrointestinal ulcers.

Onions come in many varieties: yellow, red and white. Sweet onions like Vidalia and Walla Walla have a lower sulfur content than other more pungent varieties. To minimize tears, chill onions for 30 minutes before peeling and chopping. It is best to eat them raw for their full health benefit; if you cook them, do so lightly - overcooking will destroy important enzymes.

Garlic's papery skin should be peeled off and the hard roots trimmed at the end. After you chop garlic, let it sit for 10 minutes before cooking or eating, to let the beneficial enzymes develop.

Other types of garlic and onions include shallots, garlic shoots, leeks, chives and scallions (green onions) – all are beneficial to your health for a long life and are perfect adding to recipes.

Herbs, onions and garlic add healthy, delicious flavors to most all foods.
– Patricia Bragg, N.D., Ph.D.

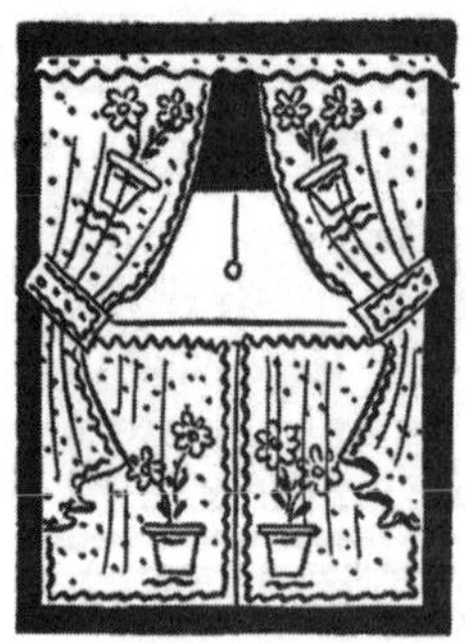

The Window-Box Herb Garden

It is not always possible to have your own herb garden, although it is very desirable both from the standpoint of variety and the quantities of herbs you can grow and because an herb garden is a delightful hobby. If you cannot have your outdoor garden because of space considerations, you need not be without a small indoor garden.

In the fall, before freezing weather begins, such culinary herbs as parsley, basil, sweet marjoram and chives may be placed in flowerpots or in a window box. Often the window box can be kept in a south window during the winter.

In the southern sections of the United States, these plants can be kept in good condition all winter long. In the window box, good soil is even more important, due to size, than in the garden plot. Here is a good mixture:

1 part sharp sand

1 part compost (available garden shops)

2-3 parts of good garden loam

Well-rotted composts contribute to rich soils and then, the rotted chicken or cow manure, sand and a small quantity of bone meal can be added. The soil should be mixed well and sifted through a coarse screen.

The window box can be any size, provided it is at least 8 inches deep. Place a layer of broken stones, about an inch in thickness, at the bottom of the box to provide for efficient drainage (be sure there are several holes in the bottom of the box to allow excess water to drain out). Do not crowd the plants. They should be watered when the top of the soil becomes dry.

By painting a window box in gay colors you have a lovely floral decoration for your window, as well as flavorful, healthy herbs for your kitchen.

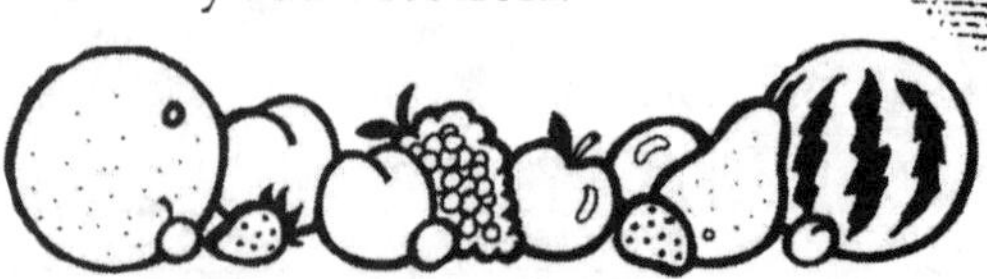

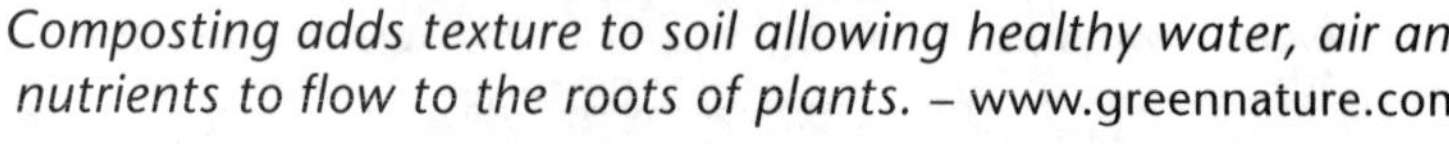

Composting adds texture to soil allowing healthy water, air and nutrients to flow to the roots of plants. – www.greennature.com

Organic Health Gardening

Good Nutrition Starts in the Ground

A chapter on gardening in a cookbook is not so strange as it appears at first glance. Food, no matter how cleverly or artfully cooked, is no better than the soil it comes from.

This is a sad day for all of modern civilization because humans are slowly losing the great vital Health from the soil they could possess. Look at China and India with thousands suffering from every form of vicious and fatal malnutrition. History tells us these were happy countries at one time, where people had an abundance to eat, and lived long and happy lives. However, somewhere in their culturing of the land, they lost the art of fertilizing; they took out crops in abundance and failed to put back the necessary minerals to produce nutritionally healthy foods. This went on for years and years until finally they "mined out" their soil. The foods the land produces are now meager, and fail to nourish and sustain the human body. Visit web: *www.organicgardening.com*

Beautiful, bountiful farms that once used to produce crops high in nutritional value, which in turn produced healthy vigorous people, animals and fowl, became barren, bare, desolate ground. Finally, with nothing growing on it to protect it from rain and wind, all the topsoil that remained has eroded away. This happened in the U.S. dust bowl years ago. That is the reason today many areas of India and China are barren wastelands, upon which nothing will grow. The cause? The topsoil – the life-producing top layer – is either devoid of minerals or disappeared. *www.Organicgardeninfo.com.*

When our forefathers arrived on the North American continent, which is now the USA, they found a most priceless treasure: a wonderfully rich nine-inch topsoil, which had taken nature millions of years to prepare. For millions of years, fallen tree leaves decomposed to create a rich soil that was powerfully saturated with minerals. Grass crops, wild weeds, wild grains and bird and animal waste produced a rich, fertile soil. It was an agricultural paradise in which the first Americans produced their crops. Today, Thanksgiving Day commemorates the abundance produced by our Pilgrim forefathers. The soil was so rich with Health and life-giving minerals that one of the most hearty and sturdy races of men and women prospered. The rich land produced the people who fought the Revolutionary War, won our freedom, and gave birth to these United States of America. It produced the pioneers who blazed a trail from the Atlantic to the Pacific Ocean—men and women with incredible physical endurance—men and women who could fight and win when the greatest of odds were against them; surviving uncharted wildernesses, intense cold, burning deserts. The makers of our republic were products of a hearty land; they were no weaklings. They were tough, vigorous pioneers who won a new country by their great physical strength.

Look at the physical record of our country today. When we were attacked at Pearl Harbor on December 7, 1941, we declared war on Japan and Germany and started to raise an army, navy and marine corps to defend ourselves. The flower of our youth willingly applied for enlistment to be patriotic. Then the shock came: we found that an amazingly large percentage of men aged 18-35 were totally unfit for any type of military service. A lot of these young men – the cream of the crop – were suffering from bad teeth, weak, mis-shapen bones, broken-down flat feet, night blindness and hundreds of crippling diseases produced by nutritional, mineral and vitamin deficiency. The same sad facts repeated themselves during Korean and Vietnam Wars and Desert Storm War to the now current unfortunate wars costing lives and billions!!!

Today, there are millions of people in our hospitals and nursing homes, which are crowded beyond capacity. Outside their walls, we have millions more crippled with arthritis, heart disease, cancer, diabetes, osteoporosis, Alzheimer's, Parkinson's, and more. (American nationwide health care costs soared over $2.5 trillion in 2010, and is expected to more than double by year 2015 according to National Coalition on Healthcare).

In this short period of history, we mined our soil instead of using organic farming. Then, we took our nutritionally poor food and refined it, further destroying most of the remaining minerals and vitamins! Many people still believe that all lettuce, for example, has the same vitamin and mineral content. This is not true. One head of lettuce may be high in both, while another may have hardly any nutritional value. This is because the mineral (and to an even larger extent, the vitamin) content of a vegetable is determined by the mineral content of the soil in which it grows. As the soil varies in health, so does the health of the plant!!!

Healthy citizens cannot be produced from eroded, dead, depleted, chemicalized soils (millions of pounds of toxic petrochemicals are dumped on American farmland each year!) that have no earthworms, natural humus or organic compost. Farmers take big crops out of the soil and put little or nothing back. Some of our soil is completely worn out. Today, all over America there are millions of acres of farmland that have been completely mined out. The

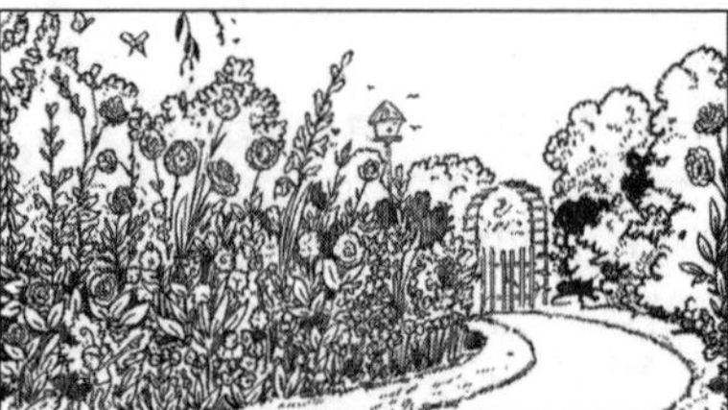

minerals are no longer in this over-chemicalized topsoil; it is depleted, . . . lifeless and dead!

In thousands of instances, the topsoil has been so badly mistreated that it has either washed away by rain or blown away by wind, and you can see the naked subsoil, which can only support certain rank, useless weeds. Few people realize that this country is slowly, but surely, moving toward the same agricultural tragedy that befell India, Africa and other countries. When what little good topsoil we have left is gone, we too shall be an impoverished sick nation.

There is a way you can personally remedy this sad situation. Begin with your family organic garden and/or help organize a community organic, mineralized, healthy vegetable garden where you can eat not only delicious, but highly mineralized foods. With a little space in your backyard, you can have a vitamin rich garden – start your own Garden of Eden!

How to Make a Compost Pile

It is very simple to make a compost pile. Just set aside a special space where you can keep all the dead leaves that fall from trees. It would be a crime to burn this rich material! Place all fruit and vegetable peelings (which are ordinarily thrown away) and lawn cuttings (grass or any other weeds and greens).

1. Create a 6′ x 6′ square.
2. Cover with a 6 inch layer of dead leaves, grass cuttings, kitchen discards, fruit and vegetable peelings.
3. Lay 2 inches of organic manure over leaves and cuttings.
4. Sprinkle thin layer of earth and ground limestone to finish.

While your compost pile is working, temperatures inside your pile will range between 140°F to 145°F. Over the next 3 to 4 months, you will have rich compost that can be worked into the soil of your vegetable garden! *www.organicgardening.com.*

By putting these rich, organic materials back into the soil, you give nature a chance to work her miracle of transferring them to your body through growing food. Reclaim your heritage of Health and well-being from the soil and food you eat.

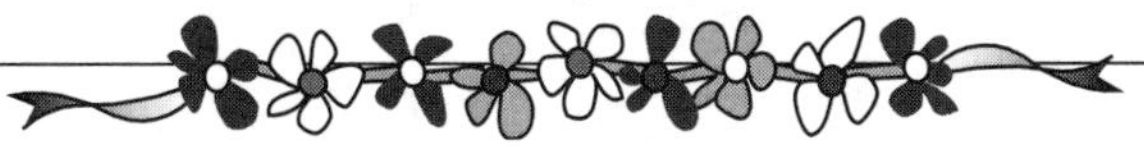

Cherish Life's Simple Pleasures

• Singing Birds • Walks in nature • Smelling the flowers • Miracle Rainbows • Letters from friends • Children's laughter • Love of family and friends • Delicious health meals • Visit with friends

Total Health for the Total Person

In a broad sense, "Total Health for the Total Person" is a combination of physical, mental, emotional, social and spiritual components. The ability of the individual to function effectively in their environment depends on how smoothly these components function as a whole. Of all the qualities that comprise an integrated personality, a well-developed, totally fit and healthy body is most desirable.

A person may be said to be totally physically fit if they can function as a total personality with efficiency and without pain or discomfort of any kind. It means having a painless, tireless, ageless body that possesses sufficient muscular strength and endurance to maintain an effective posture; successfully carry out the duties imposed by one's environment; meet emergencies satisfactorily; and enough energy for recreation and social obligations after the "work day" has ended. The total person's body also meets the requirements for his environment through efficient functioning of sensory organs, possesses the resilience to recover rapidly from fatigue, stress and strain without the aid of stimulants; enjoys natural sleep at night and wakes feeling fit and alert in the morning, prepared for a full day ahead.

Keeping the body totally fit, healthy and in excellent working order is no job for the uninformed or careless person. It requires an understanding of the body, sound health and eating practices and living a disciplined Bragg Healthy Lifestyle. The results of such a health regimen can be measured in happiness, radiant health, feeling ageless, peace of mind and a higher achievement in the joy of living!

Paul C. Bragg   Patricia Bragg

Perfect health is above gold; a sound body before riches. – Solomon

Good Health, generated by physical fitness, is the logical starting point for the pursuit of excellence in all fields of life. Physical vitality promotes mental vitality and is essential to executive achievement. – Dr. Richard E. Dutton

3 John 2 is Our Bragg Motto For You

Dear friend, I wish above all things that thou may prosper and be in health even as the soul prospers.

GO ORGANIC!
DON'T PANIC!

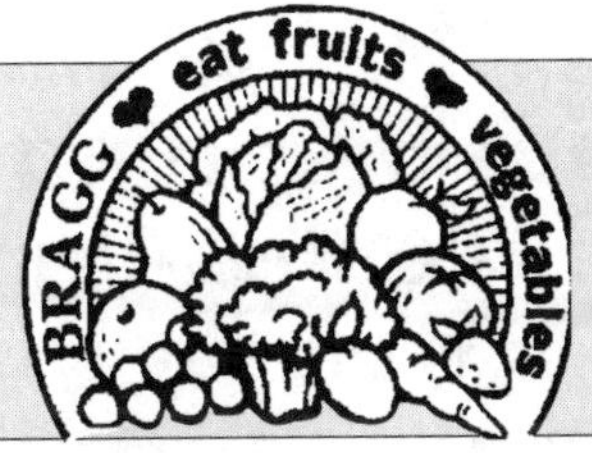

GUARD YOUR
TOTAL HEALTH

FROM THE AUTHORS

This book was written for You! It can be your passport to a healthy, long, vital life. We in the Alternative Health Therapies join hands in one common objective – promoting a high standard of health for everyone. Healthy nutrition points the way – which is Mother Nature and God's Way. This book teaches you how to work with them, not against them! Health Doctors, therapists nurses, teachers and caregivers are becoming more dedicated than ever before to keeping their patients healthy and fit. This book was written to emphasize the great needed importance of healthy lifestyle living for health and longevity, close to Mother Nature and God.

Statements in this book are scientific health findings, known facts of physiology and biological therapeutics. Paul C. Bragg practiced natural methods of living for over 80 years with highly beneficial results, knowing that they were safe and of great value. His daughter Patricia lectured and co-authored the Bragg Health Books with him and continues to carrying on The Bragg Health Crusades.

Paul C. Bragg and daughter Patricia express their opinions solely as Public Health Educators and Health Crusaders. They offer no cure for disease. Only the body has the ability to cure a person. Experts may disagree with some of the statements made in this book. However, such statements are considered to be factual, based on the long-time experience of dedicated pioneer health crusaders Paul C. Bragg and Patricia Bragg. If you suspect you have a medical problem, please always seek qualified health care professionals to help you make the healthiest, wisest and best-informed choices!

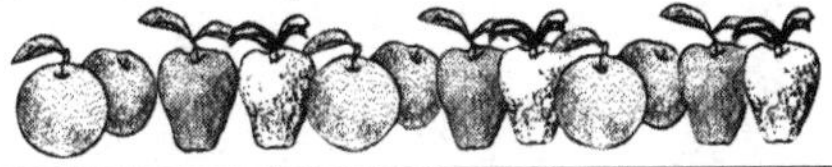

Count your blessings daily while you do your 30 to 45 minute brisk walks and exercises with these affirmations – health! strength! youth! vitality! peace! laughter! humility! understanding! forgiveness! joy! and love for eternity! and soon all these qualities will come flooding and bouncing into your life. With blessings of super health, peace and love to you, our dear friends – our readers. – Patricia Bragg, Health Crusader

The person you are today, the person you will be tomorrow, next week, next month, ten years from now – depends on what you eat. You are the sum total of the food you consume. How you look, how you feel, how you carry your years, all depends on what you eat. – Paul C. Bragg, N.D., Ph.D.

Earn Your Bragging Rights
Live The Bragg Healthy Lifestyle To Attain Supreme Physical, Mental, Emotional and Spiritual Health!

With your new awareness, understanding and sincere commitment of how to live The Bragg Healthy Lifestyle – you can now live a healthier, longer life to 120 years! *(Genesis 6:3)*

God bless you and your family and may He give you the strength, the courage and the patience to win your battle to re-enter the Healthy Garden of Eden while you are still living here on Earth with more years to enjoy it all!

With Blessings of Health, Peace, Joy and Love,

Paul and Patricia

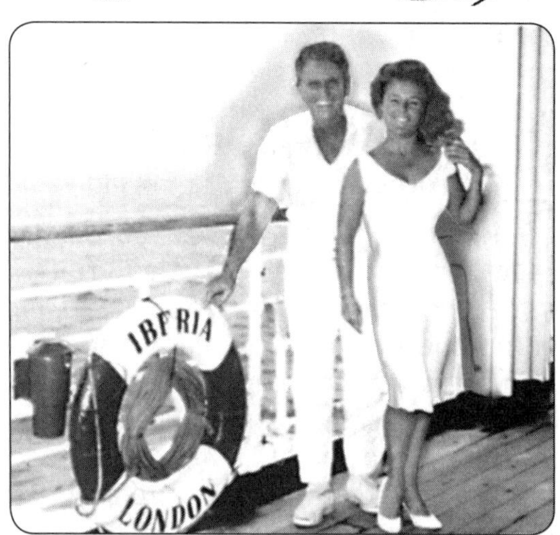

Health Crusaders Paul C. Bragg and daughter Patricia traveled the world spreading health, inspiring millions to renew and revitalize their health.

– 3 John 2

– Genesis 6:3

The Bragg books are written to inspire and guide you to health, fitness and longevity. Remember, the book you don't read won't help. So please read and reread Bragg Books and you will benefit living The Bragg Healthy Lifestyle!

Fixing Life's Flats: When your life seems a bit flat, look around for a source of leakage! Life habits, actions, words, deeds, thoughts – are they healthy and happy? Just a little leak will in time cause a tire to go flat, also your life! Check your life for leaks and stop them now! – Patricia Bragg, Health Crusader

---

Every man is the builder of a temple called his body. We are all sculptors and painters, and our material is our own flesh and blood and bones. Any nobleness and goodness begins at once to refine a man's life! – Henry David Thoreau

---

The doctor of the future will give no medicine, but will interest his patients in the care of the human frame, in diet and the cause and prevention of disease.
– Thomas Edison,genius inventor of light bulb, telephone and phonograph

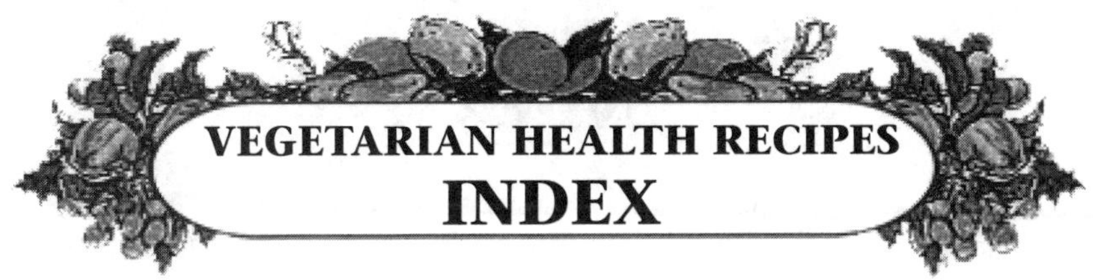

VEGETARIAN HEALTH RECIPES INDEX

A

When you sell a man a book you don't just sell him paper and ink, you sell him a whole new life! There's heaven and earth in a real book. The real purpose of books is to inspire the mind into doing its own thinking. – Christopher Morley

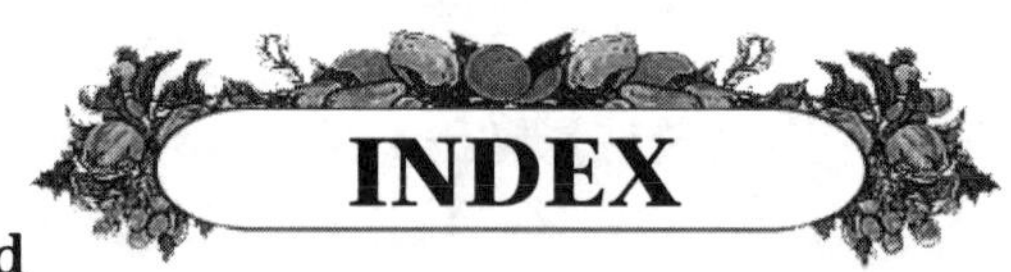

INDEX

A continued

B

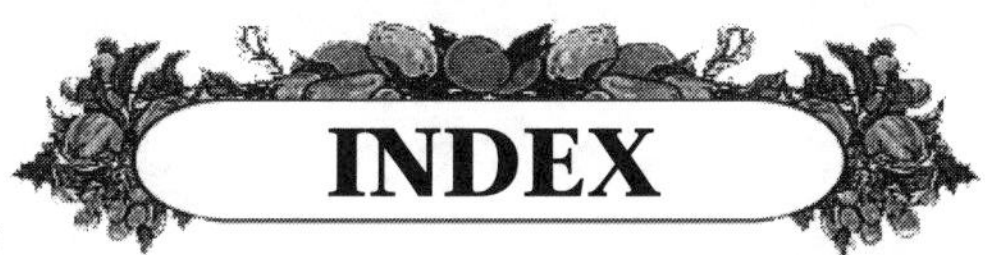

INDEX

B continued

C

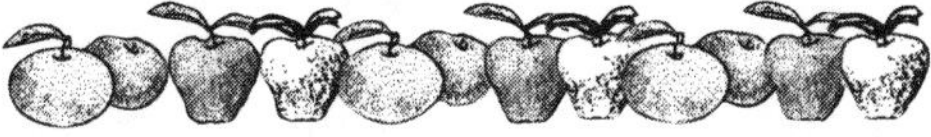

The word "vegetarian" is not derived from "vegetable," but from the Latin, homo vegetus, meaning among the Romans a strong, robust, thoroughly healthy man.

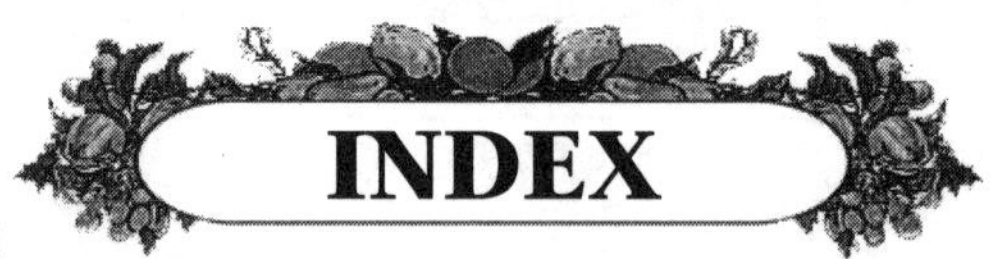

INDEX

C continued

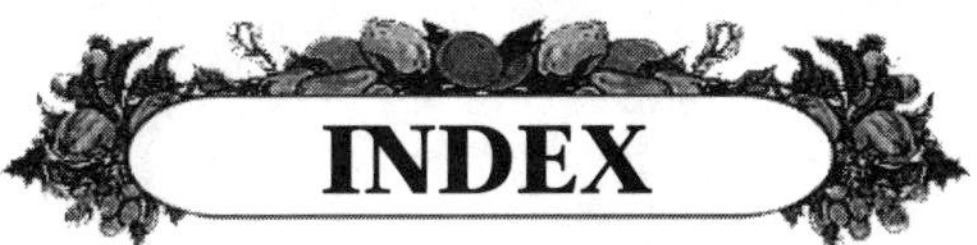

INDEX

C continued

D

INDEX

D continued

E

F

Exercise, along with healthy foods and some fasting helps maintain or restore a healthy physical balance and normal weight for a long, happy, vital life.

INDEX

F continued

G

H

I

Mother nature, time and patience are three great physicians. – Irish Proverb

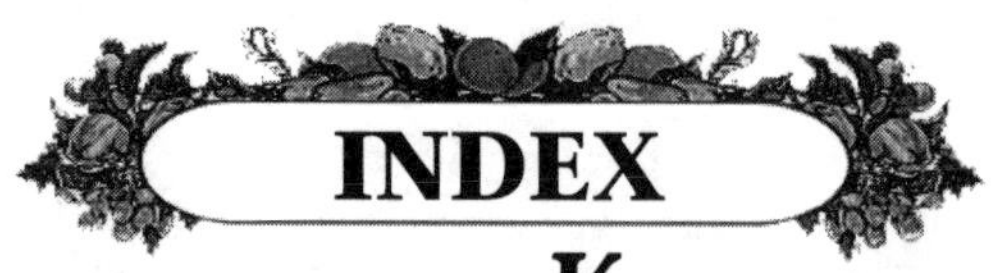

INDEX

J

K

L

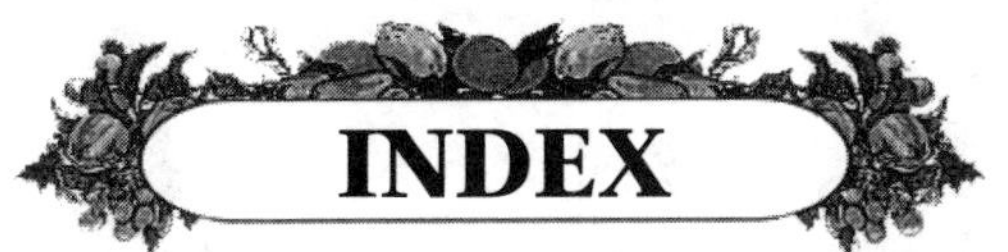

INDEX

M

N

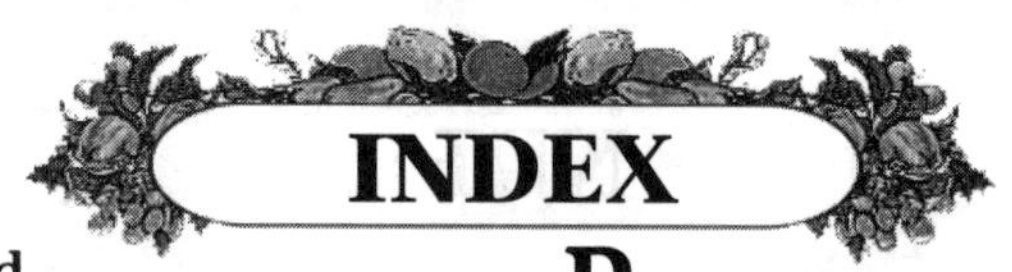

INDEX

N continued

O

P

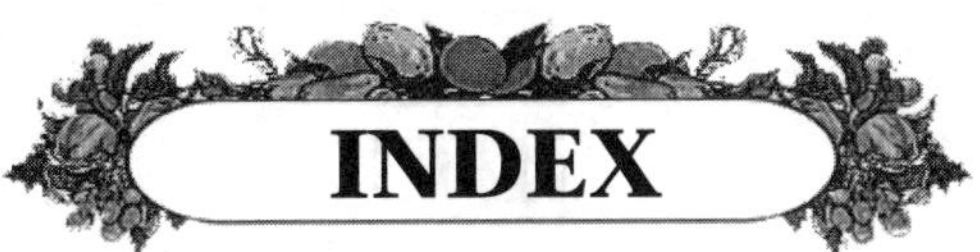

INDEX

P continued

Q

R

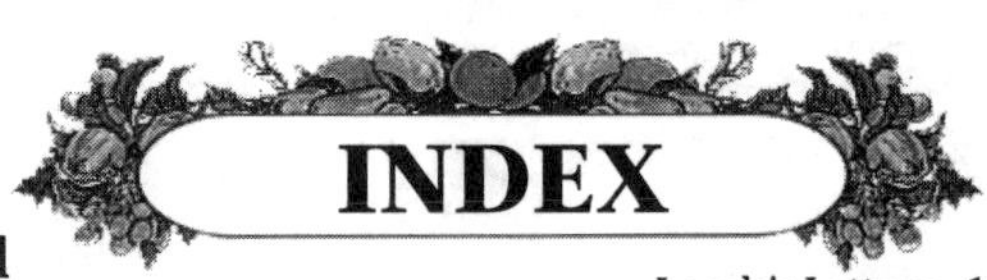

INDEX

R continued

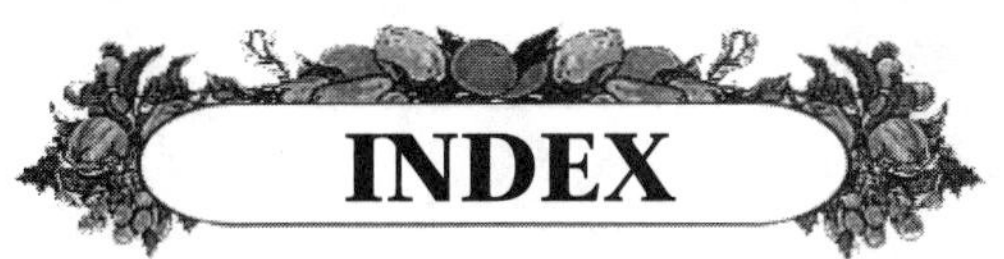

INDEX

S

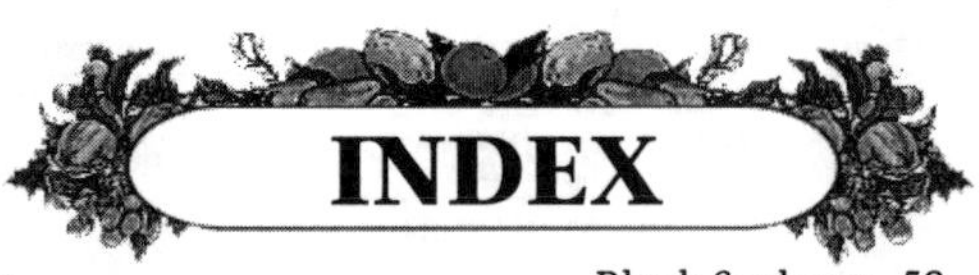

INDEX

S continued

S continued

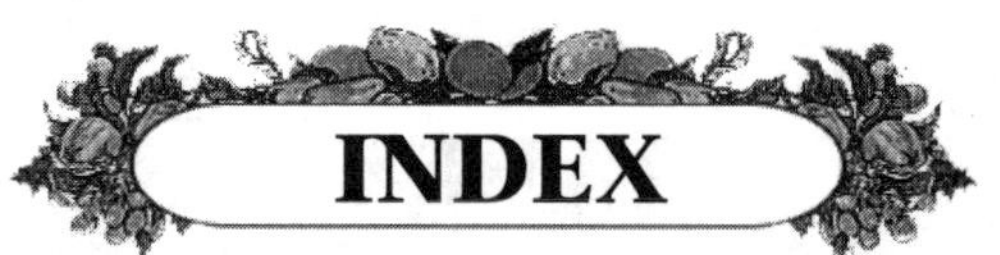

INDEX

T

U

V

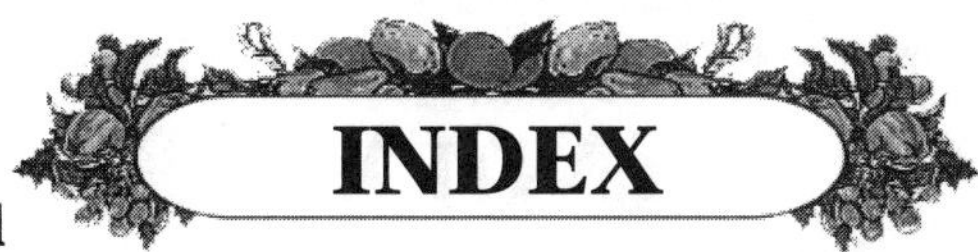

INDEX

V continued

Your Daily Habits Form Your Future

Habits can be wrong, good or bad, healthy or unhealthy, rewarding or unrewarding. The right or wrong habits, decisions, actions, thoughts, words or deeds . . . are up to you! Wisely choose your habits. They can make or break your life!

– Patricia Bragg, N.D., Ph.D., World Health Crusader

INDEX

W

Y

Z

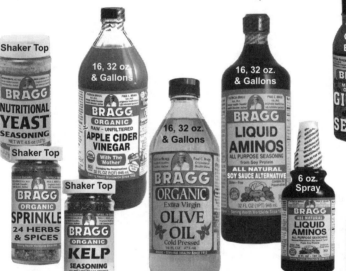

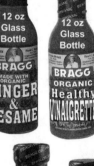

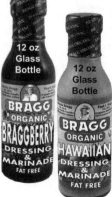

– Make copies of order form to use if Bragg Books are unavailable in your area –

BRAGG "HOW-TO, SELF-HEALTH" BOOKS

Authored by America's First Family of Health

Live Longer – Healthier – Stronger Self-Improvement Library

Qty.	BRAGG Book Titles Health Science ISBN: 978- 0-87790	Price	$ Total
	10 BRAGG Book Offer – Get Healthy, Live Longer Special – plus Free SH	only 89.00	.
	(Please see next 2 pages for book descriptions)		
______	**Apple Cider Vinegar Miracle Health System** – *(over 8 million in print)*	9.95	.
______	**Back Fitness Program** – For Pain-Free, Strong, Healthy Back	9.95	.
______	**Bragg Healthy Lifestyle – Vital Living to 120** (formerly Toxicless Diet)	9.95	.
______	**Build Powerful Nerve Force** – Increase Energy, Eliminate Fatigue, Stress, Anger, Anxiety	11.95	.
______	**Build Strong Healthy Feet** – Banish Aches & Pains, Dr Scholl said "it's the best"	9.95	.
______	**Healthy Heart** – Keep Your Heart & Cardiovascular Healthy & Fit at any age	11.95	.
______	**The Miracle of Fasting** – Bragg Bible of Health, Physical Rejuvenation & Longevity	11.95	.
______	**Super Power Breathing** – for Super Energy, Longevity, & Heal Asthma, Allergies	11.95	.
______	**Water, The Shocking Truth** – That Can Save Your Life - Learn safest water to drink	11.95	.
______	**Vegetarian Health Recipes** – 700 Delicious, Nutritious, Healthy Recipes	13.95	.
	BRAGG DVD – Enjoy BRAGG History, Lectures, Exercise Class, etc.	only 7.95	.
TOTAL COPIES	Books also available as E-books - see bragg.com Due to printing/paper costs, prices subject to change without notice.	**TOTAL BOOKS**	$.
		Books Only: CA Residents add 8.75% tax	.
		(S&H) Shipping & Handling	.
		(USA Funds Only) **TOTAL BOOKS**	$.

Please Specify: ☐ Check ☐ Money Order ☐ Credit Card

Charge To: ☐ Visa ☐ Master Card ☐ Discover

VISA MasterCard DISCOVER

Month Year

Card Expires

CVV #:

Credit Card Number

Signature

USA Shipping Please add $5 first book, $1 each additional book
USA retail book orders over $50 add $7 only

International Shipping Canada add $11 for first book. $1.50 each additional book
All other Int'l. orders add $13. $1.50 each additional book

CREDIT CARD ORDERS ONLY
CALL **(800) 446-1990**
8 am - 4 pm PST • Mon.-Fri.
OR FAX **(805) 968-1001**

Business office calls (805) 968-1020. We accept MasterCard, Discover or VISA phone orders. Please prepare order using this order form. It will speed your call and serve as your order record.
Hours: 8 am to 4 pm Pacific Time, Monday thru Friday.
• Visit our Web: www.bragg.com • e-mail: bragg@bragg.com

See & Order Bragg "Bound" Books, E-Books, & Products on www.bragg.com

Mail to: **HEALTH SCIENCE, Box 7, Santa Barbara, CA 93102 USA**

Please Print or Type – Be sure to give street & house number to facilitate delivery.

BOF 511

Name

Address Apt. No.

City State Zip

Phone ( ) e-mail

Bragg Books are available most Health & Book Stores – Nationwide

America's First Family of Health Since 1912
Founder Paul C. Bragg, Health Crusader & Originator of Health Stores
Bragg Health Books – Health Science – ISBN 978-0-87790

Fasting promotes health, longevity and normalizes weight, thru detox and healing. Helps reverse ageing.

This Bragg classic is one of the great contributions to natural healing in the world today.
– Gabriel Cousens, M.D.

In Russia we love Bragg Fasting Book and living this healthier lifestyle. It has led millions of us to the Lord. We love you and Thank You.
– Elena Troussva, Russia

978-0-87790-039-9 – $11.95

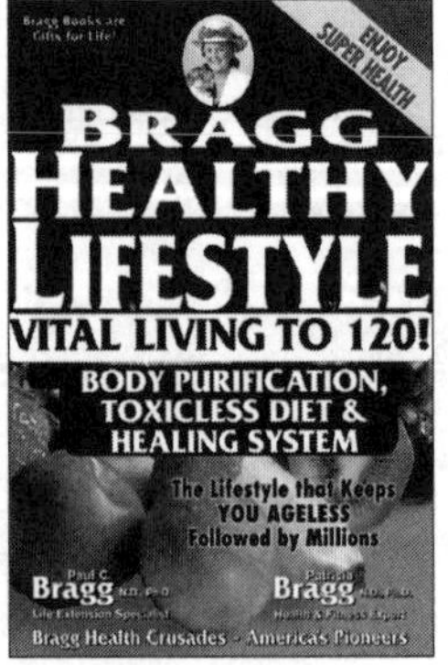

978-0-87790-008-5 – $9.95

Learn The Bragg Healthy Lifestyle that can keep you ageless, tireless and stronger by following this simple body detox and purification with natural healthy foods; enjoyed by Bragg followers worldwide!

I've known the wonderful Bragg Health Books for over 25 years. They are a blessing to me, my family and all who read them.
– Pastor Mike MacIntosh,
Horizon Christian Fellowship,
San Diego, CA

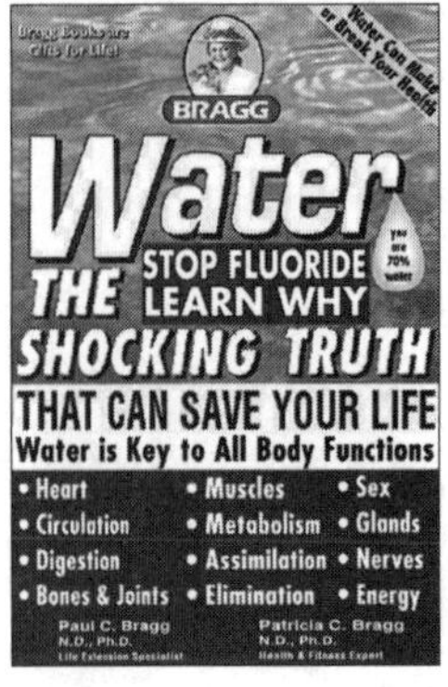

978-0-87790-065-8 – $11.95

This book can save your life. The water you drink can make or break your health! Learn what kind of water is safe, and why. This book also exposes the dangers of toxic fluoride and why it should be banned.

This Bragg Water book is a shocker! Should be required reading by everyone-schools, parents, dentists, and health professionals, etc.
– Chris Linville, M.D.

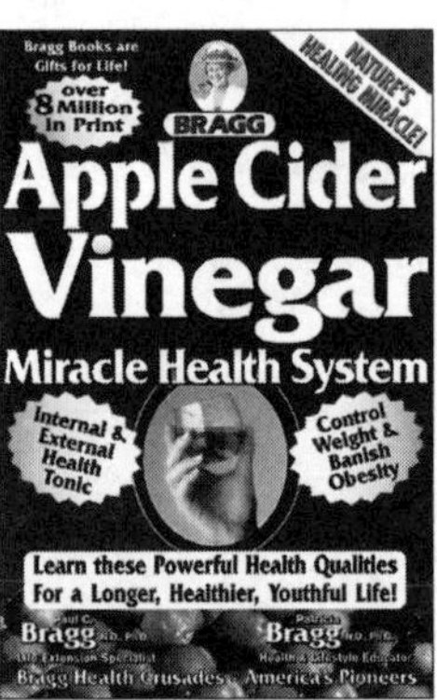

978-0-87790-100-6 – $9.95

This Best-Seller explains the powerful, miracle health benefits of raw organic apple cider vinegar. Hippocrates, Father of Medicine, in 400 B.C., treated patients with raw apple cider vinegar. Learn to use this natural antibiotic, antiseptic and powerful body healer.

Do as I do – have 3 Bragg's Apple Cider Vinegar drinks daily. 2 tsps Bragg Vinegar & raw honey in an 8 oz. glass of distilled water.
– Julian Whitaker, M.D.,
Health & Healing Newsletter

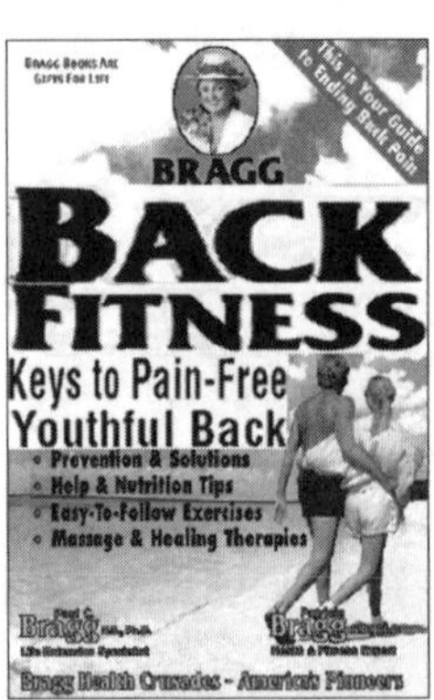

978-0-87790-057-3 – $9.95

Keys to Pain-Free, Youthful Back. Learn the Solutions, Prevention and Latest Non-Invasive Surgery and Healing Therapies. Includes Exercises, Nutrition, Health Tips & more.

I've had back and knee pain for 2 years and in one week following your health program with exercise and the Vinegar Drink, I am now completely pain free!
– Patricia Henderson

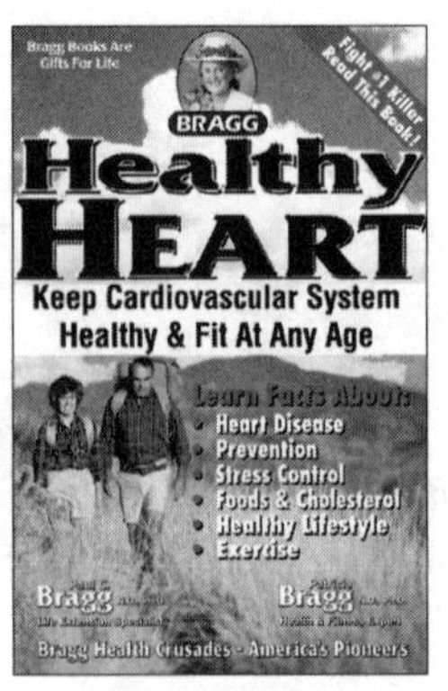

978-0-87790-097-9 – $11.95

Fight America's #1 Killer! Important info on heart disease, angina, prevention, stress reduction, exercise, diet and cholesterol. This book shows how to keep your heart strong, healthy and ageless!

I thank Paul Bragg for saving my life at 15 with The Bragg Healthy Lifestyle. I love Bragg Health Products and Bragg Health Books.
– Jack LaLanne
Health & Fitness Legend

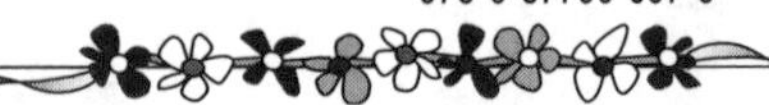

Bragg Health Books are available most Health and Book Stores or call wkdays 8am-4pm: 800-446-1990 or visit web: bragg.com

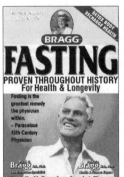

BRAGG HEALTH BOOKS ARE GIFTS FOR LIFE

Gen. 6:3 — 3 John 2

– Jack LaLanne, Bragg follower since 15 years old

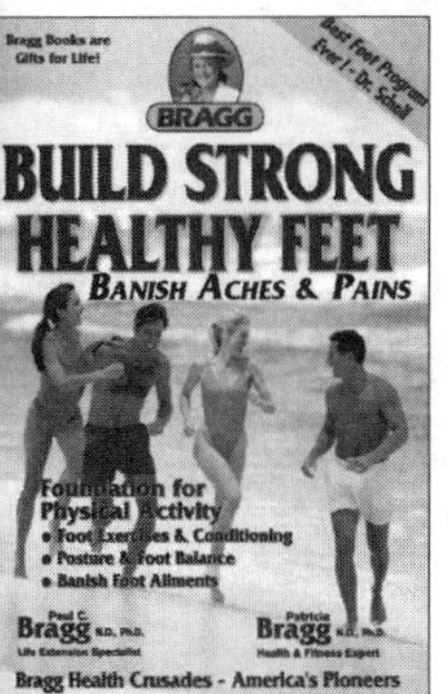

978-0-87790-077-1 – $9.95

Learn how to banish aches & pains. Read about Reflexology, Acupressure and much more. Almost all of us are born with perfect feet. It's the abuse millions give their feet that makes them cry as they limp through life - "my aching feet are killing me!" Read this book!

The Bragg Foot Program is the best. I thank Bragg Books and their wisdom for my long, active, healthy life.

– Dr. Scholl,
Famous Foot Doctor

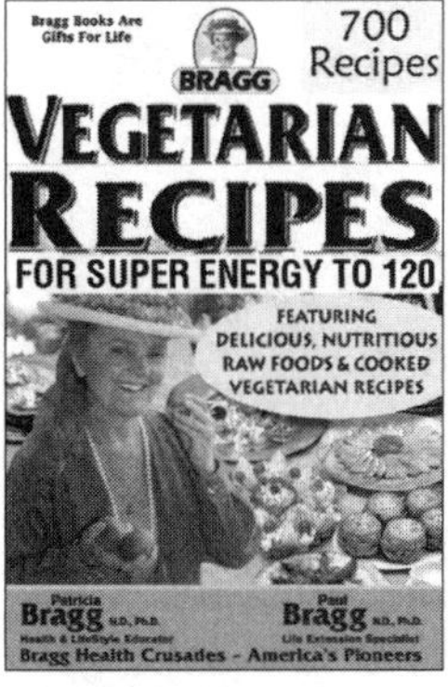

978-0-87790-027-6 – $13.95

Enjoy the worlds finest health recipes for super health and high energy that you and your family will love. Over 700 Healthy Recipes for Health, Super Energy and Longevity. 336 pages filled with delicious raw and cooked foods, vegan and vegetarian recipes.

This book shows how to eat right with nutritious recipes to maintain the body's health and fitness.

– Henry Hoegerman, M.D.

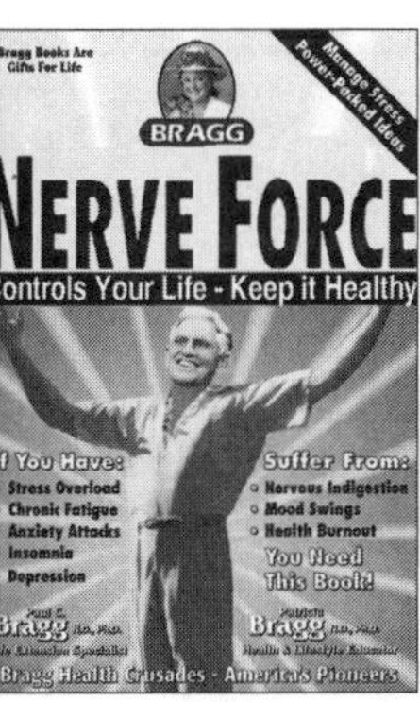

978-0-87790-093-1 – $11.95

Millions of healthy, happy followers have learned to control and increase their Vital Nerve Force Energy - the Bragg Healthy Way. Here's Prevention and Health Maintenance all in one book.

I have my life back after many years of chronic fatigue, fibromyalgia and clinical depression. I give thanks to The Bragg Health Books.

– Marilyn Mason

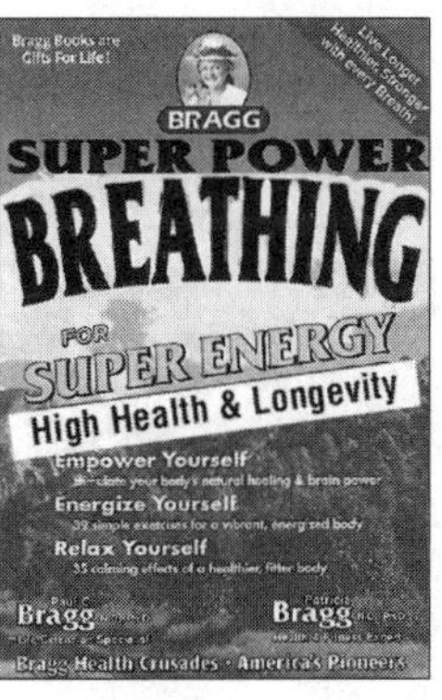

978-0-87790-120-4 – $11.95

Breathing deeply, fully and completely energizes, calms, fills you with peace and keeps you youthful. Learn Bragg Breathing Exercises for more go-power and Super Health!

Thanks to Paul Bragg and Bragg Books, my years of asthma were cured in only one month with The Bragg Super Breathing and Bragg Healthy Lifestyle Living!

– Paul Wenner
Gardenburger Creator

"I thank Paul Bragg and the Bragg Healthy Lifestyle for my healthy, long, active life." I love Bragg Books and Health Products."
– Jack LaLanne, Bragg follower to 96 1/2 years

I have followed "The Bragg Healthy Lifestyle for years and it teaches you to take control of your health and build a healthy future."
– Mark Victor Hansen, Co-Producer *Chicken Soup for the Soul* Series

"Thanks to Bragg Books for my conversion to the healthy way."
– James F. Balch, M.D.
Co-Author of – *Prescription for Nutritional Healing*

"Bragg Books have been a blessing to our family and the TBN family of loyal viewers"
– Evangelist Dwight Thompson - *Co-Host TBN "Praise The Lord"*

If Bragg Books are unavailable in your area you may order:
on-line at: www.bragg.com or see Bragg book list.
Bragg Book Special: All 10 books for only $89 Postpaid.

Bragg Organic Health Products available most Health Stores & Grocery Health Depts Nationwide

BRAGG Organic Raw APPLE CIDER VINEGAR

With The Mother . . . Nature's Delicious, Healthy Miracle

HAVE AN APPLE HEALTHY LIFE!

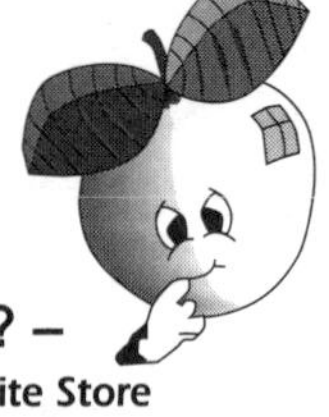

– IF ? –

Your Favorite Store doesn't carry Bragg Products & Books - Ask them to Contact their Distributor to stock them!

Or they can Call Bragg at

1-800-446-1990

Weekdays 8-4pm

Voted the BEST by Customers & Chefs

BRAGG ORGANIC RAW – UNFILTERED APPLE CIDER VINEGAR With The 'Mother'

16oz, 32oz Gallons

INTERNAL BENEFITS:

- Helps Normalize & Control Weight
- Rich in Miracle Potassium & Enzymes
- Natural Antibiotic. Germ & UTI Fighter
- Helps Eliminate Toxins & Body Sludge
- Improves Digestion & Helps Balances pH
- Relieves Sore, Dry Throats & Food Poisoning
- Helps Remove Artery Plaque & Infections
- Helps Fight Arthritis & Stiffness

EXTERNAL BENEFITS:

- Helps Promote Youthful, Healthy Body
- Helps Promote & Maintain Healthy Skin
- Soothes Sunburn, Bites & Rashes
- Helps Relieve Dandruff & Itching Scalp
- Helps Heal Acne, Pimples & Shingles
- Soothes Aching Joints & Muscles

BRAGG ALL NATURAL LIQUID AMINOS

Healthy Seasoning with 16 Amino Acids – Healthy Alternative to Tamari & Soy Sauce

BRAGG LIQUID AMINOS – Taste you love, Nutrition you need...a family favorite for over 88 years. Delicious and nutritious life-renewing protein from healthy certified non-GMO soybeans only. Add to or spray over casseroles, tofu, soups, sauces, gravies, rice, beans, potatoes, veggies, even popcorn, etc. Also ideal "pick-me-up" broth at work, home or gym. Healthy replacement for Tamari, Worchestershire and Soy Sauce. Start today add 16 vital Amino Acids to your daily diet for healthy living – the easy BRAGG LIQUID AMINOS Way!

16oz, 32oz, Gallons 6 oz Spray

BRAGG LIQUID AMINOS SEASONING ALL NATURAL SOY SAUCE ALTERNATIVE

SPRAY or DASH brings NEW TASTE DELIGHTS! PROVEN & ENJOYED BY MILLIONS.

America's Healthiest All-Purpose Seasoning

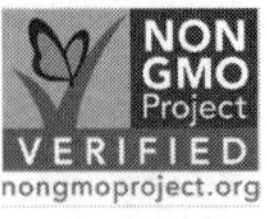

Spray or Dash of Bragg Aminos Brings New Taste Delights to Season:

• Tofu	• Dressings	• Rice/Beans
• Stir-frys	• Soups	• Wok foods
• Tempeh	• Poultry	• Gravies
• Sauces	• Fish	• Meats
• Veggies	• Casseroles	• Popcorn
• Salads	• Potatoes	• Macrobiotics

Pure Soybeans and Purified Water Only:

- No Added Sodium
- No Coloring Agents
- No Preservatives
- Not Fermented
- No Chemicals
- No Additives
- No Wheat & No Gluten

BRAGG ORGANIC EXTRA VIRGIN OLIVE OIL

Delicious, Extra Virgin, Unrefined, First Cold-Pressed

AWARD WINNING!

BRAGG ORGANIC Extra Virgin OLIVE OIL Cold Pressed

16oz, 32oz, Gallons

BRAGG ORGANIC OLIVE OIL – is made from 100% organically grown Arbequina Olives that continually provides the best quality and flavor. A heart healthy oil that's an antioxidant, oleic acid and vitamin E rich that helps to normalize cholesterol and blood pressure. It has a delicious, smooth body with a light after taste, adding the finest flavor and aroma to salads, vegetables, pastas, pestos, sauces, sautés, potatoes and most foods – even popcorn. Also used world-wide as a skin beauty tonic. In 400 BC the Father of Medicine, Hippocrates, used and wrote about olive oil's great health benefits.

– Here's other Bragg Healthy Products for your Taste Delights:

★ **Bragg Sprinkle** (24 herbs & spices)
★ **Bragg Organic Kelp Seasoning**
★ **Bragg Healthy Salad Dressings:**
★ **Vinaigrette** ★ **Ginger/Sesame**
★ **Hawaiian** ★ **Braggberry**

BRAGG OLIVE OIL VINAIGRETTE OR MARINADE

1/3 cup Bragg Organic Extra Virgin Olive Oil
1/2 cup Bragg Organic Apple Cider Vinegar
1/2 tsp Bragg Liquid Aminos (All Purpose Seasoning)
1/4 tsp Bragg Sprinkle (24 herbs & spices)
1 to 2 tsps raw Honey — 1 to 2 Garlic cloves, mince
1/2 tsp fresh Ginger, grate — Mix All Ingredients Together

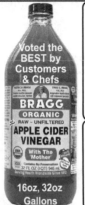

– Order form to copy and use if products unavailable in your area –

BRAGG ORGANIC APPLE CIDER VINEGAR

SIZE	PRICE		UPS SHIPPING & HANDLING For USA	$ Amount
16 oz.	$ 3.29	each	S/H – Please add $9. for 1st bottle and $1.50 each additional bottle	.
16 oz.	$ 36.00	Special Case /12	S/H Cost by Time Zone: CA $12. PST/MST $14. CST $22. EST $25	.
32 oz.	$ 5.29	each	S/H – Please add $10. for 1st bottle – $2. each additional bottle	.
32 oz.	$ 58.00	Special Case /12	S/H Cost by Time Zone: CA $17. PST/MST $20. CST $35. EST $38	.
1 gal.	$ 16.49	each	S/H – 1st bottle: CA $10. PST/MST $10. CST $13. EST $15 – $6. each add'l bottle	.
1 gal.	$ 57.00	Special Case /4	S/H Cost by Time Zone: CA $17. PST/MST $20. CST $34. EST $37	.

BRAGG Vinegar is a food and not taxable

BRAGG VINEGAR $	.
(S&H) Shipping & Handling	.
TOTAL $	.

BRAGG LIQUID AMINOS

SIZE	PRICE		UPS SHIPPING & HANDLING For USA	$ Amount
6 oz.	$ 3.59	each	S/H – Please add $9. for 1st 3 bottles – $1.50 each additional bottle	.
6 oz.	$ 78.00	Special Case /24	S/H Cost by Time Zone: CA $10. PST/MST $11. CST $17. EST $19	.
16 oz.	$ 4.69	each	S/H – Please add $9. for 1st bottle – $1.50 each additional bottle	.
16 oz.	$ 51.00	Special Case /12	S/H Cost by Time Zone: CA $12. PST/MST $14. CST $22. EST $25	.
32 oz.	$ 7.69	each	S/H – Please add $9. for 1st bottle and $2. each additional bottle	.
32 oz.	$ 84.00	Special Case /12	S/H Cost by Time Zone: CA $17. PST/MST $20. CST $35. EST $38	.
1 gal.	$ 28.39	each	S/H – 1st bottle: CA $10. PST/MST $10. CST $13. EST $15 – $6. each add'l bottle	.
1 gal.	$ 99.00	Special Case /4	S/H Cost by Time Zone: CA $17. PST/MST $20. CST $34. EST $37	.

BRAGG Aminos & Olive Oil are foods and not taxable

BRAGG AMINOS $	.
(S&H) Shipping & Handling	.
TOTAL $	.

BRAGG ORGANIC OLIVE OIL

SIZE	PRICE		UPS SHIPPING & HANDLING For USA	$ Amount
16 oz.	$ 10.99	each	S/H – Please add $9. for 1st bottle – $1.50 each additional bottle	.
16 oz.	$ 120.00	Special Case /12	S/H Cost by Time Zone: CA $12. PST/MST $14. CST $22. EST $25	.
32 oz.	$ 17.89	each	S/H – Please add $10. for 1st bottle and $2. each additional bottle	.
32 oz.	$ 196.00	Special Case /12	S/H Cost by Time Zone: CA $17. PST/MST $20. CST $35. EST $38	.
1 gal.	$ 62.69	each	S/H – 1st bottle: CA $10. PST/MST $10. CST $13. EST $15 – $6. each add'l bottle	.
1 gal.	$ 219.00	Special Case /4	S/H Cost by Time Zone: CA $17. PST/MST $20. CST $34. EST $37	.

BRAGG OLIVE OIL $	.
(S&H) Shipping & Handling	.
TOTAL $	.

Please Specify: ☐ Check ☐ Money Order ☐ Cash
Charge to: ☐ Visa ☐ Master Card ☐ Discover

Credit Card Number:______________________ Card Expires: ____/____ month / year

VISA MasterCard DISCOVER

Signature:______________________

Business office calls (805) 968-1020. We accept MasterCard, Discover & VISA phone orders. Please prepare order using order form. It speeds your call and serves as order record. Hours: 8 to 4 pm Pacific Time, Monday thru Friday.

CREDIT CARD ORDERS
CALL **(800) 446-1990**
8 am-4 pm PST • Mon.-Fri.
OR FAX **(805) 968-1001**

• Visit our Web: www.bragg.com • e-mail: bragg @ bragg.com

Mail to: **HEALTH SCIENCE, Box 7, Santa Barbara, CA 93102 USA** BOF 511

Please Print or Type – Be sure to give street & house number to facilitate delivery.

Name ____________________

Address ____________________ **Apt. No.** _____

City __________ **State** _____ **Zip** _____

Phone ( ) __________ **e-mail** __________

Bragg Health Products available most Health Stores & Grocery Health Depts Nationwide

Bragg Organic Products available Health Stores & Grocery Health Depts Nationwide

BRAGG HEALTHY SALAD DRESSINGS

ORGANIC HEALTHY VINAIGRETTE

This Bragg Healthy Organic Vinaigrette Dressing makes a salad special with its tasty, tangy flavor. A zesty blend of Bragg Organic Extra Virgin Olive Oil, Bragg Organic Apple Cider Vinegar, Bragg Liquid Aminos, garlic, and onion, raw honey and delicious organic herbs. This unique taste brings you a healthy dressing with the Bragg's best tradition of healthy eating and healthy living.

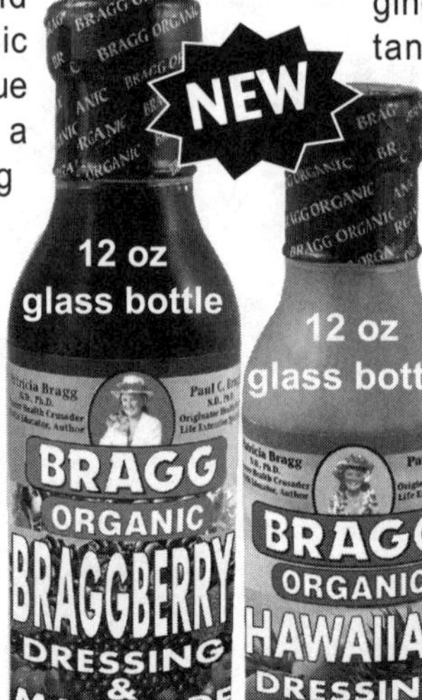

Made with Organic GINGER & SESAME

This Bragg Healthy Dressing is based on the delicious flavors of our famous Bragg Liquid Aminos and ginger's sweet and tangy taste. Great on salads and veggies, brings you the best of Bragg tradition of healthy eating and living.

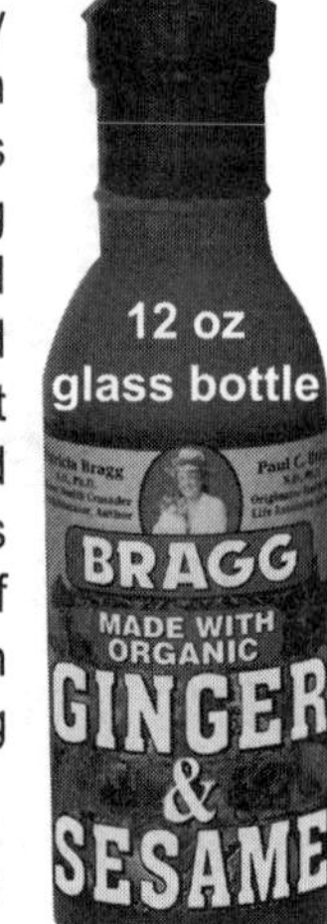

BRAGGBERRY Dressing & Marinade

Brings new taste treats, with Blueberries, Raspberries, Acai, Goji and Grape. Low-fat and natural antioxidants. All of the best of Bragg's tradition of healthy eating and living.

BRAGG HAWAIIAN Dressing & Marinade

Brings Taste of Aloha to salads, veggies, stir-frys and other healthy foods. Unlock Hawaiian secret flavors you will love with Bragg Natural Delicious and Tasty Hawaiian Dressing and Marinade.

America's Healthiest All-Purpose Seasonings

BRAGG SPRINKLE
ORGANIC 24 HERBS & SPICES

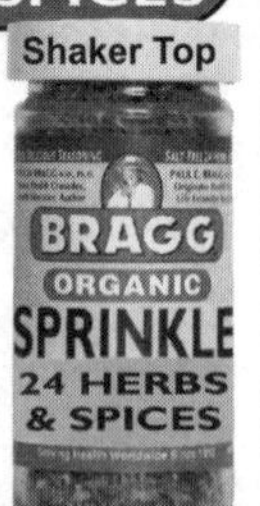

This old favorite is now available again. Bragg Sprinkle was created in 1931 by Paul C. Bragg, Health Pioneer & Originator Health Food Stores. Organic Sprinkle adds new healthy, delicious flavors to most recipes & meals. It's salt-free with no additives, preservatives or fillers.

BRAGG ORGANIC KELP SEASONING

Shaker Top

This original Organic Kelp Seasoning made from sun-dried Organic Pacific Ocean Sea Kelp, combined with 24 all natural herbs and spices. It's a healthy, delicious seasoning for almost all recipes and meals and is specially suited for low-sodium diets.

NEW

BRAGG Delicious Nutritional Yeast Seasoning

Nutritionally designed to help meet nutritional needs of vegetarians, vegans and anyone wanting a good source of B12, B-Complex Vitamins. It's "cheese-like" flavor makes it a delicious, healthy seasoning.

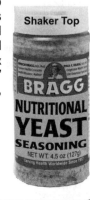

- Gluten-Free • Non-GMO
- No Salt • No Sugar • No Dairy
- No Artificial Colors & Preservatives
- No Brewery Products
- No Candida Albicans
- Vegetarian & Kosher Certified

You are what you eat, drink, breathe, think, say & do. – Patricia Bragg, ND, PhD.

– Order form to copy and use if unavailable in your area –

BRAGG SPRINKLE – 24 Herbs & Spices Seasoning

SIZE	PRICE		UPS SHIPPING & HANDLING For USA	$ Amount
1.5 oz.	$ 4.69	each	S/H – Please add $9. for 1st 3 bottles and $1. each additional bottle	.
1.5 oz.	$ 51.00	Special Case /12	S/H Cost by Time Zone: CA $9. PST/MST $9. CST $10. EST $12.	.

BRAGG Sprinkle Seasoning is a food and not taxable

BRAGG SPRINKLE $	.
(S&H) Shipping & Handling	.
TOTAL $	.

BRAGG ORGANIC SEA KELP

2.7 oz.	$ 4.69	each	S/H – Please add $9. for 1st 3 bottles and $1. each additional bottle	.
2.7 oz.	$ 51.00	Special Case /12	S/H Cost by Time Zone: CA $9. PST/MST $9. CST $10. EST $12.	.

BRAGG Kelp Seasoning is a food and not taxable

BRAGG KELP $	.
(S&H) Shipping & Handling	.
TOTAL $	.

BRAGG NUTRITIONAL YEAST

4.5 oz.	$ 6.29	each	S/H – Please add $9. for 1st 3 bottles and $1. each additional bottle	.
4.5 oz.	$ 69.00	Special Case /12	S/H Cost by Time Zone: CA $9. PST/MST $9. CST $10. EST $12.	.

BRAGG Nutritional Yeast Seasoning is a food and not taxable

BRAGG YEAST $	.
(S&H) Shipping & Handling	.
TOTAL $	.

BRAGG SALAD DRESSINGS

✱ BRAGG GINGER & SESAME SALAD DRESSING

12 oz.	$ 5.49	each	S/H – Please add $9. for 1st bottle and $1.25 each additional bottle	.
12 oz.	$ 60.00	Special Case /12	S/H Cost by Time Zone: CA $11. PST/MST $12. CST $19. EST $22	.

✱ BRAGG ORGANIC VINAIGRETTE SALAD DRESSING

12 oz.	$ 5.49	each	S/H – Please add $9. for 1st bottle and $1.25 each additional bottle	.
12 oz.	$ 60.00	Special Case /12	S/H Cost by Time Zone: CA $11. PST/MST $12. CST $19. EST $22	.

✱ BRAGG BRAGGBERRY DRESSING & MARINADE

12 oz.	$ 5.49	each	S/H – Please add $9. for 1st bottle and $1.25 each additional bottle	.
12 oz.	$ 60.00	Special Case /12	S/H Cost by Time Zone: CA $11. PST/MST $12. CST $19. EST $22	.

✱ BRAGG HAWAIIAN DRESSING & MARINADE

12 oz.	$ 5.49	each	S/H – Please add $9. for 1st bottle and $1.25 each additional bottle	.
12 oz.	$ 60.00	Special Case /12	S/H Cost by Time Zone: CA $11. PST/MST $12. CST $19. EST $22	.

BRAGG Salad Dressings/Marinades are foods and not taxable

BRAGG SALAD DRESSINGS $	.
(S&H) Shipping & Handling	.
TOTAL $	.

Payment Method:

☐ Check ☐ Money Order ☐ Cash **Charge To:** ☐ Visa ☐ Master Card ☐ Discover

Credit Card Number:____________________ Card Expires:____/____ month / year

Signature:____________________

MasterCard VISA DISCOVER

Business office calls (805) 968-1020. We accept MasterCard, Discover & VISA phone orders. Please prepare order using order form. It speeds your call and serves as order record. Hours: 8 to 4 pm Pacific Time, Monday thru Friday. • Visit our Web: www.bragg.com • e-mail: bragg @ bragg.com

CREDIT CARD ORDERS
CALL **(800) 446-1990**
8 am - 4 pm PST • Mon.- Fri.
OR FAX **(805) 968-1001**

Mail to: **HEALTH SCIENCE, Box 7, Santa Barbara, CA 93102 USA** BOF 511

Please Print or Type – Be sure to give street & house number to facilitate delivery.

• ____________________
Name

• ____________________ • ______
Address **Apt. No.**

• __________ • ______ • ______
City **State** **Zip**

• ( ) __________ • __________
Phone **e-mail**

Bragg Products available most Health Stores & Grocery Health Depts Nationwide

BRAGG Organic Health Drinks available most Health Stores & Grocery Health Depts Nationwide

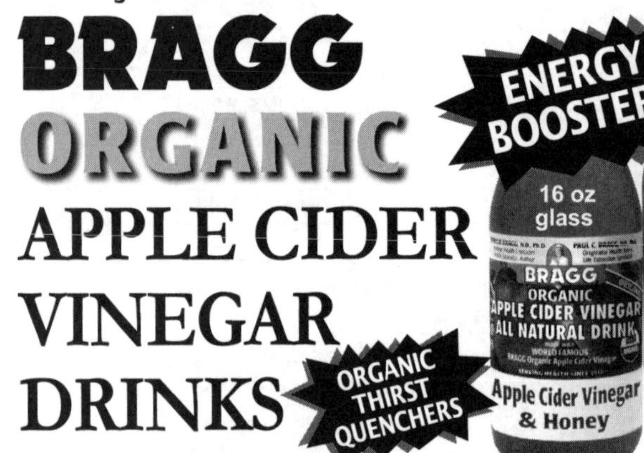

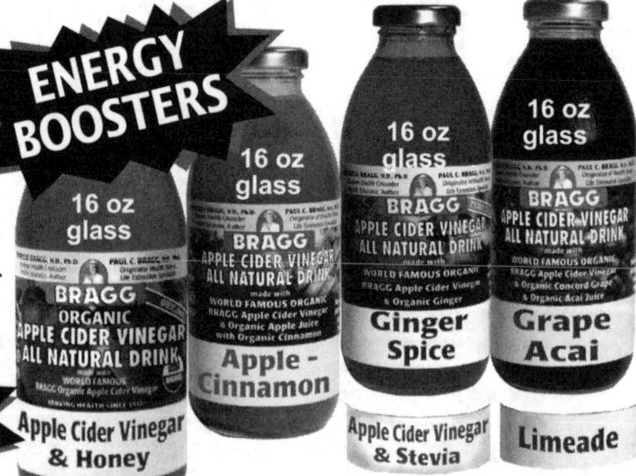

Each contains two 8 oz. servings

Enjoy Healthy Goodness and Taste of BRAGG Organic Apple Cider Vinegar in Energizing, Refreshing Health Drinks.

Made with "World Famous" Bragg Organic Apple Cider Vinegar & Organic Raw Honey

Delicious, ideal pick-me-up for home, work, gym or sports. Perfect taken as healthy thirst quencher & energy booster.

6 DeliciousChoices:

- **Apple Cider Vinegar & Honey**
- **Apple Cider Vinegar & Sweet Stevia**
- **Apple-Cinnamon** • **Ginger Spice**
- **Concord Grape-Acai** • **Limeade**

- Based on Paul & Patricia Bragg's Original Recipe
- Natural Goodness of Bragg Organic Apple Cider Vinegar
- Sweetened with Organic Honey or Organic Natural Stevia
- Great-Tasting, Healthy Refreshing Drinks
- Great for a Quick Energy Boost
- Convenient Pre-mixed Drinks (two 8-oz. servings per bottle)
- Certified Organic and Kosher Certified
- Try Drinks Today! Your Body and You will Love them!

USDA ORGANIC

Discover the Power of BRAGG Organic Apple Cider Vinegar.

In 400 BC Hippocrates, the Father of Medicine, used Apple Cider Vinegar for its amazing natural detox cleansing, healing, and energizing qualities. Hippocrates prescribed ACV mixed with honey for its health properties.

BRAGGZYME®

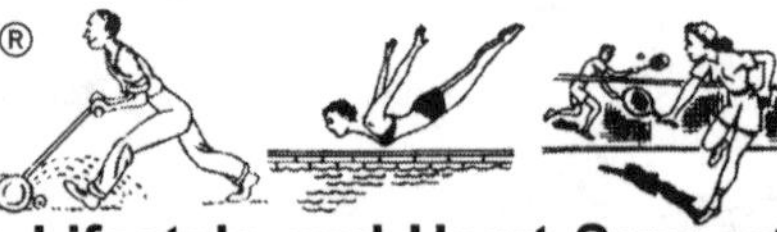

Powerful Systemic Enzymes for Active Lifestyle and Heart Support

Dr. Paul C. Bragg, the first to introduce enzyme supplements in 1931. Now Bragg Health Science is proud to introduce most advanced systemic enzyme supplement, Braggzyme – that contains powerful 500mg Complex Formula (Nattokinase, Serrapeptase, Bromelain, Papain, Protease and Lipase) and Co-Q10.

BRAGGZYME™ Superior Systemic Enzymes provide nutritional and cardiovascular support you need to help maintain a normal inflammatory response and maintain safe fibrin levels for a healthy cardiovascular system.* Braggzyme contains no animal derivatives, no artificial flavors, no artificial coloring, no yeast and no wheat.

NEW

120 Veg. Caps

BRAGGZYME
SUPERIOR SYSTEMIC ENZYMES
120 CAPSULES

- Enzyme support for back, joints, muscles, tendons and immune system.*
- Boost energy levels – infuses life-giving oxygen to every cell in body.*
- Nutritional support to help maintain a normal inflammatory response.*
- Helps eliminate dangerous fibrin levels for a healthier blood flow.*
- 4,500 Fibrinolytic Units (FU) per cap to help normalize healthy fibrin levels.*
- Helps keep your hands and feet and entire body warm.*
- Helps keep your memory and brain more sharp.*
- 100% Safe, All Natural Vegetarian Formula in Veg. caps.

*These statements have not been evaluated by the Food & Drug Administration. This product is not intended to diagnose, treat, cure, or prevent any disease.

– Order form to copy and use if unavailable in your area –

BRAGG ORGANIC APPLE CIDER VINEGAR DRINKS

FLAVORS SIZE	PRICE	QTY	CASE PRICE	QTY	$ Amount
Original Apple Cider Vinegar & Honey - 16 oz	$2.19		$24.00		.
ACV with Ginger - Spice - 16 oz	$2.19		$24.00		.
ACV with Apple - Cinnamon - 16 oz	$2.19		$24.00		.
ACV with Concord Grape - Acai - 16 oz	$2.19		$24.00		.
Apple Cider Vinegar & Sweet Stevia - 16 oz	$2.19		$24.00		.
Apple Cider Vinegar Limeade - 16 oz	$2.19		$24.00		.

BRAGG ORGANIC APPLE CIDER VINEGAR DRINKS are Foods and are not taxable

BRAGG VINEGAR DRINK $	.
(S&H) Shipping & Handling	.
TOTAL $	.

SHIPPING CHART FOR ACV DRINKS

number of bottles	CA	PST/MST	CST	EST
1-2 bottles	$8.00	$8.00	$9.00	$12.00
3-4 bottles	$8.00	$9.00	$11.00	$13.00
5-6 bottles	$9.00	$9.00	$13.00	$15.00
7-12 bottles	$11.00	$13.00	$21.00	$24.00
Special Case/12	$11.00	$13.00	$21.00	$24.00

Please call around to Health & Grocery Stores first, because many are now selling Bragg Products.

BRAGGZYME – Systemic Enzymes

SIZE	PRICE		UPS SHIPPING & HANDLING For USA	$ Amount
120 cap	$ 43.95	each	S/H – Please add $9. for 1st 3 bottles and $1. each additional bottle	.
120 cap	$ 483.00	Special Case /12	S/H Cost by Time Zone: CA $9. PST/MST $10. CST $11. EST $12.	.

on Braggzyme CA Residents only pay tax

for BRAGGZYME only CA Residents add 8.75% TAX $	.
(S&H) Shipping & Handling	.
TOTAL $	.

Payment Method:

☐ Check ☐ Money Order ☐ Cash

Charge To: ☐ Visa ☐ Master Card ☐ Discover

Credit Card Number:______________________________ Card Expires:____/____ month / year

Signature:______________________________

VISA MasterCard DISCOVER

Business office calls (805) 968-1020
We accept MasterCard, Discover & VISA
Phone orders please prepare order using order forms, as it speeds up your call and serves as your order record.
Hours: 8 to 4 pm Pacific Time, Monday thru Friday.
• Visit Web: www.bragg.com • e-mail: bragg @ bragg.com

CREDIT CARD ORDERS
CALL **(800) 446-1990**
8 am - 4 pm PST • Mon.-Fri.
OR FAX **(805) 968-1001**

Mail to: **HEALTH SCIENCE, Box 7, Santa Barbara, CA 93102 USA**
Please Print or Type – Be sure to give street & house number to facilitate delivery. BOF 511

• Name

• Address • Apt. No.

• City • State • Zip

• ( ) Phone • e-mail

Bragg Products available most Health Stores & Grocery Health Depts Nationwide

– Make copies when needed for mailing in. –

Send for Free Health Bulletins

Patricia wants to keep in touch with you, your relatives and friends about the latest Health, Nutrition and Longevity Discoveries. Please enclose one stamp for each USA name listed or visit *www.bragg.com* and sign up for literature.

With Blessings of Health, Peace and Thanks

Please make copy, then print clearly and mail to:

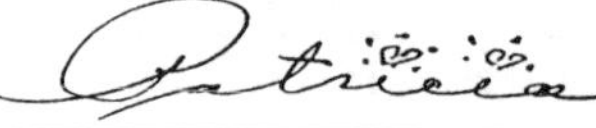

BRAGG HEALTH CRUSADES, Box 7, Santa Barbara, CA 93102

Name

Address Apt. No.

City State Zip

Phone ( ) e-mail

Name

Address Apt. No.

City State Zip

Phone ( ) e-mail

Name

Address Apt. No.

City State Zip

Phone ( ) e-mail

Name

Address Apt. No.

City State Zip

Phone ( ) e-mail

Name

Address Apt. No.

City State Zip

Phone ( ) e-mail

Bragg Health Crusades spreading health worldwide since 1912

PAUL C. BRAGG, N.D., Ph.D.

Life Extension Specialist • World Health Crusader
Lecturer and Advisor to Olympic Athletes, Royalty and Stars
Originator of Health Food Stores & Founder of Health Movement Worldwide

"The Bragg Health and Fitness Way of Life"
Works Wonders for Millions!

Paul C. Bragg, Father of the Health Movement in America, had vision and dedication. This dynamic Health Crusader for worldwide health and fitness is responsible for more *firsts* in the history of the Health Movement than any other individual.

Bragg's amazing pioneering achievements the world now enjoys:

- Bragg originated, named and opened the first Health Food Store in America.
- Bragg Health Crusades pioneered the first Health Lectures across America and he inspired followers to open Health Food Stores across America and also worldwide.
- Bragg was the first to introduce pineapple juice and then tomato juice to America.
- He introduced Juice Therapy in America by importing the first hand-juicers.
- He was the first to introduce and distribute honey and date-sugar nationwide.
- He pioneered Radio Health Programs from Hollywood 3 times daily in 1920's - 1930's.
- Bragg and daughter Patricia pioneered a Health TV show from Hollywood to spread The Bragg Health Crusade on their show, *Health and Happiness.* It included exercises, health recipes, visual demonstrations and guest appearances by famous, health-minded people.
- Bragg opened the first health restaurants and the first health spas in America.
- He created and produced the first health products and then made them available nationwide: herbal teas, health beverages and oils, seven-grain cereals and crackers, vitamins, calcium and mineral supplements, wheat germ, whey, digestive enzymes from papaya, sundried fruits, raw nuts, herbs and kelp seasonings, amino acids from soybeans, health candies and health cosmetics. Bragg inspired others to follow (Schiff, Gardenburger, Shaklee, TwinLabs, Trader Joe's, GNC, Herbalife, etc.) and now there are thousands of health stores & health items available worldwide!

Crippled by TB as a teenager, Bragg developed his own eating, breathing and exercising program to rebuild his body into an ageless, tireless, pain-free citadel of glowing, super health. He excelled in running, swimming, biking, progressive weight training and mountain climbing. He made an early pledge to God, in return for his renewed health, to spend the rest of his life showing others the road to super health. He honored his pledge! Paul Bragg's health pioneering made a difference worldwide.

A legend and beloved health crusader to millions, Bragg was the inspiration and personal health and fitness advisor to top Olympic Stars from 4 time swimming Gold Medalist Murray Rose to 4 time track Gold Medalist Betty Cuthbert of Australia, his relative (pole-vaulting Gold Medalist) Don Bragg, and countless others. The Hulk, Lou Ferrigno, went from puny to super shape. Jack LaLanne, the original TV Fitness King, says, *"Bragg saved my life at age 15 when I attended the Bragg Crusade in Oakland, California."* From the earliest days, Bragg advised the greatest Hollywood Stars and Giants of American Business, JC Penney, Del E. Webb, Dr. Scholl and Conrad Hilton are just a few who he inspired to long, successful, healthy, active lives!

Dr. Bragg changed the lives of millions worldwide in all walks of life with the Bragg Health Crusades, Books, Radio and TV appearances. (See and hear Bragg on the web.)

BRAGG HEALTH CRUSADES, Box 7, SANTA BARBARA, CA 93102 USA • www.bragg.com

PATRICIA BRAGG, N.D., Ph.D.
Health Crusader & Angel of Health & Healing

Author, Lecturer, Nutritionist, Health & Lifestyle Educator to World Leaders, Hollywood Stars, Singers, Athletes, etc. & Millions

Patricia is a 100% health crusader with a lifetime dedication passion like her father, Paul C. Bragg, world renowned health authority. Patricia has won international fame on her own. She conducts Bragg Health & Fitness Seminars & Lectures for Conventions & Schools, Women's, Men's, Youth & Church Groups world-wide. She promotes Bragg Healthy Lifestyle Living & "How-To, Self-Health" Books on Radio & TV Talk Shows throughout the English-speaking world. Consultants to Presidents & Royalty, to Stars of Stage, Screen & TV & to Champion Athletes, Patricia & her father co-authored The Bragg Health Library of Instructive, Inspiring Books that promote a healthier lifestyle, for a long, healthy, happy life.

Patricia herself is the symbol of health, perpetual youthfulness & natural femininity, radiant & super energy. She is a living & sparkling example of her & her father's healthy lifestyle precepts & this she loves sharing world-wide.

A fifth-generation Californian on her mother's side, Patricia was reared by The Bragg Natural Health Method from infancy. In school, she not only excelled in athletics, she won honors for her studies & counseling. She is an accomplished musician & dancer, tennis player & mountain climber. Patricia is a popular gifted Health Teacher, a dynamic personality & perfect Talk Show Guest on Radio & TV Shows where she regularly spreads the simple, easy-to-follow Bragg Healthy Lifestyle for everyone of all ages. Patricia's been on the covers of many magazines as her health message is needed & well received by millions.

Man's body is his vehicle through life, his earthly temple & the Creator wants us filled with joy & health for a long, fulfilled life. The Bragg Crusades of Health & Fitness (3 John 2) has carried her around the world over 30 times – spreading physical, emotional, mental & spiritual health & joy. Health is our birthright & Patricia teaches how to prevent the destruction of our health from man-made wrong lifestyle habits of living.

Patricia's been a Health Consultant to American Presidents, British Royalty, to Champion Triathletes *(She wrote 600 page Tri-Health Fitness Manual),* Betty Cuthbert, Australia's "Golden Girl" (16 world records & 4 Olympic track gold medals), & New Zealand's Olympic Track & Triathlete Star, Allison Roe. Among those who follow her advice are some of Hollywood's top Stars from Clint Eastwood to ever-youthful singing group – The Beach Boys, Singing Stars of Metropolitan Opera & top Ballet Stars, etc. Patricia's message is of world-wide appeal & well received by people of all ages, nationalities & walks-of-life. Those who follow The Bragg Healthy Lifestyle & attend The Bragg Crusades world-wide are living testimonials . . . like ageless, super athlete, Jack LaLanne, who at age 15 went from sickness to Total Fitness & Health!

Patricia inspires you to Renew, Rejuvenate and Revitalize your Life with "The Bragg Healthy Lifestyle" Books and Health Crusades worldwide. Millions have benefitted from these life-changing events with a longer, healthier and happier life! She loves to share with your community, organization, church groups, etc. Also, she is a perfect radio and TV talk show guest to spread the message of healthy lifestyle living. See and hear Patricia on the web: bragg.com For radio interview & lecture requests write or e-mail: **patricia@bragg.com**
BRAGG HEALTH CRUSADES, BOX 7, SANTA BARBARA, CA 93102, USA